TESTING STATISTICAL HYPOTHESES OF EQUIVALENCE

TESTING STATISTICAL HYPOTHESES OF EQUIVALENCE

Stefan Wellek

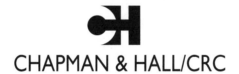

CHAPMAN & HALL/CRC

A CRC Press Company

Boca Raton   London   New York   Washington, D.C.

Library of Congress Cataloging-in-Publication Data

Wellek, Stefan.
    Testing statistical hypotheses of equivalence / by Stefan Wellek.
        p. cm.
    Includes bibliographical references and index.
    ISBN 1-58488-160-7 (alk. paper)
    1. Statistical hypothesis testing. I. Title.

QA277 .W46 2002
519.5′6—dc21   2002031307

Visit the CRC Press Web site at www.crcpress.com

© 2003 by Chapman & Hall/CRC Press LLC

No claim to original U.S. Government works
International Standard Book Number 1-58488-160-7
Library of Congress Card Number 2002031307
Printed in the United States of America 1 2 3 4 5 6 7 8 9 0
Printed on acid-free paper

To Brigitte,
Anne and Felix

Contents

Preface

Roughly speaking, equivalence tests provide the adequate answer to the most natural question of how to proceed in a traditional two-sided testing problem if it turns out that primary interest is in verifying rather than rejecting the null hypothesis. Put in more technical terms, equivalence assessment deals with a particular category of testing problems characterized by the fact that the alternative hypothesis specifies a sufficiently small neighbourhood of the point in the space of the target parameter which indicates perfect coincidence of the distributions to be compared.

The relevance of inferential procedures which, in the sense of this notion, enable one to "prove the null hypothesis" for many areas of applied statistical data analysis, is obvious enough. A particularly striking phenomenon which demonstrates the real need for such methods, is the adherence of generations of authors to using the term "goodness-of-fit tests" for methods which are actually tailored for solving the reverse problem of establishing absence or lack of fit. From a "historical" perspective (the first journal article on an equivalence test appeared as late as in the sixties of the twentieth century), the interest of statistical researchers in equivalence assessment was almost exclusively triggered by the introduction of special approval regulations for so-called generic drugs by the Food and Drug Administration (FDA) of the U.S. as well as the drug regulation authorities of many other industrial countries. Essentially, these regulations provide that the positive result of a test, which enables one to demonstrate with the data obtained from a so-called comparative bioavailability trial the equivalence of the new generic version of a drug to the primary manufacturer's formulation, shall be accepted as a sufficient condition for approval of the generic formulation to the market. The overwhelming practical importance of the entailed problems of bioequivalence assessment (drugs whose equivalence with respect to the measured bioavailabilities can be taken for granted, are termed "bioequivalent" in clinical pharmacology literature), arises mainly out of quantity: Nowadays, at least half of the prescription drug units sold in the leading industrial countries are generic drugs that have been approved to be marketed on the basis of some bioequivalence trial.

However, bioequivalence assessment is by no means the only medical application of equivalence testing methods of considerable interest. In fact, considerations of equivalence play an increasingly important role in the design and analysis of genuine clinical trials of therapeutic methods for the treatment of diseases which by ethical reasons cannot be investigated in a study involving a negative control (in particular placebo). Such active or positive control therapeutic trials are frequently designed as one-sided equivalence trials, and that is one of the reasons why the present book contains also a chapter on tests for problems where the alternative hypothesis specifies that the experimental treatment is not relevantly inferior to the reference treatment.

The core of this monograph deals with methods of testing for equivalence in the strict, i.e., two-sided sense. The spectrum of specific two-sided equivalence testing problems it covers ranges from the one-sample problem with normally distributed observations of fixed known variance (which will serve as the basis for the derivation of asymptotic equivalence tests for rather complex multiparameter and even semi- and nonparametric models), to problems involving several dependent or independent samples and multivariate data. A substantial part of the testing procedures presented here satisfy rather strong optimality criteria which is to say that they maximize the power of detecting equivalence uniformly over a large class of valid tests for the same (or an asymptotically equivalent) problem. In equivalence testing, the availability of such optimal procedures seems still more important than in testing conventional one- or two-sided hypotheses. The reason is that even those equivalence tests which can be shown to be uniformly most powerful among all valid tests of the same hypotheses, turn out to require much higher sample sizes in order to maintain some given bounds on both types of error risks than do ordinary one- or two-sided tests for the same statistical models, unless one starts from an extremely liberal specification of the equivalence limits.

The theoretical basis of the construction of such optimal tests for interval hypotheses has been laid within the mathematical statistics literature already in the nineteen fifties. However, up to now the pertinent results have only rarely been exploited in the applied, in particular the biostatistical literature on equivalence testing. In a mathematical appendix to this book, they will be presented in a coherent way and supplemented with a corollary which allows great simplification of the computation of the critical constants of optimal equivalence tests under suitable symmetry restrictions. An additional appendix contains a listing of all computer programs supplied at the URL http://www.zi-mannheim.de/wktsheq for facilitating as much as possible the routine application of all testing procedures discussed in the book. Most of the concrete numerical examples given in the text for purposes of illustrating the individual methods, are taken from the author's own field of application, i.e., from medical research.

The book can be used in several ways depending on the reader's interests and level of statistical training. Chapter 1 gives a general introduction to the topic and should at least be skimmed by readers of any category. Chapter 2 deals with what is called in the clinical trials literature testing for noninferiority and is mainly intended for readers with strong interests in practical applications of the methods. In particular, the algorithm presented there for the computation of sample sizes required in the Fisher-type exact test for one-sided equivalence should be of considerable practical use in the planning of noninferiority trials with binary outcome. Readers of the same category should profitably skip Chapter 3 except for the section on confidence interval inclusion. In contrast, if primary interest is in a systematic account of equivalence testing procedures and their mathematical basis, then it has to be recommended not only to go through this chapter in full detail but to supplement its reading by referring extensively to part A of the Appendix.

Apart from occasional cross-references, all remaining chapters (and even individual sections of them) can be read independently of each other. The material they contain is to provide the working statistician of any background and level of sophistication with a sufficiently rich repertoire of efficient solutions to specific equivalence testing problems frequently encountered in the analysis of real data sets. Except for Section 4.4 which introduces no additional testing procedure, Chapters 4–9 should even be suited for serving as a procedure reference book in the field of equivalence testing. In order to keep the page count within reasonable limits, the coverage of this book is confined to methods for samples of fixed size. Fully and group sequential methods for equivalence testing problems are left out of account.

All in all, one of the following alternative guides to the book should be followed:

A) [for readers primarily interested in practical applications]

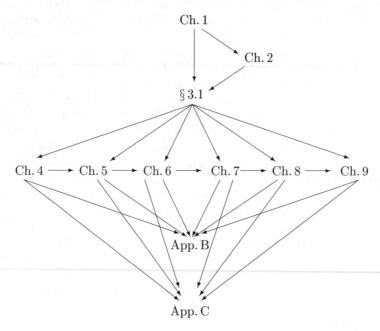

B) [for the reader particularly interested in theory and mathematical background]

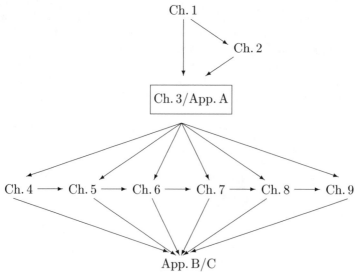

I have many people to thank for helping me in the endeavour of preparing this book, without being able to make mention here of more than a few of them. Niels Keiding played an initiating role, not only by encouraging me to make the material contained in a book on the same topic I had published in 1994 in German accessible to an international readership, but also by bringing me in contact with Chapman & Hall/CRC. Cooperation with the staff of this publisher proved remarkably smooth and constructive, and I am particularly grateful to Kirsty Stroud as the managing editor for her continued understanding of the difficulties of an author involved in many other activities, with meeting a fixed deadline for the delivery of his manuscript. The former vice-president of Gustav Fischer Verlag Stuttgart, Dr. Wolf D. von Lucius, is gratefully acknowledged for having given his permission to utilize in part the content of my book of 1994. Last but not least, there are also two people from the staff in my department at the Central Institute of Mental Health at Mannheim to whom I owe a debt of gratitude: Mireille Lukas typeset the bulk of the text in LaTeX with impressive expertise, and Peter Ziegler generated the majority of the figures contained in the book, writing suitable programs in *SAS/GRAPH*.

Mannheim
July 2002   STEFAN WELLEK

CHAPTER 1

Introduction

1.1 Demonstration of equivalence as a basic problem of applied statistics

It is a basic fact well known to every statistician that in any hypotheses testing problem there is an inherent logical asymmetry concerning the roles played by the two statements (traditionally termed null and alternative hypotheses) between which a decision shall be taken on the basis of the data collected in a suitable trial or experiment: Any valid testing procedure guarantees that the risk of deciding erroneously in favour of the alternative does not exceed some prespecified bound whereas the risk of taking a wrong decision in favour of the null hypothesis can typically be as high as 1 minus the significance level (i.e., 95% in the majority of practical applications). On the other hand, from an experimental or clinical researcher's perspective, there seems little reason why he should not be allowed to switch his views towards the problem under consideration and define what he had treated as the null hypothesis in a previous study, as the hypothesis of primary interest in a subsequent trial.

If, as is so often the case in practice, the "traditional" formulation of the testing problem has been a two-sided one specifying equality of the effects of, say, two treatments under the null hypothesis, then such a switch of research interest leads to designing a study which aims at proving absence of a difference between both treatment effects. In biostatistics, any trial which is run with the purpose of demonstrating nonexistence of (relevant) differences between two (or maybe more) treatments in the broadest sense, is called an equivalence trial. Typically, the rigorous construction of a testing procedure for the confirmatory analysis of an equivalence trial requires rather heavy mathematical machinery. Nevertheless, the basic idea leading to a logically sound formulation of an equivalence testing problem and the major steps making up an appropriate statistical decision procedure can be illustrated by an example as simple as the following.

Example 1.1

Of an antihypertensive drug which has been in successful use for many years, a new generic version has recently been approved to the market and started to be sold in the pharmacies at a price undercutting that of the reference formulation (R) by about 40%. A group of experts in hypertensiology doubt the clinical relevance of existing data showing the *bio*equivalence of the generic to the reference formulation, notwithstanding the fact that these data had been accepted by the drug regulation authorities as sufficient for approving the new formulation. Accordingly, the hypertensiologists agree to launch into a clinical trial aiming at establishing the *therapeutic* equivalence of the new formulation of the drug. Instead of recruiting a control group of patients to be treated with R, one decides to base the assessment of the therapeutic equivalence of the new formulation on comparison to a fixed responder rate of 60% obtained from long-term experience with formulation R. Out of $n = 125$ patients eventually recruited for the current trial, 56% showed a positive response in the sense of reaching a target diastolic blood pressure below 90 mmHg. Statistical assessment of this result was done by means of a conventional binomial test of the null hypothesis that the probability p, say, of obtaining a positive response in a patient given the generic formulation, equals the reference value $p_{\circ} = .60$, versus the two-sided alternative $p \neq p_{\circ}$. Since the significance probability (*p*-value) computed in this way turned out to be as high as .41, the researchers came to the conclusion that the therapeutic equivalence of the generic to the reference formulation could be taken for granted implying that the basic requirement for switching to the new formulation whenever confining the costs of treatment is an issue, was satisfied.

Unfortunately, it follows from the logical asymmetry between null and alternative hypothesis mentioned at the beginning that such kind of reasoning misses the following point of fundamental importance: "Converting" a traditional two-sided test of significance by inferring equivalence of the treatments under comparison from a nonsignificant result of the former, generally fails to yield a valid testing procedure. In a word: *A nonsignificant difference must not be confused with significant homogeneity.* Even in the extremely simple setting of the present example, i.e., of a one-arm trial conducted for the purpose of establishing (therapeutic) equivalence of a single treatment with regard to a binary success criterion, correct inference requires the application of a testing procedure exhibiting genuinely new features.

(i) First of all, it is essential to notice that the problem of establishing the alternative hypothesis of *exact* equality of the responder rate p associated with the generic formulation of the drug, to its reference value $p_{\circ} = .60$ by means of a statistical test admits no sensible solution (the reader interested in the logical basis of this statement is referred to § 1.2). The natural way around this difficulty consists of *introducing a region of values of p close enough to the target value $p_{\circ}$ for considering the deviations practically irrelevant.* For the moment, let us specify this region as the interval $(p_\circ - .10\,,\, p_\circ + .10) = (.50\,,\, .70)$. Hence, by equivalence of p to $p_\circ$ we eventually mean a weakened form of identity specifying equality except for ignorable differences.

(ii) The closer the observed responder rate X/n comes up to the target rate $p_\circ = .60$, the stronger the evidence in favour of equivalence provided by the available data. Thus, a reasonable test for equivalence of p to $p_\circ$ will use a decision rule of the following form: The *null hypothesis of inequivalence is rejected if and only if* the difference $X/n - p_\circ$ *between the observed and the target responder rate falls between suitable critical bounds*, say c_1 and c_2, such that c_1 is some negative and c_2 some positive real number, respectively.

(iii) Optimally, the rejection region of the desired test, i.e., the set of possible outcomes of the trial allowing a decision in favour of equivalence, should be defined in such a way that the associated requirement on the degree of closeness of the observed responder rate X/n to the reference rate $p_\circ$ is as weak as possible without increasing the risk of an erroneous equivalence decision over α, the prespecified level of significance (chosen to be .05 in the majority of practical applications).

(iv) As follows from applying the results to be presented in §4.3 with $p_\circ \mp .10$ as the *theoretical* range of equivalence and at level $\alpha = 5\%$, the optimal critical bounds to $X/n - p_\circ$ to be used in a test for equivalence of p to $p_\circ = .60$ based on a random sample of size $n = 125$ are given by $c_1 = -2.4\%$ and $c_2 = 3.2\%$, respectively. Despite the considerable size of the sample recruited to the trial, the rejection interval for $X/n - p_\circ$ corresponding to these values of c_1 and c_2 is pretty narrow, and the observed rate 56% of responders falls relatively far outside giving $X/n - p_\circ = -4.0\%$. Consequently, at significance level 5%, the data collected during the trial do not contain sufficient evidence in favour of equivalence of the generic to the reference formulation in the sense of $|p - p_\circ| < .10$.

The confirmatory analysis of experimental studies, clinical trials etc. which are performed in order to establish equivalence of treatments is only one out of many inferential tasks of principal importance which can adequately be dealt with only by means of methods allowing to establish the (suitably enlarged) null hypothesis of a conventional two-sided testing problem. Another category of problems for which exactly the same holds true, refers to the verification of statistical model assumptions of any kind. Notwithstanding the traditional usage of the term "goodness-of-fit test" obscuring the fact that the testing procedures subsumed in the associated category are tailored for solving the reverse problem of establishing lack of fit, in the majority of cases it is much more important to positively demonstrate the compatibility of the model with observed data. Thus, if a goodness-of-fit test is actually to achieve what is implied by its name, then it has to be constructed as an equivalence test in the sense that a positive result supports the conclusion that the true distribution from which the data have been taken, except for minor discrepancies, coincides with the distribution specified by the model.

The primary objective of this book is a systematic and fairly comprehensive account of testing procedures for problems such that the *alternative* hypothesis specifies a sufficiently *small neighbourhood* of the point in the space of the target parameter (or functional) which indicates perfect coincidence of the probability distributions under comparison. As will become evident from the numerical material presented in the subsequent chapters, the sample sizes required in an equivalence test in order to achieve a reasonable power typically tend to be considerably larger than in an ordinary one- or two-sided testing procedure for the same setting unless the range of tolerable deviations of the distributions from each other is chosen so wide that even distributions exhibiting pronounced dissimilarities would be declared "equivalent". This is the reason why in equivalence testing optimization of the procedures with respect to power is by no means an issue of purely academic interest but a necessary condition for keeping sample size requirements within the limits of practicality. The theory of hypotheses testing as developed in the fundamental work of Lehmann (1986) provides in full mathematical generality methods for the construction of optimal procedures for four basic types of testing problems covering equivalence problems in the sense of the present monograph as well. Converting these general results into explicit decision rules suitable for routine applications will be a major concern in the chapters to follow.

1.2 Formalization of the statistical notion of equivalence

As explained in nontechnical terms in the previous section, equivalence problems are distinguished from conventional testing problems by the form of the hypotheses to be established by means of the data obtained from the experiment or study under analysis. Typically [for an exception see § 9.3], the hypotheses formulation refers to some real-valued parameter θ which provides a sensible measure of the degree of dissimilarity of the probability distributions involved. For example, in the specific case of a standard parallel group design used for the purpose of testing for equivalence of two treatments A and B, an obvious choice is $\theta = \mu_1 - \mu_2$ with μ_1 and μ_2 denoting a measure of location for the distribution of the endpoint variable under A and B, respectively. The equivalence hypothesis whose compatibility with the data one wants to assess, specifies that θ is contained in a suitable neighbourhood around some reference value $\theta_\circ$ taken on by θ if and only if the distributions under comparison are exactly equal. This neighbourhood comprises those values of θ whose distance from $\theta_\circ$ is considered compatible with the notion of equivalence for the respective setting.

It will be specified as an open interval throughout with endpoints denoted by $\theta_\circ - \varepsilon_1$ and $\theta_\circ + \varepsilon_2$, respectively. Of course, both ε_1 and ε_2 are positive constants whose numerical values must be assigned a priori, i.e., without knowledge of the data under analysis. Specifically, in the case of the simple parallel group design with $\theta = \mu_1 - \mu_2$, the usual choice of $\theta_\circ$ is $\theta_\circ = 0$, and the equivalence interval is frequently chosen symmetrical about $\theta_\circ$, i.e., in the form $(-\varepsilon, \varepsilon)$.

Accordingly, in this book, our main objects of study are statistical decision procedures which define a valid statistical test at some prespecified level $\alpha \in (0, 1)$ of the *null hypothesis*

$$H : \theta \leq \theta_\circ - \varepsilon_1 \quad \text{or} \quad \theta \geq \theta_\circ + \varepsilon_2 \tag{1.1a}$$

of nonequivalence, versus the *equivalence assumption*

$$K : \theta_\circ - \varepsilon_1 < \theta < \theta_\circ + \varepsilon_2 \tag{1.1b}$$

as the alternative hypothesis. Such a decision rule has not necessarily to exhibit the form of a significance test in the usual sense. For example, it can and will [see § 9.3.3] also be given by a Bayes rule for which there is additional evidence that the "objective probability" of a false decision in favour of equivalence will never exceed the desired significance level α. Bayesian methods for which we cannot be sure enough about this property taken for crucial from the frequentist point of view, are of limited use in the present context as long as the regulatory authorities to which drug approval applications based on equivalence studies have to be submitted, keep insisting on the maintenance of a prespecified significance level in the classical sense.

It is worth noticing that an equivalence hypothesis of the general form (1.1b) will never be the same as the null hypothesis $H_0 : \theta = \theta_\circ$ of the corresponding two-sided testing problem, irrespective of what particular positive values are assigned to the constants ε_1 and ε_2. In other words, switching attention from an ordinary two-sided to an equivalence testing problem entails not simply an exchange of both hypotheses involved but in addition a more or less far-reaching modification of them. Replacing the nondegenerate interval K of (1.1b) by the singleton $\{\theta_\circ\}$ would give rise to a testing problem admitting of no worthwhile solution at all. In fact, in all families of distributions being of interest for concrete applications, the rejection probability of any statistical test is a *continuous* function of the target parameter θ. But continuity of the power function $\theta \mapsto \beta(\theta)$, say, clearly implies, that the test can maintain level α on $\{\theta \neq \theta_\circ\}$ only if its power against $\theta = \theta_\circ$ exceeds α neither. Consequently, if we tried to test the null hypothesis $\theta \neq \theta_\circ$ against the alternative $\theta = \theta_\circ$, we would not be able to replace the trivial "test" rejecting the null hypothesis independently of the data with probability α, by a useful decision rule.

1.3 Major fields of application of equivalence tests

1.3.1 Comparative bioequivalence trials

It was not until the late nineteen sixties that statistical researchers started to direct some attention to methods of testing for equivalence of distributions in the sense made precise in the previous section. In this initial phase, work on equivalence assessment was almost exclusively triggered by the introduction of special approval regulations for so-called generic drugs by the Food and Drug Administration (FDA) of the U.S. as well as the drug regulation authorities of many other industrialized countries. Loosely speaking, a generic drug is an imitation of a specific drug product of some primary manufacturer that has already been approved to the market and prescribed for therapeutic purposes for many years but is no longer protected by patent. As a matter of course, with regard to the biologically active ingredients, every such generic drug is chemically identical to the original product. However, the actual biological effect of a drug depends on a multitude of additional factors referring to the whole process of the pharmaceutical preparation of the drug. Examples of these are

- chemical properties and concentrations of excipients
- kind of milling procedure
- choice of tablet coatings
- time and strength of compression applied during manufacture.

For the approval of a generic drug, the regulatory authorities do not require evidence of therapeutic efficacy and tolerability based on comparative clinical trials. Instead, it is considered sufficient that in a trial on healthy volunteers comparing the generic to the original formulation of the drug, the hypothesis of absence of relevant differences in basic pharmacokinetic characteristics (called "measures of bioavailability") can be established. If this is the case, then the generic drug is declared equivalent with respect to biovailability or, for short, bioequivalent to the original formulation.

Assessment of bioequivalence between a new and a reference formulation of some drug is still by far the largest field of application for statistical tests of the type this book focusses upon, and can be expected to keep holding this position for many years to come. The overwhelming importance of the problem of bioequivalence assessment has to do much more with economic facts and public health policies than with truly scientific interest: During the last decade, the market share of generic drugs has been rising in the major industrial countries to levels ranging between 43% (U.S., 1996) and 67.5% (Germany, 1993)! From the statistical perspective, the field of bioequivalence assessment is comparatively narrow. In fact, under standard model assumptions [to be made explicit in Ch. 9], the confirmatory analysis of a prototypical bioequivalence study reduces to a comparison of two Gaussian distributions. In view of this it is quite misleading that equivalence testing is still more or less identified with *bio*equivalence assessment by many (maybe even the majority) of statisticians. As will hopefully become clear enough from further reading of the present monograph, problems of equivalence assessment are encountered in virtually every context where the application of the methodology of testing statistical hypotheses makes any sense at all. Accordingly, it is almost harder to identify a field of application of statistics where equivalence problems play no or at most a minor role, than to give reasons why they merit particular attention in some specific field.

1.3.2 Clinical trials involving an active control

In medical research, clinical trials which involve an active (also called positive) control make up the second large category of studies commonly analyzed by means of equivalence testing methods. An active rather than negative control (typically placebo) is used in an increasing number of clinical trials referring to the treatment of diseases for which well-established therapeutic strategies of proven efficacy and tolerability already exist. Under such circumstances it would be clearly unethical to leave dozens or hundreds of patients suffering from the respective disease without any real treatment until the end of the study. What has to be and is frequently done instead, is replacing the traditional negative control by a group to which the best therapy having been in use up to now, is administered. Usually, it is not realistic to expect then that the group which is given the new treatment will do still better than the control group with respect to efficacy endpoints. In return, the experimental therapy is typically known in advance to have much better tolerability so that its use can and should be recommended as soon as there is convincing evidence of equivalent efficacy. A particularly important example are trials of modifying adjuvant chemotherapy regimes well established in oncology, by reducing dosages and/or omitting the most toxic of the substances used. For such a reduced regime, superiority with respect to tolerability can be taken for granted without conducting any additional trial at all, and it is likewise obvious that demonstrating merely noninferiority with regard to efficacy would entail a valuable success.

In the clinical trials methodology literature, it has sometimes been argued (cf. Windeler and Trampisch, 1996) that tests for equivalence in the strict, i.e., two-sided sense are *generally* inappropriate for an active control study and should always be replaced by one-sided equivalence tests of the kind considered in Chapter 2. In contrast, we believe that there are several convincing points (not to be discussed in detail here) for the view that the question whether a one- or a two-sided formulation of the equivalence hypothesis eventually to be tested is the appropriate one, should be carefully discussed with the clinicians planning a specific active control trial rather than decided by biostatistical decree once and for all.

An undisputed major difference between clinical trials involving an active control, and comparative bioavailability studies (the consensus about the adequacy of two-sided equivalence tests for the confirmatory analysis of the latter has never been seriously challenged) refers to the structure of the distributions which the variables of primary interest typically follow: Quite often, the analysis of an active control trial has to deal with binomial proportions [→ §§ 2.3., 6.5] or even empirical survivor functions computed from partially censored observations [→ § 6.6] rather than with means and variances determined from samples of normally distributed observations.

1.3.3 Preliminary tests for checking assumptions underlying other methods of statistical inference

Looking through statistical textbooks of virtually all kinds and levels of sophistication, it is hard to find any which does not give at least some brief account of methods for checking the assumptions that the most frequently used inferential procedures have to rely upon. All of them approach this basic problem from the same side: The testing procedures provided are tests of the null hypothesis that the assumptions to be checked hold true, versus the alternative hypothesis that they are violated in one way or the other. Since the aim a user of such a preliminary test commonly has in mind is to give evidence of the correctness of the required assumptions, one cannot but state that the usual approach is based on an inadequate formulation of the hypotheses. It is clear that equivalence tests in the sense of § 1.2 are exactly the methods needed for finding a way around this logical difficulty so that another potentially huge field of applications of equivalence testing methods comes within view.

One group of methods needed in this context are of course tests for goodness rather than lack of fit since they allow in particular the verification of parametric distributional assumptions of any kind. Other important special cases covered by the methods presented in subsequent chapters refer to restrictions on nuisance parameters in standard linear models such as

- homoskedasticity [→ §§ 6.4, 7.4]
- additivity of main effects [→ § 8.3.1]
- identity of carryover effects in crossover trials [→ § 8.3.2]

1.4 Choosing the main distributional parameter

Except for single-parameter problems, the scientific relevance of the result of an equivalence testing procedure highly depends on a careful and sensible choice of the target parameter θ [recall (1.1a), (1.1b) of p. 5] in terms of which the hypotheses have been formulated. The reason is that, in contrast to the corresponding conventional testing problems with the common boundary of null and alternative hypothesis being given by zero, equivalence problems remain generally not invariant under redefinitions of the main distributional parameter. A simple, yet practically quite important example which illustrates this fact, is the two-sample setting with binomial data. If we denote the two unknown parameters in the usual way, i.e., by p_1 and p_2, and define δ and ρ as the difference $p_1 - p_2$ and the odds ratio $p_1(1 - p_2)/((1 - p_1)p_2)$, respectively, then the null hypotheses $\delta = 0$ and $\rho = 1$ correspond of course to exactly the same subset in the space $[0, 1] \times [0.1]$ of the primary parameter (p_1, p_2). On the other hand, the set $\{(p_1, p_2)| -\delta_1 < \delta < \delta_2\}$ will be different from $\{(p_1, p_2)|1 - \varepsilon_1 < \rho < 1 + \varepsilon_2\}$ for *any* choice of the constants $0 < \delta_1, \delta_2 < 1$ and $0 < \varepsilon_1 < 1, \varepsilon_2 > 0$ determining the equivalence limits under both specifications of the target parameter.

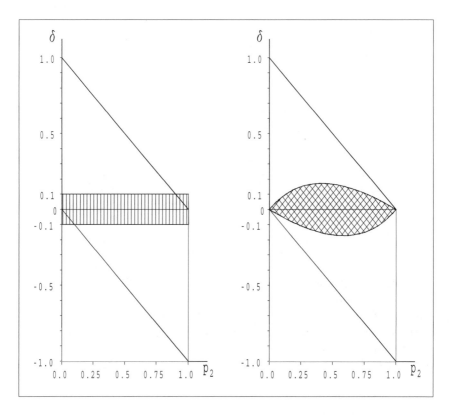

Figure 1.1 *Equivalence hypotheses in terms of the difference between both responder rates [left] and the odds ratio [right] as regions in the $p_2 \times \delta$-plane with $\delta = p_1 - p_2$. [Rhomboid $\hat{=}$ set of possible values of (p_2, δ).]*
(From Wellek and Hampel, 1999, with kind permission by Wiley-VCH.)

On the one hand, there are no mathematical or otherwise formal criteria leading to a unique answer to the question about the appropriate choice of the parameter of main interest for purposes of formulating equivalence hypotheses for a given model or setting. On the other, this is by no means a matter of purely subjective taste but in numerous cases there are convincing arguments for preferring a specific parametrization to an alternative one, with the discrimination between the difference of the responder rates and the odds ratio in the binomial two-sample setting giving an interesting case in point. Although simplicity and ease of interpretability even for the mathematically less educated user clearly speak in favour of the difference δ, plotting the regions corresponding to the two equivalence hypotheses $-\delta_1 < \delta < \delta_2$ and $1 - \varepsilon_1 < \rho < 1 + \varepsilon_2$ as done in Figure 1.1, shows to the contrary that defining equivalent binomial distributions in terms of $p_1 - p_2$ entails a serious logical flaw: Whereas the hypothesis of equivalence with respect to the odds ratio corresponds to a proper subset of the parameter space for (p_2, δ), the range of δ-coordinates of points equivalent to 0 in the sense of the first hypothesis formulation, is distinctly beyond the limits imposed by the side conditions $-p_2 \leq \delta \leq 1 - p_2$, for all sufficiently small and large values of the baseline responder rate p_2. This fact suggests that the choice $\theta = \delta$, notwithstanding its popularity in the existing literature on equivalence testing with binomially distributed data [for a selection of pertinent references see § 2.3.3] leads to an ill-considered testing problem.

Another special case whose importance for practical work can hardly be overestimated since, under standard parametric modelling, bioequivalence assessment with data from two-period crossover studies reduces to it, concerns the comparison of two Gaussian distributions with common but unknown variance on the basis of independent samples. Denoting, as usual, the two expected values and the common standard deviation by μ_1, μ_2 and σ, respectively, the predominant approach starts from the choice $\theta = \mu_1 - \mu_2$ although there are clear reasons why setting $\theta = (\mu_1 - \mu_2)/\sigma$ yields a much more sensible measure of distance between the distributions to compare in the setting of the two-sample t-test: It is an elementary fact (whose implications are given due attention in Lehmann, 1986, § 5.3) that, given any whatever large value of $|\mu_1 - \mu_2|$, both distributions become practically indistinguishable if σ is large enough, whereas the areas under the corresponding densities are next to disjoint if σ approaches zero. At the same time, focussing on the standardized rather than the raw difference between the means, facilitates the step to be discussed in some more detail in the subsequent section: Even in discussions with clinical researchers caring little for statistical subtleties, presentation of a handful of graphs usually suffices to reach a consensus that $|\mu_1 - \mu_2|/\sigma \geq 1$ is incompatible with the notion of equivalence of two Gaussian distributions, and so on.

Interestingly enough, under some circumstances, a thoughtful discussion of the question how the target parameter for defining the equivalence region should most appropriately be chosen, will even lead to the conclusion that the equivalence testing problem originally in mind should better be replaced by an ordinary one-sided testing problem. An example of this kind arises in bioequivalence studies of which one knows (or feels justified to assume) that no period effects have to be taken into account (Anderson and Hauck, 1990; Wellek, 1990/1993a) [see also Ch. 9.3 of the present book].

1.5 Numerical specification of the limits of equivalence

The first question which arises when we want to reach a decision on what numerical values shall be assigned to the equivalence limits $\theta_\circ - \varepsilon_1$, $\theta_\circ + \varepsilon_2$ defining the hypotheses in a testing problem of the form (1.1), is whether or not the equivalence interval has to be symmetric about the reference value $\theta_\circ$. More often than not it seems reasonable to answer this in the affirmative, although virtually all procedures presented in the chapters following the next allow full flexibility in that respect. Perhaps the still best known example of a whole area of application for methods of establishing equivalence in a nonsymmetric sense is bioequivalence assessment along the former FDA guidelines. Before the 1992 revision of its guidance for bioequivalence studies, the FDA strongly recommended to use the specifications $\theta_\circ - \varepsilon_1 = 2\log(.80) \approx -.446$, $\theta_\circ + \varepsilon_2 = 2\log(1.20) \approx .365$ for the maximally tolerable shift between the Gaussian distributions eventually to compare. Essentially, the corresponding interval is the log-transform of what is customarily called the 80 to 120% range for the ratio of the true drug formulation effects. In the revised version of the guidelines, the latter has been replaced with the range 80–125%.

With regard to the question whether it is advisable for the statistician to give general recommendations concerning the form of the equivalence interval, we take the same position as on the one- versus two-sidedness controversy in the context of active control trials [recall § 1.3.2]: This is a point for careful discussion with the researcher planning an individual study and should not made subject to fixed general rules. Instead, full generality should be aimed at in developing the pertinent statistical methods so that we can provide the experimental or clinical researcher with a range of options sufficiently large for allowing him to cover the question he really wants to answer by means of his data.

Even if the problem has been symmetricized by introducing the restriction $\varepsilon_1 = \varepsilon_2 = \varepsilon$ in (1.1a) and (1.1b), coming to an agreement with the experimenter about a specific numerical value to be assigned to the only remaining constant determining the equivalence interval, is not always easy. The following table is intended to give some guidance for some of the most frequently encountered settings:

Table 1.1 *Proposals for choosing the limits of a symmetrical equivalence interval in some standard settings*

(Serial No.)	Setting	Target Parameter or Functional	Reference Value	Tolerance ε: Strict	Liberal
				Choice	
(i)	Sign test	$p_+ = P[D > 0]^{\dagger)}$	1/2	.10	.20
(ii)	Mann-Whitney	$\pi_+ = P[X > Y]^{\ddagger)}$	1/2	.10	.20
(iii)	Two binomial samples	$\log \rho =$ $\log\left[\frac{p_1(1-p_2)}{(1-p_1)p_2}\right]$	0	.41	.85
(iv)	Paired t-Test	δ/σ	0	.25	.50
(v)	Two-Sample t-Test	$(\mu_1 - \mu_2)/\sigma$	0	.36	.74
(vi)	Two Gaussian distr., comparison of var.	$\log(\sigma_1/\sigma_2)$	0	.41	.69

$\dagger)$ $D \equiv$ intraindividual difference for a randomly chosen observational unit

$\ddagger)$ $X, Y \equiv$ independent observations from different distributions

Here are some reasons motivating the above suggestions:

→ (i),(ii): Everyday experience shows that most people will rate probabilities of medium size differing by no more than 10%, as rather similar; 20% or more is usually considered indicating a different order of magnitude in the same context.

→ (iii): Assuming that the reference responder rate is given by $p_2 = 1/2$, straightforward steps of converting inequalities show the condition $-\varepsilon < p_1 - p_2 < \varepsilon$ to be equivalent to $|\log \rho| < \log(\frac{1+2\varepsilon}{1-2\varepsilon}) \equiv \varepsilon_{\tilde{\rho}}$. According to this relationship, the choices $\varepsilon = .10$ and $\varepsilon = .20$ [recall (i)] correspond to $\varepsilon_{\tilde{\rho}} = \log(12/8) = .4055 \approx .41$ and $\varepsilon_{\tilde{\rho}} = \log(14/6) = .8473 \approx .85$, respectively.

→ (iv): Under the Gaussian model $D \sim \mathcal{N}(\delta, \sigma^2)$, we can write:

$$1/2 - \varepsilon < p_+ \equiv P[D > 0] < 1/2 + \varepsilon$$
$$\Leftrightarrow \quad \Phi^{-1}(1/2 - \varepsilon) < \delta/\sigma < \Phi^{-1}(1/2 + \varepsilon)$$
$$\Leftrightarrow \quad -\Phi^{-1}(1 - (1/2 - \varepsilon)) < \delta/\sigma < \Phi^{-1}(1/2 + \varepsilon)$$
$$\Leftrightarrow \quad -\Phi^{-1}(1/2 + \varepsilon) < \delta/\sigma < \Phi^{-1}(1/2 + \varepsilon)$$

where Φ^{-1} denotes the quantile function for the standard normal distribution. Hence, the choice $\varepsilon = .10$ and $\varepsilon = .20$ in case (i) corresponds here to $\varepsilon = \Phi^{-1}(.60) = .2529$ and $\varepsilon = \Phi^{-1}(.70) = .5240$, respectively.

$\rightarrow$ (v): Analogously, relating (ii) to the special case $X \sim \mathcal{N}(\mu_1, \sigma^2)$, $Y \sim \mathcal{N}(\mu_2, \sigma^2)$, yields the first in the following chain of inequalities:

$$1/2 - \varepsilon < \Phi((\mu_1 - \mu_2)/\sqrt{2}\sigma) < 1/2 + \varepsilon$$
$$\Leftrightarrow \quad \Phi^{-1}(1/2 - \varepsilon) < (\mu_1 - \mu_2)/\sqrt{2}\sigma < \Phi^{-1}(1/2 + \varepsilon)$$
$$\Leftrightarrow \quad -\sqrt{2}\,\Phi^{-1}(1/2 + \varepsilon) < (\mu_1 - \mu_2)/\sigma < \sqrt{2}\,\Phi^{-1}(1/2 + \varepsilon).$$

Thus, the choices suggested for (ii) are this time equivalent to setting $\varepsilon = \sqrt{2}\,\Phi^{-1}(.60) = .3577$ and $\varepsilon = \sqrt{2}\,\Phi^{-1}(.70) = .7411$, respectively.

$\rightarrow$ (vi): Unlike (ii) – (v), this setting cannot be related in a natural way to case (i). The suggested values of ε, except for rounding to two significant decimals, are equivalent to the requirements $2/3 < \sigma_1/\sigma_2 < 3/2$ and $1/2 < \sigma_1/\sigma_2 < 2$, respectively. The latter seem again plausible for common statistical sense.

CHAPTER 2

Methods for one-sided equivalence problems

2.1 Objective of a one-sided equivalence trial and formulation of hypotheses

The inferential problems to be treated in the present chapter share two basic properties with equivalence testing problems in the strict sense as introduced in § 1.2. In the first place, they likewise arise from modifying the hypotheses making up some customary type of testing problem very frequently arising in routine data analysis. In the second place, modification of hypotheses again entails the introduction of a region in the space of the target distributional parameter θ within which the difference between the actual value of θ and its reference value $\theta_\circ$ is considered practically irrelevant. However, there remains one crucial difference of considerable importance for the correct interpretation of the results eventually established by means of the corresponding testing procedures, as well as the mathematical treatment of the testing problems: The region of tolerable discrepancies between θ and $\theta_\circ$ is now bounded to below only whereas excesses in value of θ over $\theta_\circ$ of arbitrary magnitude are considered acceptable or even desirable. In other words, in a study of the type which the testing procedures to be discussed here are tailored for, the aim is to make it sufficiently sure that the experimental treatment A, say, is not substantially inferior to some standard treatment B, without ruling out the possibility that A may even do considerably better than B. In contrast, for an equivalence trial in the strict sense made precise in the previous chapter, the idea is constitutive that one may encounter hypo- as well as hyperefficacy of the new as compared to the standard treatment and that protecting oneself against both forms of a substantial dissimilarity between A and B is a definite requirement.

Formally speaking, the crucial difference between equivalence testing and testing for absence of substantial inferiority is that in the latter type of problem the right-hand boundary $\theta_\circ + \varepsilon_2$ of the equivalence interval is replaced with $+\infty$ or, in cases where the parameter space Θ of θ is bounded to the right itself, by $\theta^* = \sup \Theta$. The corresponding hypotheses testing problem reads

$$H_1 : \theta \leq \theta_\circ - \varepsilon \quad \text{versus} \quad K_1 : \theta > \theta_\circ - \varepsilon \tag{2.1}$$

with sufficiently small $\varepsilon > 0$. Testing problems of this general form differ from ordinary one-sided problems only by shifting the common boundary of the hypotheses away from $\theta_\circ$ by $-\varepsilon$. Nevertheless, numerous authors (among many others see Dunnet and Gent, 1977; Mehta, Patel and Tsiatis, 1984) use the term equivalence test also for decision procedures yielding a valid test for H_1 versus K_1 as defined in (2.1). Although this is clearly at variance with the primary meaning of the concept of equivalence we adopt essentially the same usage terming testing problems of the form (2.1) one-sided equivalence problems in the sequel. The term "noninferiority problem" which got rather fashionable in the recent clinical trials literature (see, e.g., Röhmel, 1998; Steinijans et al., 1998) seems not really appropriate since in the ordinary one-sided testing problem obtained by setting $\varepsilon = 0$ in (2.1), the alternative hypothesis likewise specifies superiority of the experimental over the standard treatment.

From a mathematical point of view, the direction of the shift of the common boundary of an ordinary one-sided testing problem does not matter. In fact, approaches well suited for the construction of tests for one-sided equivalence in the sense of (2.1) can also be used for the derivation of tests for one-sided problems with a boundary of hypotheses shifted to the right, and vice versa. If θ keeps denoting a meaningful measure for the extent of superiority of a new treatment A over some standard treatment B and $\theta = \theta_\circ$ indicates identity in effectiveness of both treatments, testing $\theta \leq \theta_\circ + \varepsilon$ versus $\theta > \theta_\circ + \varepsilon$ rather than $\theta \leq \theta_\circ - \varepsilon$ versus $\theta > \theta_\circ - \varepsilon$ makes sense whenever one wants to ensure that a significant result of the corresponding test indicates that replacing A by B entails a relevant improvement. As pointed out by Victor (1987) this holds true for the majority of clinical trials aiming at giving evidence of treatment differences rather than equivalence.

2.2 Standard solution for location parameter families

Whenever the target parameter θ is a measure of the shift in location of the distributions of interest, shifting the common boundary of a pair of one-sided hypotheses produces a testing problem which is new only when we look at the concrete meaning of a positive decision in favour of the alternative. From a purely statistical point of view, no more than a trivial modification of the usual test for the corresponding conventional problem $\theta \leq \theta_\circ$ versus $\theta > \theta_\circ$ is required. Subsequently we describe the rationale behind this modification in some detail for the case of comparing two treatments A and B on the basis of paired and of independent samples of univariate observations, respectively.

2.2.1 Paired observations

The data to be analyzed in any trial following the basic scheme of paired comparisons consists of random pairs (X, Y), say, such that X and Y gives the result of applying treatment A and B to the same arbitrarily selected observational unit. Except for the treatment, the conditions under which X and Y are taken are supposed to be strictly balanced allowing the experimenter to interpret the intra-subject difference $D = X - Y$ as quantifying in that individual case the superiority in effectiveness of treatment A as compared to B. In this setting, speaking of a location problem means to make the additional assumption that in the underlying population of subjects, any potential difference between both treatments is reflected by a shift θ in the location of the distribution of D away from 0 leaving the distributional shape per se totally unchanged. In absence of any treatment difference at all, let this distribution be given by some continuous cumulative distribution function (cdf) $F_\circ : \mathbb{R} \to [0, 1]$ symmetric about zero. For the time being, we do not specify whether the baseline cdf has some known form (e.g., $F_\circ = \Phi(\cdot/\sigma)$ with Φ denoting the standard normal cdf), or is allowed to vary over the whole class of all continuous cdf's on the real line being symmetric about zero [$\to$ nonparametric one-sample location problem, cf. Randles and Wolfe (1979), Ch. 10)].

Regarding the full data set, i.e., the sample $(X_1, Y_1), \ldots, (X_n, Y_n)$ of all n pairs of measurements obtained under both treatments, statistical inference is based on the following assumptions about the corresponding intraindividual differences $D_i = X_i - Y_i$:

(a) The vector $(D_1, \ldots, D_n)$ is independent and identically distributed (iid) ;

(b) $P[D_i \le d] = F_\circ(d - \theta)$ for arbitrary $z \in \mathbb{R}$ and all $i = 1, \ldots, n$, with $F_\circ(-d) = 1 - F_\circ(d) \, \forall d$ and θ denoting the parameter of interest. (By convention, positive values of θ are assumed to indicate a tendency towards "better" results under treatment A as compared to B).

Now, the general form of the rejection region of a test at level α for the traditional one-sided testing problem $H_1^\circ : \theta \le 0$ versus $K_1^\circ : \theta > 0$ [$\to$ (2.1), specialized to the case that $\theta_\circ = 0$, $\varepsilon = 0$] is well known to be given by

$$\left\{ T(D_1, \ldots, D_n) > c_\alpha \right\}$$

where $T(\cdot)$ denotes a suitable real-valued function of n arguments (usually called the test statistic), and c_α the upper 100α percentage point of the distribution of the random variable $(D_1, \ldots, D_n)$ under $\theta = 0$. If we change the directly observed intra-subject differences D_i to $\tilde{D}_i = D_i + \varepsilon$, then the modified sample $(\tilde{D}_1, \ldots, \tilde{D}_n)$ obviously satisfies again (a) and (b), provided the parameter θ is likewise shifted introducing the transform $\tilde{\theta} = \theta + \varepsilon$. Furthermore, the testing problem $H_1 : \theta \leq -\varepsilon$ versus $K_1 : \theta > -\varepsilon$ we are primarily interested in, is clearly the same as the ordinary one-sided problem $\tilde{\theta} \leq 0$ versus $\tilde{\theta} > 0$ relating to the transformed intra-subject differences $\tilde{D}_i$. Hence, in the present setting we obtain the desired test for the one-sided equivalence problem H_1 vs. K_1 simply by using the rejection region of the test for the associated nonshifted null hypothesis in terms of the observations shifted the same distance as the common boundary of the hypotheses but in the opposite direction. The test obtained in this way rejects the null hypothesis $H_1 : \theta \leq -\varepsilon$ [$\rightarrow$ relevant inferiority] if and only if we find that $T(D_1 + \varepsilon, \ldots, D_n + \varepsilon) > c_\alpha$ where $T(\cdot)$ and c_α are computed in exactly the same way as before.

Example 2.1

We illustrate the approach described above by reanalyzing the data from a study (Miller et al., 1990) of possible effects of the fat substitute olestra on the absorption of highly lipophilic oral contraceptives. The sample recruited for this trial consisted of 28 healthy premenopausal women. During the verum phase, each subject consumed 18 gm/day olestra for 28 days while taking a combination of norgestrel (300μg) and ethinyl estradiol (30μg) as an oral contraceptive. Blood samples were taken on days 12 to 14 of the cycle and analyzed for ethinyl and estradiol concentrations. For the placebo phase, the experimental and measurement procedure was exactly the same as for verum except for replacing olestra with conventional triglycerides at each meal. Table 2.1 gives the individual results for norgestrel and the maximum concentration C_{max} as the pharmacokinetic parameter of interest.

According to the general objective of the trial, let us aim at establishing that the consumption of olestra does not reduce the bioavailability of norgestrel (as measured by C_{max}) to a relevant extent. Further, let us define θ as denoting the population median of the distribution of the intra-subject differences $D_i = X_i - Y_i$ with $\varepsilon = 1.5$ as the limit of relevance, and base the confirmatory analysis of the data on the Wilcoxon signed rank statistic. Then, the computational steps which have to be carried out in order to test for one-sided equivalence are as follows.

Table 2.1 *Maximal concentrations of norgestrel (ng/ml) in the sera of 28 women while consuming olestra (X_i) and meals containing ordinary triglycerides (Y_i), respectively [$\tilde{D}_i = D_i + \varepsilon$; $\tilde{R}_i^+$ = rank of the ith subject with respect to $|\tilde{D}_i|$; $\varepsilon = 1.5$]*

i	X_i	Y_i	$\tilde{D}_i$	$\tilde{R}_i^+$	i	X_i	Y_i	$\tilde{D}_i$	$\tilde{R}_i^+$
1	6.03	6.62	0.91	12	15	11.81	11.19	2.12	21
2	5.62	6.78	0.34	5	16	8.72	9.55	0.67	9
3	6.93	6.85	1.58	18	17	7.01	5.53	2.98	26
4	5.86	8.09	−0.73	11	18	7.13	6.71	1.92	20
5	8.91	9.18	1.23	15	19	6.56	6.53	1.53	17
6	5.86	7.47	−0.11	1	20	4.22	5.39	0.33	4
7	9.43	9.90	1.03	13	21	4.13	4.92	0.71	10
8	5.30	4.29	2.51	22	22	6.57	9.92	−1.85	19
9	4.99	3.80	2.69	24	23	8.83	10.51	−0.18	2
10	6.12	7.01	0.61	8	24	9.05	10.15	0.40	6
11	12.45	9.53	4.42	28	25	9.31	9.55	1.26	16
12	5.48	6.39	0.59	7	26	7.67	8.95	0.22	3
13	6.04	4.63	2.91	25	27	7.66	6.63	2.53	23
14	8.32	5.54	4.28	27	28	5.45	8.01	−1.06	14

(i) For each $i = 1, \ldots, 28$, the shifted intra-subject difference $\tilde{D}_i$ [→ Table 2.1, 4th column] and the rank $\tilde{R}_i^+$ with respect to $|\tilde{D}_i|$ [→ Table 2.1, 5th column] have to be determined.

(ii) Denoting the sum of ranks of subjects with a positive sign of $\tilde{D}_i$ by $\tilde{V}_s^+$, the value of this modified signed rank statistic is computed to be $\tilde{V}_s^+ = 359$.

(iii) Under $\theta = -\varepsilon = -1.5$, $\tilde{V}_s^+$ has an asymptotic normal distribution with expected value $E_0(\tilde{V}_s^+) = n(n+1)/4 = 28 \cdot 29/4 = 203$ and variance $Var_0(\tilde{V}_s^+) = n(n+1)(2n+1)/24 = 1928.5$. Hence, the usual approximation with continuity correction gives the *p*-value (observed significance probability) $p_{obs} = \Phi[(203-359+.5)/\sqrt{1928.5} = \Phi[-3.5410] = .0002$.

   In view of the order of magnitude of the significance probability obtained in this way, the decision of the modified signed rank test for one-sided equivalence is positive even at the 1% level in the present case. In other words, the results of the study performed by Miller and coworkers (1990) contain sufficient evidence in favour of the hypothesis that the consumption of olestra does not lead to a relevant decrease of the bioavailability of norgestrel.

2.2.2 Two independent samples

If a comparative study of two treatments A and B follows the parallel group design, the data set to be analyzed consists of values of $m + n$ mutually independent random variables $X_1, \ldots, X_m, Y_1, \ldots, Y_n$. By convention, it is assumed that the X_i are observed in subjects who are given treatment A whereas the Y_j relate to the other treatment, i.e., to B. In this setting, the location model implies that any possible treatment difference can be represented by means of the relationship $X_i \overset{\mathrm{d}}{=} Y_j + \theta$ where, as usual (cf. Randles and Wolfe, 1979, §1.3), the symbol "$\overset{\mathrm{d}}{=}$" indicates identity of the distributions of the two random variables appearing on its left- and right-hand side, respectively. In other words, in the case of the parallel group design the location model assumes that the distributions associated with the two treatments have exactly the same shape implying that distribution A can be generated by shifting all individual values making up distribution B the same distance $|\theta|$ to the right (for $\theta > 0$) or left (for $\theta < 0$). Making this idea mathematically precise leads to specifying the following assumptions about the two distributions under comparison:

(a*) The complete data vector $X_1, \ldots, X_m, Y_1, \ldots, Y_n$ is independent, and all X_i and Y_j have the same continuous distribution function F and G, respectively.

(b*) There exists a real constant θ such that $F(x) = G(x - \theta)$ for all $x \in \mathbb{R}$.

Reduction of the one-sided equivalence problem $H_1 : \theta \leq -\varepsilon$ vs. $K_1 : \theta > -\varepsilon$ to the corresponding ordinary one-sided testing problem $\tilde{\theta} \leq 0$ vs. $\tilde{\theta} > 0$ proceeds here along analogous lines as in the case of paired observations discussed in the previous subsection. To start with, one has to select a suitable test for the nonshifted hypothesis which rejects if and only if one has $T(X_1, \ldots, X_m, Y_1, \ldots, Y_n) > c_\alpha$, where the test statistic $T(\cdot)$ is a real-valued function of $m + n$ arguments and c_α stands for the upper 100α percentage point of the distribution of $T(X_1, \ldots, X_m, Y_1, \ldots, Y_n)$ under $\theta = 0$. As before, this test has to be carried out with suitable transforms $\tilde{X}_i$ and $\tilde{Y}_j$, say, of the primary observations X_i and Y_j, given by $\tilde{X}_i = X_i + \varepsilon$ (for $i = 1, \ldots, m$) and $\tilde{Y}_j = Y_j$ (for $j = 1, \ldots, n$), respectively. In view of the close analogy to the paired observations case, illustration of the approach by another numerical example is dispensable. Its implementation gets particularly simple in the parametric case with $F(x) = \Phi((x - \theta)/\sigma)$, $G(y) = \Phi(y/\sigma)$ and T chosen to be the ordinary two-sample t-statistic: One has just to replace $\bar{x} - \bar{y}$ by $\bar{x} - \bar{y} + \varepsilon$ in the numerator of T then and proceed exactly as usual in all remaining steps.

2.3 Exact two-sample tests for binomial distributions

2.3.1 Exact Fisher type test for one-sided equivalence with respect to the odds ratio

One of the most obvious and important examples of a setting which is definitely not accessible to the translation-based approach to one-sided equivalence testing discussed in the previous section, is that of a two-arm trial with a binary endpoint, i.e., an outcome-variable taking on only two possible values conveniently labelled "response" and "nonresponse". Without loss of statistical information, the data obtained from a trial of this type can be reduced to the frequencies of responders and nonresponders observed in both treatment arms. The latter are conveniently arranged in a table of the well-known 2×2 layout. In order to fix notation, a generic contingency table of that type is displayed below.

By assumption, X has a binomial distribution with parameters m, p_1 [short-hand notation: $X \sim \mathcal{B}(m, p_1)$] and is independent of $Y \sim \mathcal{B}(n, p_2)$. As to parametrization of the corresponding family of joint distributions of (X, Y), we adopt the view supported by the arguments given in § 1.4 that the odds ratio $\rho = p_1(1-p_2)/(1-p_1)p_2$ provides a more adequate measure of dissimilarity of the two distributions under comparison than the difference

Table 2.2 *Contingency table for the analysis of a two-arm trial with binary outcome-variable*

Treat-ment	Response +	−	Σ
A	X (p_1)	$m - X$ $(1 - p_1)$	m (1.00)
B	Y (p_2)	$n - Y$ $(1 - p_2)$	n (1.00)
Σ	S	$N - S$	N

$\delta = p_1 - p_2$ between the responder rates in the underlying populations. Accordingly, we are seeking for a suitable test of

$$H_1 : \rho \leq 1 - \varepsilon \quad \text{versus} \quad K_1 : \rho > 1 - \varepsilon \tag{2.2}$$

with some fixed $0 < \varepsilon < 1$.

An optimal solution to this problem can be derived by way of generalizing the construction behind the exact test usually named after R.A. Fisher (1934, § 21.02) for homogeneity of $\mathcal{B}(m, p_1)$ and $\mathcal{B}(n, p_2)$. Like the latter, the optimal [precisely: uniformly most powerful unbiased (UMPU) – see Lehmann (1986, pp. 154-155)] test for (2.2) is based on the conditional distribution of X given the realized value $s \in \{0, 1, \ldots, N\}$ of the "column total" $S = X + Y$. The conditional p-value $p(x|s)$ of the number x of responders counted in treatment arm A has to be computed by means of a probability distribution which, following Harkness (1965), is usually named extended hypergeometric distribution (cf. Johnson, Kotz and Kemp, 1992, § 6.11). In this conditional distribution, any possible value of X is an integer x such that $\max \{0, s - n\} \leq x \leq \min\{s, m\}$. For any such x the precise formula for the conditional p-value reads

$$p(x|s) = \sum_{j=x}^{m} \binom{m}{j} \binom{n}{s-j} (1 - \varepsilon)^j \Bigg/$$
$$\sum_{j=\max\{0,s-n\}}^{\min\{s,m\}} \binom{m}{j} \binom{n}{s-j} (1 - \varepsilon)^j . \quad (2.3)$$

Except for trivial cases like $s = 1$ or $x = m$, this formula is tractable for manual computations only if both sample sizes are very small. On the other hand, writing a program for the extended hypergeometric distribution is hardly more than a routine exercise, and the SAS system provides an intrinsic function (named **probhypr** – see SAS, 1999, p. 489) for the exact computation of the corresponding cdf.

Fortunately, the computational tools which can be made use of when applying the UMPU test for one-sided equivalence of two binomial distributions with respect to the odds ratio, go considerably beyond the availability of an algorithm for computing significance probabilities. In fact, both the power of the test against arbitrary specific alternatives, and sample sizes required for maintaining some prespecified power, are accessible to exact computational methods as well. Naturally, both of these tasks are much more demanding conceptually no less than technically than mere computation of exact conditional p-values. An algorithm for exact power computations will be outlined first.

Let us keep both sample sizes m, n fixed and denote by $(p_1^*, p_2^*) \in (0, 1)^2$ any point in the region corresponding to the alternative hypothesis K_1 of (2.2). By definition, the power of the test based on (2.3) against (p_1^*, p_2^*) equals the *nonconditional* rejection probability, given the true distribution of X and Y is $\mathcal{B}(m, p_1^*)$ and $\mathcal{B}(n, p_2^*)$, respectively. In view of this, for *each* possible value $s = 0, 1, \ldots, N$ of the column total $S = X + Y$, the critical value $k_\alpha(s)$, say, of the test has to be determined. Adopting the convention that, conditional on $\{S = s\}$, the rejection region be of the form $\{X > k_\alpha(s)\}$, $k_\alpha(s)$ is obviously given as the smallest integer x such that $\max\{0, s - n\} \le x \le \min\{s, m\}$ and $p(x + 1|s) \le \alpha$. Furthermore, it is essential to observe that the test holds its (rather strong) optimality property only if in each conditional distribution of X the prespecified significance level $\alpha \in (0, 1)$ is exactly attained rather than only maintained in the sense of not exceeding it. In view of the discreteness of all distributions involved, this typically requires that on the boundary of the critical region $\{X > k_\alpha(s)\}$, i.e., for $X = k_\alpha(s)$ a randomized decision in favour of the alternative hypothesis is taken with probability $\gamma(s) = [\alpha - p(k_\alpha(s) + 1 \mid s)]/[p(k_\alpha(s) \mid s) - p(k_\alpha(s) + 1 \mid s)]$. Although randomized decisions between statistical hypotheses are hardly acceptable for real applications, it seems reasonable to carry out the power calculations both for the randomized and the ordinary nonrandomized version of the test defined by accepting on the boundary of the rejection regions *always* H_1. In fact, given some specific alternative (p_1^*, p_2^*) of interest, the rejection probability of the randomized version of the test is an upper bound to the power attainable in any other conditional test of (2.1). Accordingly, it provides precise information about the maximum improvement which might be achieved by deriving more sophisticated nonrandomized versions of the test [see below, pp. 25-27].

The conditional power of the randomized test is given by

$$\beta(p_1^*, p_2^*|s) =$$

$$\frac{\displaystyle\sum_{j=k_\alpha(s)+1}^{\min\{s,m\}} \binom{m}{j}\binom{n}{s-j}\rho_*^{\,j} + \gamma(s)\binom{m}{k_\alpha(s)}\binom{n}{s-k_\alpha(s)}\rho_*^{\,k_\alpha(s)}}{\displaystyle\sum_{j=\max\{0,s-n\}}^{\min\{s,m\}} \binom{m}{j}\binom{n}{s-j}\rho_*^{\,j}}, \quad (2.4)$$

with $\rho_* = p_1^*(1 - p_2^*)/(1 - p_1^*)p_2^*$.

In order to compute its nonconditional power against the arbitrarily fixed specific alternative (p_1^*, p_2^*), we have to integrate the functions $s \mapsto \beta(p_1^*, p_2^*|s)$ with respect of the distribution of S. Unfortunately, the latter is simply of binomial form again only if (p_1^*, p_2^*) lies on the diagonal of the unit square. Whenever we select a parameter combination with $p_1^* \ne p_2^*$, the distribution of S must be computed from scratch by means of convolution.

The Fortran program bi2ste1 supplied at http://www.zi-mannheim.de/wktsheq implements this algorithm for sample sizes m, n with $m+n \le 2000$ and arbitrary choices of $\alpha, \varepsilon, p_1^*$ and p_2^*. In order to guarantee high numerical accuracy of the results, it uses (like the other Fortran programs to be found at the same URL) fourfold precision in floating-point arithmetic throughout. Nevertheless, execution time is reasonable even for very large sample sizes (≤ 15sec on a DEC Personal Workstation DPW 500). Unavoidably, the computational effort entailed in determining sample sizes required to guarantee some prespecified power β^* is much higher. The program `bi2ste2` which has been constructed for that purpose, is based on an iteration algorithm whose efficiency strongly depends on a sensible choice of the initial values we let the iteration process start from. In determining the latter, the exact nonconditional power $\beta(p_1^*, p_2^*)$ is approximated by the conditional power $\beta(p_1^*, p_2^* | \tilde{s}(m, n))$ where $\tilde{s}(m, n)$ denotes the integer closest to the expected value $mp_1^* + np_2^*$ of S.

Example 2.2

To provide an illustration of the Fisher type exact test for one-sided equivalence of two binomial distributions with respect to the odds ratio, we will use some part of the data from a comparative phase-IV trial of two antibiotics administered to treat streptoccal pharyngitis (Scaglione, 1990). At the time the trial was launched, clarithromycin was an experimental drug of which one knew from animal experiments that its toxicity was considerably weaker than that of the classical macrolid antibiotic erythromycin used as the reference medication. Hence, with regard to therapeutic efficacy, one-sided equivalence with erythromycin could have been considered a sufficient argument for preferring the new macrolid in the treatment of streptococcal infections.

Table 2.3 *Successes and failures observed when treating β hemolytic streptococcal pharyngitis in patients less than 65 years of age by means of clarithromycin (A) and erythromycin (B), respectively*

Treat-ment	Response favourable	Response nonfavour.	Σ
A	98 (92.45%)	8 (7.55%)	106 (100.0%)
B	97 (90.65%)	10 (9.35%)	107 (100.0%)
Σ	195	18	213

Specifying $\varepsilon = .50$ in (2.2), we find with the data of Table 2.3 by means of the *SAS* function mentioned in connection with the general formula for computing the p-value in the test under consideration $[\to (2.3)]$ that $p(98|195) = 1 - \mathtt{probhypr}(213,106,195,97,.50) = .049933$. Thus, at the 5% level of significance, the data of the trial allow the conclusion that the odds of a favourable response to clarithromycin do not fall by more than 50% as compared to those of a positive outcome after administering erythromycin. For the power of the UMPU test at level $\alpha = .05$ against the observed alternative $(p_1^*, p_2^*) = (.9245, .9065)$ [$\leftarrow$ relative frequencies of favourable responses shown in Table 2.3], the Fortran program $\mathtt{bi2ste1}$ gives the result $\beta = .579960 \approx 58\%$. Omitting randomized decisions and keeping the nominal value of α equal to the target significance level, the power drops to $.505559 \approx 51\%$. Accordingly, about every second two-arm trial using a binary endpoint and sample sizes $m = 106, n = 107$ will lead to a rejection of the null hypothesis $\varrho \le .50$ if the true values of the binomial parameters are 90.65% ($\leftrightarrow$ Treatment B) and 92.45% ($\leftrightarrow$ Treatment A), and the test is applied in its conservative nonrandomized version. The sample sizes required in a balanced trial to raise the power of the randomized test against the same specific alternative to 80%, are computed to be $m = n = 194$ by means of $\mathtt{bi2ste2}$.

2.3.2 On improved nonrandomized conditional tests

The loss of power entailed by dispensing with randomized decisions in performing the exact conditional test described in 2.3.1 can be dismissed as irrelevant for practical applications only as long as the sample sizes are fairly large. In small samples this conservatism can assume extreme proportions, and that is the reason why even in the case of the traditional null hypothesis $p_1 - p_2 \le 0$ corresponding to the choice $\varepsilon = 0$ in (2.2), the test obtained by conditioning on $S = X + Y$ has been criticized in the literature almost from the beginning (cf. Pearson, 1947). Of the numerous approaches suggested in more recent years to finding a way around this difficulty (for an up-to-date review see Martín Andrés, 1998), the most interesting for our present purposes seem those which do not alter the basic conditional structure of the test. In fact, the conditional distributions of X given S constitute a one-parameter family depending on (p_1, p_2) only via the odds ratio ϱ chosen as the target parameter for defining one-sided equivalence of the underlying distributions $\mathcal{B}(m, p_1)$ and $\mathcal{B}(n, p_2)$. In addition, there are numerous theoretical arguments supporting the conditional approach to any testing problem which refers to a multiparameter exponential family of distributions (for the special case under consideration, an exhaustive description of these reasons is given by Little, 1989). Essentially, two different approaches to constructing improved nonrandomized versions of the conditional test described in 2.3.1 deserve to be taken into consideration:

(i) The first approach which was proposed by McDonald et al. (1977;1981) [for the case $\varepsilon = 0$, i.e., the traditional null hypothesis $p_1 \leq p_2$], starts with arranging the set $\{k_\alpha(s) \,|\, s = 0, 1, \ldots, N\}$ of all critical bounds to X in ascending order with respect to their unconditional rejection probabilities maximized over H_1. Afterwards, the union of all N conditional rejection regions in the sample space of X is successively enlarged by adding in that order as many boundary points as possible without raising the size of the test (i.e., the maximum of the rejection probability taken over the null hypothesis) over the significance level α.

(ii) The other approach follows a strikingly simple idea which was first exploited (again for the classical formulation of the testing problem) by Boschloo (1970). The usual nonrandomized version of the UMPU test is carried out at an increased nominal significance level $\alpha^* > \alpha$ determined iteratively by maximization over the set of all nominal levels which are admissible in the sense of keeping the size of the resulting test below α.

The most important difference between the two approaches is that (i) produces rejection regions containing points of the sample space whose conditional p-value is larger than that of some or even several points retained in the acceptance region. Our preference for the second approach is mainly motivated by the fact that it lacks this rather counter-intuitive property. Moreover, for the practical implementation of Boschloo's technique one can rely on tables of an extremely simple and compact form since, given both sample sizes, the boundary of the hypotheses and the target level, the nonrandomized test modified according to (ii) is uniquely determined by just one additional constant, viz. α^*.

All values of α^* displayed in Table 2.4 have been computed by means of the Fortran program bi2ste3. The program can be used for determining maximally raised nominal levels for arbitrary additional combinations of $\alpha, \varepsilon, m, n$ as long as the sum N of both sample sizes does not exceed 2000. Actually, each α^* given in the above table represents a nondegenerate interval of nominal levels over which the size of the test remains constant. Of course, it makes no difference if one specific point in that interval is replaced with some other value producing a test of identical size. All what really matters is maximization of the size subject to the condition that the latter must not exceed the prespecified significance level (except for differences small enough for being neglected in practice).

Table 2.4 *Nominal significance levels and sizes of improved conditional tests for (2.2) maintaining the 5%-level, for $\varepsilon = 1/3$, $1/2$ and $m = n = 10, 25, 50, 100, 200$ [Number in ( ): size of the nonrandomized test at nominal level $\alpha = .05$]*

ε	n	α^*	Size	
1/3	10	.08445	.04401	(.02118)
"	25	.09250	.05083	(.02728)
"	50	.07716	.04991	(.02790)
"	75	.06295	.04997	(.03797)
"	100	.06064	.05006	(.03915)
"	200	.05974	.05015	(.04108)
1/2	10	.10343	.04429	(.02869)
"	25	.07445	.05064	(.03049)
"	50	.06543	.04999	(.03551)
"	75	.06810	.05053	(.03584)
"	100	.06468	.05040	(.03761)
"	200	.05992	.04970	(.04344)

2.3.3 Short review of approaches using alternative parametrizations

Although there are large fields of application (epidemiology being perhaps the most important of them) where considerations of odds ratios play a predominant role, not a few users of equivalence testing methods prefer to look at the difference $\delta = p_1 - p_2$ between both binomial parameters, notwithstanding the logical difficulties encountered in defining equivalence in terms of this apparently more intuitive measure of treatment effect [recall p. 8]. Keeping in line with this tendency, the literature contains numerous contributions dealing with the problem of testing $H_1^\delta : p_1 - p_2 \leq -\delta_0$ vs. $K_1^\delta : p_1 - p_2 > -\delta_0$ [with some fixed $\delta_0 > 0$] instead of (2.2) (among many others see Makuch and Simon, 1978; Blackwelder, 1982; Rodary, Com-Nougue and Tournade 1989; Roebruck and Kühn, 1995; Chan, 1998; Chan and Zhang, 1999). This is a special case of the general problem of testing

$$H_1^g : g(p_1, p_2) \leq g(1/2, 1/2) - \varepsilon \quad \text{vs.} \quad K_1^g : g(p_1, p_2) > g(1/2, 1/2) - \varepsilon \quad (2.5)$$

where $g : (0, 1) \times (0, 1) \to \mathbb{R}$ denotes any fixed transformation of the full parameter space into the real line which is constant on the diagonal and strictly increasing (decreasing) in its first (second) argument.

Under the additional assumption that g is totally differentiable with g_1', g_2' as its two first-order partial derivatives, it seems reasonable to base a test for (2.5) on Wald's statistic (cf. Rao, 1973, §6e.3) which in the present setting admits the simple explicit representation

$$W_g(X,Y) =$$

$$\frac{g(\hat{p}_1, \hat{p}_2) - g(1/2, 1/2) + \varepsilon}{[(g_1'(\hat{p}_1, \hat{p}_2))^2 \hat{p}_1(1 - \hat{p}_1)/m + (g_2'(\hat{p}_1, \hat{p}_2))^2 \hat{p}_2(1 - \hat{p}_2)/n]^{1/2}}, \quad (2.6)$$

where $\hat{p}_1$ and $\hat{p}_2$ denotes as usual the relative frequency of "successes" observed under treatment A and B, respectively. In order to construct a nonconditional test of exact level α based on (2.6) one has to determine the smallest $w \in \mathbb{R}$ such that $\sup_{(p_1,p_2) \in H_1^g} P_{p_1,p_2}[W_g(X,Y) > w] \leq \alpha$ and use this w as a critical constant. As long as simple explicit formulas are available for both partial derivatives of g, adopting this technique (the basic idea behind it goes back to Suissa and Shuster, 1985) is a straight-forward exercise. However, even on a high-speed computer, determination of the critical constant $w_g(\varepsilon, \alpha)$, say, of a test of that type with satisfactory numerical accuracy will be a very time-consuming process except for very small sample sizes m and n. The reason is that it is in general not sufficient to restrict maximization of the rejection probability $P_{p_1,p_2}[W_g(X,Y) > w_g(\varepsilon; \alpha)]$ to the boundary $\partial H_1^g = \{(p_1,p_2) \mid g(p_1,p_2) = g(1/2,1/2) - \varepsilon\}$ of H_1^g. In fact, except for parametrizations g satisfying rather strong addi-tional conditions (as derived by Röhmel and Mannsmann, 1999a), the full size $\sup_{(p_1,p_2) \in H_1^g} P_{p_1,p_2}[W_g(X,Y) > w_g(\varepsilon; \alpha)]$ of the rejection region under consideration will be greater than the value found by maximization over ∂H_1^g only. Some of the exact nonconditional tests for one-sided equivalence of two binomial distributions studied in the literature provide control over the significance level only in this weaker sense (for a recent example see Chan 1998; 1999 and the comment by Röhmel and Mannsmann, 1999b on the first of those papers).

CHAPTER 3

General approaches to the construction of tests for equivalence in the strict sense

3.1 The principle of confidence interval inclusion

The most popular and frequently used approach to problems of equivalence testing in the strict (i.e., two-sided) sense is still that which starts from interval estimation. The principle of confidence interval inclusion was originally introduced in a rather inconspicuous paper (written in the form of a Letter to the Editor of a pharmaceutical journal) by W. Westlake (1972). Since that time, it has been discussed in at least three different versions by numerous authors (among many others, see Metzler, 1974; Westlake, 1976, 1979b, 1981; Steinijans and Diletti, 1983, 1985; Mau, 1988; Hauschke, Steinijans, and Diletti, 1990) dealing almost exclusively with *bio*equivalence assessment ($\rightarrow$ Ch. 9) as the only worthwhile field of applying such methods. Our exposition of the approach concentrates on that version which is most efficient with regard to the power of the corresponding testing procedures.

Let $\underline{\theta}(\mathbf{X}; \alpha)$ and $\bar{\theta}(\mathbf{X}; \alpha)$ denote a lower and upper confidence bound for θ at the *same one-sided* confidence level $1 - \alpha$. In the symbols used for these confidence bounds (and similarly for test statistics), $\mathbf{X}$ represents the collection of all observations obtained in terms of the experiment or study under current analysis, i.e., a random vector of dimension at least as large as the sum of all sample sizes involved [e.g., in an ordinary parallel group design for a trial of two treatments one has $\mathbf{X} = (X_1, \ldots, X_m, Y_1, \ldots, Y_n)$]. Then, according to the confidence interval inclusion principle, we get a valid test for equivalence in the sense of (1.1b) [$\rightarrow$ p. 5] by way of rejecting the null hypothesis $H : \theta \leq \theta_\circ - \varepsilon_1$ or $\theta \geq \theta_\circ + \varepsilon_2$ if and only if the random interval $\left(\underline{\theta}(\mathbf{X}; \alpha), \bar{\theta}(\mathbf{X}; \alpha) \right)$ is completely covered by the equivalence interval $(\theta_\circ - \varepsilon_1, \theta_\circ + \varepsilon_2)$ specified by our alternative hypothesis K. Of course, this means that the interval inclusion test decides in favour of equivalence provided both inequalities $\underline{\theta}(\mathbf{X}; \alpha) > \theta_\circ - \varepsilon_1$ and $\bar{\theta}(\mathbf{X}; \alpha) < \theta_\circ + \varepsilon_2$ are satisfied simultaneously.

To be sure, under the assumptions made explicit in the previous paragraph, the two-sided confidence level of the interval $\left(\underline{\theta}(\mathbf{X}; \alpha), \bar{\theta}(\mathbf{X}; \alpha) \right)$ is just $1 - 2\alpha$. Nevertheless, the equivalence test based upon it has always significance level α rather than 2α. The proof of this important fact is almost trivial and requires just a few lines: Let θ be any point in the parameter space belonging to the left-hand part of H such that we have $\theta \leq \theta_\circ - \varepsilon_1$. By definition, the event that the interval inclusion test rejects can be written $\{\theta_\circ - \varepsilon_1 < \underline{\theta}(\mathbf{X}; \alpha), \bar{\theta}(\mathbf{X}; \alpha) < \theta_\circ + \varepsilon_2\}$. Hence, for $\theta \leq \theta_\circ - \varepsilon_1$, an error of the first kind can only occur if we find $\underline{\theta}(\mathbf{X}; \alpha) > \theta$ which means that the corresponding one-sided confidence region $(\underline{\theta}(\mathbf{X}; \alpha), \infty)$ fails to cover the true value of θ. By construction of $\underline{\theta}(\mathbf{X}; \alpha)$, this happens in at most $100\alpha\%$ of the applications of the corresponding confidence procedure so that we have in fact $P_\theta[\text{type-I error}] \leq \alpha$ for all $\theta \leq \theta_\circ - \varepsilon_1$. A completely analogous argument shows that for any $\theta \geq \theta_\circ + \varepsilon_2$, we have $P_\theta[\text{type-I error}] \leq P_\theta[\bar{\theta}(\mathbf{X}; \alpha) \leq \theta] \leq \alpha$. For all remaining points in the parameter space, i.e., for $\theta_\circ - \varepsilon_1 < \theta < \theta_\circ + \varepsilon_2$, there is nothing to show because rejecting H will be a correct decision then. Although the mathematical reasoning required for establishing the validity of interval inclusion tests based on confidence intervals at level $(1 - 2\alpha)$ is so simple, most of the earlier work on the approach (see Westlake, 1981) used intervals of two-sided confidence level $1 - \alpha$ yielding unnecessarily conservative testing procedures. (Nonequal tails confidence intervals at level $1 - \alpha$ for which the associated equivalence tests do not suffer from such a marked conservatism, are constructed in the paper of Hsu et. al., 1994.)

Another fact of considerable importance for a proper understanding of the confidence interval inclusion principle was first pointed out by Schuirmann (1987) for the special case of the setting of the two-sample t-test. Generally, any interval inclusion test for equivalence as defined above is logically equivalent to a combination of two one-sided tests. In fact, it is obvious from its definition that an interval inclusion test decides in favour of equivalence if and only if both the test of $\theta \leq \theta_\circ - \varepsilon_1$ vs. $\theta > \theta_\circ - \varepsilon_1$ based on $\underline{\theta}(\mathbf{X}; \alpha)$, and that of $\theta \geq \theta_\circ + \varepsilon_2$ vs. $\theta < \theta_\circ + \varepsilon_2$ using $\bar{\theta}(\mathbf{X}; \alpha)$ as the test statistic, can reject its null hypothesis [$\rightarrow$ "double one-sided testing procedure"].

For the setting of the two-sample t-test with $\theta = \mu_1 - \mu_2$ and $\theta_\circ = 0$, the $(1 - 2\alpha)$−confidence interval $(\underline{\theta}(\mathbf{X}; \alpha), \bar{\theta}(\mathbf{X}; \alpha))$ introduced above is symmetric about the pivot $\hat{\theta} = \bar{X} - \bar{Y}$ rather than 0. In Westlake (1976) it was argued that applying the interval inclusion rule with confidence intervals nonsymmetric with respect to 0 is unsuitable whenever we deal with a symmetric equivalence hypothesis specifying that $|\theta| = |\mu_1 - \mu_2| < \varepsilon$. Adopting this point of view would imply that the test be based on a $(1-\alpha)$-confidence interval of the form $(\bar{Y} - \bar{X} - C_\alpha, \bar{X} - \bar{Y} + C_\alpha)$ with C_α denoting a suitable real-valued random variable such that $\bar{X} - \bar{Y} + C_\alpha > 0$. However, on closer examination it becomes obvious that this suggestion relates the symmetry requirement to the wrong object. In fact, assuming two samples from homoskedastic Gaussian distributions, the testing problem $|\mu_1 - \mu_2| \geq \varepsilon$ vs. $|\mu_1 - \mu_2| < \varepsilon$ as such turns out to exhibit a clear-cut symmetry structure in that it remains invariant against treating the Y's as making up the first rather than the second of the two samples [formally: against the transformation $(x_1, \ldots, x_m, y_1, \ldots, y_n) \mapsto (y_1, \ldots, y_n, x_1, \ldots, x_m)$]. In such a case, the well-accepted principle of invariance (cf. Cox and Hinkley, 1974, § 2.3 (vi); Lehmann, 1986, Ch. 6) requires that we use a decision rule leading to the same conclusion irrespective of whether or not the samples are labelled in the original manner. It is easy to check that the test based on the symmetric confidence interval $(\bar{Y} - \bar{X} - C_\alpha, \bar{X} - \bar{Y} + C_\alpha)$ lacks this invariance property. In fact, $(\bar{Y} - \bar{X} - C_\alpha, \bar{X} - \bar{Y} + C_\alpha)$ is included in the equivalence interval $(-\varepsilon, \varepsilon)$ if and only if there holds $\bar{X} - \bar{Y} + C_\alpha < \varepsilon$, and the latter inequality is obviously not equivalent to $\bar{Y} - \bar{X} + C_\alpha < \varepsilon$. On the other hand, the test based on the shortest $(1 - 2\alpha)$-confidence interval symmetric about $\bar{X} - \bar{Y}$ rejects if and only if it happens that $|\bar{X} - \bar{Y}| < \varepsilon - S(X_1, \ldots, X_m, Y_1, \ldots, Y_n) \cdot t_{m+n-2;1-\alpha}$ where $S(X_1, \ldots, X_m, Y_1, \ldots, Y_n) = \sqrt{1/m + 1/n} \cdot [(\sum_{i=1}^{m}(X_i - \bar{X})^2 + \sum_{j=1}^{n}(Y_j - \bar{Y})^2)/(m+n-2)]^{1/2}$ and $t_{m+n-2;1-\alpha}$ denotes the upper 100α percentage point of a central t-distribution with $m + n - 2$ degrees of freedom. In view of $S(X_1, \ldots, X_m, Y_1, \ldots, Y_n) = S(Y_1, \ldots, Y_n, X_1, \ldots, X_m)$, the condition for rejecting nonequivalence is the same as $|\bar{Y} - \bar{X}| < \varepsilon - S(Y_1, \ldots, Y_n, X_1, \ldots, X_m) \cdot t_{m+n-2;1-\alpha}$. In other words, the nonsymmetric confidence interval leads to a symmetric test, and vice versa.

If we assume the common variance of the two normal distributions under comparison to be a known constant with respect to which all observations in both samples have been standardized, then the test of $H : |\mu_1 - \mu_2| \geq \varepsilon$ vs. $K : |\mu_1 - \mu_2| < \varepsilon$ based on shortest $(1 - 2\alpha)$-confidence intervals rejects if and only if we have

$$|\bar{X} - \bar{Y}| < \varepsilon - u_{1-\alpha} \cdot \sqrt{m^{-1} + n^{-1}} , \qquad (3.1)$$

where $u_{1-\alpha} = \Phi^{-1}(1 - \alpha)$. Trivially, condition (3.1) defines a nonempty region in the sample space only if the bound $\varepsilon - u_{1-\alpha} \cdot \sqrt{m^{-1} + n^{-1}}$ represents a positive real number which is true only for sufficiently large sample sizes m, n. For example, in the balanced case $m = n$ with $\varepsilon = .25$ and $\alpha = .05$, (3.1) corresponds to a test which will never be able to reject nonequivalence unless the number n of observations available in both groups is at least 87. At first sight, this example seems to be fatal for the interval inclusion principle as a *general* approach to constructing equivalence tests. In fact, it refers to an extremely regular setting since the distribution of the sufficient statistic $(\bar{X}, \bar{Y})$ belongs to a two-parameter exponential family and the distribution of the test statistic $(\bar{X}, \bar{Y})$ is absolutely continuous for any parameter constellation (μ_1, μ_2). Nevertheless, even if the common sample size is as large as 86, the testing procedure given by (3.1) is still poorer than the trivial level-α "test" deciding independently of the data in favour of equivalence whenever in some external random experiment an event of probability α happens to get realized. On the other hand, as will be shown in § 4.5, this is well compatible with the fact that for sample sizes exceeding the minimum value of 87 sufficiently far, decision rule (3.1) yields a test which is practically indistinguishable from the optimal solution to exactly the same testing problem.

3.2 Bayesian tests for equivalence

From the Bayesian viewpoint, problems of testing for equivalence exhibit no peculiarities at all, neither conceptually nor technically. All that is needed as soon as the target parameter θ and the limits $\theta_\circ - \varepsilon_1, \theta_\circ + \varepsilon_2$ of the equivalence range have been fixed, is a joint prior distribution $\pi(\cdot)$, say, of all unknown parameters contained in the underlying statistical model. The Bayesian test for equivalence of θ with $\theta_\circ$ rejects if the posterior probability of the equivalence interval $(\theta_\circ - \varepsilon_1, \theta_\circ + \varepsilon_2)$ with respect to this prior is computed to be larger than a suitably lower bound which is customarily set equal to the complement of the nominal significance level. In other words, given the prior distribution $\pi(\cdot)$, the Bayesian test for equivalence uses the decision rule*:

Reject nonequivalence if and only if
$$\pi^{\theta|\mathbf{X}=\mathbf{x}}(\theta_\circ - \varepsilon_1, \, \theta_\circ + \varepsilon_2) \geq 1 - \alpha. \qquad (3.2)$$

For the sake of eliminating subjectivism entailed by selecting the prior in an arbitrary way, relying on so-called noninformative priors has much to recommend it. By definition, a noninformative prior is a (maybe improper) uniform distribution of the model parameters involved or of suitable parametric functions. Although there is still considerable controversy about the theoretical foundation of the concept (cf. Berger, 1985, § 3.3; Cox and Hinkley, 1974, § 10.4), there is a useful pragmatic rule for determining a noninformative prior which has been extensively exploited in many applications of Bayesian inference (see in particular the landmark monograph of Box and Tiao, 1973). The rule was first proposed by Jeffreys (1961) and states that $\pi(\cdot)$ is (approximately) noninformative if it is defined by a density (with respect to Lebesgue measure) taken proportional to the square root of the determinant of the information matrix.

For illustration, let us consider the setting of the paired t-test with the intra-subject differences $D_i = X_i - Y_i$ as the data eventually to be analyzed and the expected value δ of the D_i as the parameter of interest. This is

---

* Using extra symbols for parameters treated as random variables rather than constants seems dispensable here. It becomes clear from the context which version is actually intended.

a case in which the posterior distribution of the target parameter with respect to the noninformative "reference prior" admits a simple explicit representation. As shown, e.g., in Lindley (1970, pp. 36-7) and Box and Tiao (1973, §2.4), given the observed values $\bar{d}$ and s_D of the mean $\bar{D}$ and standard deviation S_D of the D_i, $n^{1/2}(\delta - \bar{d})/s_D$ has a posterior distribution then which is central t with the usual number $n - 1$ of degrees of freedom. Hence, the posterior probability of the equivalence interval specified by the alternative hypothesis whose limits are this time denoted by δ_1, δ_2 can be written

$$\pi^{\delta | \mathbf{D} = \mathbf{d}}(\delta_1, \delta_2) = F_{n-1}^T(n^{1/2}(\delta_2 - \bar{d})/s_D) - F_{n-1}^T(n^{1/2}(\delta_1 - \bar{d})/s_D) \quad (3.3)$$

where $F_{n-1}^T(\cdot)$ stands for the cdf of a central t-distribution with $n-1$ degrees of freedom. Suppose specifically that we obtained $\bar{d} = .16$, $s_D = 3.99$ in a sample of size $n = 23^\dagger$ and that $\delta_1 = -1.75$, $\delta_2 = 1.75$ have been chosen as equivalence limits for δ. Then, evaluating the expression on the right-hand side of (3.3) by means of the SAS (1999, pp. 502-3) function probt gives for the posterior probability of (δ_1, δ_2):

$$\pi^{\delta | \mathbf{D} = \mathbf{d}}(-1.75, 1.75) =$$

$$F_{22}^T(23^{1/2}(1.75 - .16)/3.99) - F_{22}^T(23^{1/2}(-1.75 - .16)/3.99) =$$
$$F_{22}^T(1.911121) - F_{22}^T(-2.295749) = .965447 - .015796 = .949651.$$

Hence, at the nominal level $\alpha = 0.05$, for this specific data set the Bayesian test (3.2) with respect to the reference prior distribution of (δ, σ_D) would not be able to reject nonequivalence in the sense of $|\delta| \geq 1.75$.

It is worth noticing that in situations where Bayesian credible intervals coincide with classical confidence intervals, the test obtained by applying decision rule (3.2) is the same as the interval inclusion test with confidence limits at one-sided confidence level $1 - \alpha/2$ rather than $1 - \alpha$. Recalling the correspondence between interval inclusion tests and double one-sided tests for equivalence, this suggests that for the sake of avoiding overconservatism, the double one-sided Bayesian test given by the decision rule

Reject nonequivalence if and only if

$$\pi^{\theta | \mathbf{X} = \mathbf{x}}(\theta_\circ - \varepsilon_1, \infty) \geq 1 - \alpha \text{ and } \pi^{\theta | \mathbf{X} = \mathbf{x}}(-\infty, \theta_\circ + \varepsilon_2) \geq 1 - \alpha \quad (3.4)$$

should generally be preferred to the "direct" Bayesian equivalence test (3.2). In the numerical example introduced before, the posterior probabilities of the two infinite intervals to be intersected in order to get the equivalence interval itself, are computed to be $\pi^{\delta | \mathbf{D} = \mathbf{d}}(-1.75, \infty) = 1 - F_{22}^T(-2.295749)$ $= 1 - .015796 = .984204$, $\pi^{\delta | \mathbf{D} = \mathbf{d}}(-\infty, 1.75) = F_{22}^T(1.911121) = .965447$. Since with $\alpha = .05$, both of these values exceed the critical lower bound $1 - \alpha$, the double one-sided Bayesian test (3.4), in contrast to the direct

---

† The source of these data is a pilot study (described in some more detail in Example 5.3, p. 81) of the temporal stability of the capillary flow in the brain of rabbits.

Bayesian decision rule (3.2), leads to a positive result which reflects its improved power.

As any technique of Bayesian inference, the approach to equivalence testing given by (3.2) or (3.4) is attractive not only for its conceptual simplicity, but likewise for its high flexibility with respect to reparametrizations of the problem. Like the prior, the posterior distribution is determined jointly for all unknown parameters of the model under analysis. Hence, it can easily be calculated for any sufficiently regular function of the primary parameters by means of the well-known transformation theorem for probability densities (cf. Bickel and Doksum, 1977, § 1.2). In order to illustrate this technique, we keep considering the paired t-test setting and demonstrate how to compute the posterior density of the standardized expected difference $\theta = \delta/\sigma_D$ assuming the same prior distribution of (δ, σ_D) which underlies formula (3.2). For that purpose, the following results (to be found again in the book of Box and Tiao, 1973, pp. 95-6) are needed:

1) The conditional posterior distribution of δ given σ_D is $\mathcal{N}(\bar{d}, \sigma_D{}^2/n)$ [i.e., Gaussian with mean $\bar{d}$ and variance $\sigma_D{}^2/n$].

2) The marginal posterior distribution of σ_D is that of $s_D(n-1)^{1/2}/X_{n-1}$ with $X_{n-1}^2 \sim \chi_{n-1}^2$ [= central χ^2-distribution with $n-1$ degrees of freedom].

From 1) and 2), it follows that the joint posteriori density of (δ, σ_D) can be written:

$$f(\delta, \sigma_D \mid \mathbf{D} = \mathbf{d}) = (n^{1/2}/\sigma_D)\,\varphi(n^{1/2}(\delta - \bar{d})/\sigma_D)\,\big(\Gamma((n-1)/2)\big)^{-1} \times$$
$$\big((n-1)s_D{}^2\big)^{(n-1)/2}\,2^{(3-n)/2}\sigma_D{}^{-n}\,\exp\big\{-((n-1)/2)\,(s_D/\sigma_D)^2\big\} \quad (3.5)$$

with $\Gamma(\cdot)$ and $\varphi(\cdot)$ denoting the gamma and the standard Gaussian density function, respectively. (3.5) leads to the following expression for the posterior probability of the hypothesis $\theta_1 < \theta < \theta_2$ with $\theta = \delta/\sigma_D$ and arbitrarily fixed equivalence limits $-\infty < \theta_1 < \theta_2 < \infty$:

$$\pi^{\theta \mid \mathbf{D} = \mathbf{d}}(\theta_1, \theta_2) = \int_0^\infty \Big[\big(\Phi(n^{1/2}(\theta_2\sigma_D - \bar{d})/\sigma_D) - \Phi(n^{1/2}(\theta_1\sigma_D - \bar{d})/\sigma_D)\big) \times$$
$$\big(\Gamma((n-1)/2)\big)^{-1}\big((n-1)s_D{}^2\big)^{(n-1)/2}\,2^{(3-n)/2}\,\sigma_D{}^{-n} \times$$
$$\exp\big\{-((n-1)/2)\,(s_D/\sigma_D)^2\big\}\Big]\,d\sigma_D. \quad (3.6)$$

The integral on the right-hand side of equation (3.6) can be evaluated by means of a suitable quadrature rule to any desired degree of numerical accuracy. A numerical method which serves remarkably well with integrals of that type is Gaussian quadrature (cf. Davis and Rabinowitz, 1975, § 2.7). The error entailed by truncating the interval of integration from above at some point c_0 can be made smaller than any prespecified

$\varepsilon_\circ > 0$ [e.g., $\varepsilon_\circ = 10^{-6}$] by choosing $c_\circ > \sqrt{(n-1)s_D{}^2/\chi^2_{n-1\,;\,\varepsilon_\circ}}$ with $\chi^2_{n-1\,;\,\varepsilon_\circ}$ denoting the $100\varepsilon_\circ$-percentage point of a central χ^2-distribution with $n-1$ degrees of freedom. The SAS macro `postmys` to be found at http://www.zi-mannheim.de/wktsheq implements this computational approach using a grid of 96 abscissas (for a table of all constants involved in 96-point Gaussian quadrature see Abramowitz and Stegun, 1965, p. 919). In the specific case $n = 23$, $\bar{d} = .16$, $s_D = 3.99$ used for illustration once more, it gives for the posterior probability of the equivalence region $\{(\delta,\sigma_D)\,|\,-0.5 < \delta/\sigma_D < 0.5\}$ the value $\pi^{\theta|\mathbf{D}=\mathbf{d}}(-0.5, 0.5) = .981496$. Hence, with these data the Bayesian test for equivalence with respect to δ/σ_D leads to the same decision as the optimal frequentist testing procedure to be discussed in §5.3 (see in particular p. 81).

Clearly, the most crucial issue to be raised in discussing the suitability of the decision rules (3.2) and (3.4) concerns the point that in the corresponding test maintenance of the prespecified significance level in the classical sense cannot generally be taken for granted. Since the latter is still considered an indispensable property of any procedure to be relied upon for confirmatory purposes by the majority of the users of statistical methodology [in particular, the regulatory authorities deciding upon the eventual success of drug development projects], it seems advisable to check Bayesian decision rules from a frequentist perspective as carefully as possible before adopting them for real applications. Unfortunately, deriving sufficient conditions for the validity of Bayesian tests with regard to the risk of a type-I error is still more difficult a task in the case of equivalence than that of conventional one-sided hypotheses. In fact, the results obtained by Casella and Berger (1987) for the latter cannot be exploited for establishing the validity of Bayesian equivalence tests even if attention is restricted to simple location-parameter problems decomposed into two one-sided problems by replacing (3.2) with (3.4). The reason is that the results proved by Casella and Berger require symmetry of the density of the data about the common boundary of null and alternative hypothesis, and it can easily be shown that there exists no proper probability density which is symmetric about two different points [viz., $\theta_\circ - \varepsilon_1$ and $\theta_\circ + \varepsilon_2$].

An abstract concept which proves worthwhile as a starting-point for investigations into possible relationships between Bayesian and frequentist tests for equivalence is that of a confidence distribution as introduced by Cox (1958) and exploited for a systematic discussion of the interval inclusion approach to equivalence testing by Mau (1987; 1988). Roughly speaking, a confidence distribution is defined to be a random probability measure [depending in some mathematically clear-cut way on the data under analysis] such that its quantiles give confidence bounds to the parameter θ of interest. Whenever the posterior distribution of θ admits a representation as a realization of a random measure of that type, both versions (3.2) and

(3.4) of a Bayesian rule for deciding between equivalence and existence
of relevant differences coincide with interval inclusion rules as introduced
in the previous section and hence share with them the property of being
valid with regard to the type-I error risk. Unfortunately, representability
of Bayesian posterior as frequentist confidence distributions turns out to
be a highly restrictive condition. In fact, from a practical point of view,
it provides hardly more than a characterization in abstract terms of situations where the distributions of the data (typically after suitable reductions
by sufficiency) belong either to a location family $(P_\theta)_{\theta \in \mathbb{R}}$, a scale family
$(P_\sigma)_{\sigma > 0}$, or a location-scale family $(P_{\theta,\sigma})_{(\theta,\sigma) \in \mathbb{R} \times \mathbb{R}_+}$, and the prior is the
usual reference prior defined by an improper density proportional to 1 or
σ^{-1}, respectively. However, for most models involving only a location or
a scale parameter or both, there exist well-established methods of interval
estimation and even optimal tests for equivalence are comparatively easy
to implement. In view of this, the possibility of establishing the validity
of a Bayesian test for equivalence by way of verifying that the posterior
distribution involved satisfies the definition of an observed confidence distribution is mainly of theoretical and conceptual interest. Moreover, for
purposes of proving the validity of equivalence tests using decision rule
(3.4) with a suitable noninformative reference prior, an alternative method
exists which avoids detailed comparative inspections of the underlying posterior distributions. It is obtained by exploiting the theory of right-invariant
Haar densities and provides, at least potentially, a more versatile tool than
the approach via paralleling posterior and confidence distributions since it
covers transformation families of any kind (for a detailed exposition of this
theory see Berger, 1985, § 6.6).

Additional results on sufficient conditions for the validity of Bayesian
equivalence tests are derived in the thesis of Kloos (1996). They are based
on the concept of so-called conjugate families of the second kind and cover
cases where the Bayesian decision rule (3.4) is applied in connection with
suitable informative prior distributions. Again, the class of models and priors allowed according to these conditions is rather small so that we refrain
from discussing them here in more detail. In a later chapter [→ § 9.3] the
reader will become acquainted with an instance of a Bayesian construction
of an equivalence test for which there is no other way of ensuring its validity
but via direct numerical determination of the maximum rejection probability taken over the respective null hypothesis. Nevertheless, we will see that
the method serves quite satisfactorily the purpose of filling an important
gap in the repertoire of useful frequentist solutions to equivalence testing
problems of considerable practical relevance.

Notwithstanding the considerable, sometimes even insurmountable difficulties encountered in proving that a Bayesian testing procedure satisfies at
the same time basic frequentist criteria, the proportion of Bayesian contributions to the literature on statistical methods for equivalence assessment

has been substantial all along. This has especially been true in the field of the analysis of comparative bioavailability trials. A representative selection of influential papers on Bayesian methods of bioequivalence assessment is constituted of Selwyn, Dempster and Hall (1981), Rodda and Davis (1986), Flühler et al. (1983), Selwyn and Hall (1984), and Racine-Poon et al. (1987).

3.3 The classical approach to deriving optimal parametric tests for equivalence hypotheses

In the classical theory of hypotheses testing, statistical tests are derived as solutions to optimization problems arising from the endeavour to maximize the power over a class of alternative decision procedures chosen as large as possible. Ideally, this class contains the totality of all tests of the null hypothesis under consideration which maintain the prespecified significance level, and maximization of power can be achieved uniformly over the whole subset of the parameter space specified by the alternative hypothesis. In the majority of situations occurring in practice, the class of testing procedures to be taken into consideration must be restricted by means of supplementary criteria to be imposed in addition to that of validity with respect to the type-I error risk. The most useful of them are based on the principle of sufficiency and invariance, respectively. The basic mathematical results which the construction of such optimal testing procedures for equivalence hypotheses relies upon, are presented in due rigour and generality in § A.1 of the Appendix. Hence, it suffices to give in the present section a brief outline of the basic techniques available for purposes of carrying out optimal constructions of tests for equivalence.

As is the case in the treatment of traditional one- or two-sided problems, the natural starting-point of the classical approach to the construction of testing procedures is given by settings where the possible distributions of the data form a one-parameter family of sufficiently regular structure. When dealing with interval hypotheses, the suitable way of making this regularity precise is based on the concept of total positivity whose fundamental importance for the theory of statistical decision procedures has been demonstrated in a series of frequently cited papers and an encyclopedic monograph by Karlin (1956; 1957a,b; 1968). For purposes of deriving optimal one-sided tests, the assumption of monotone likelihood ratios (or, equivalently, of strict total positivity of order 2) proves mathematically natural. In contrast, in order to ensure the existence of optimal tests for equivalence, families of distributions are required whose densities are STP_3 (strictly totally positive of order 3 - see Definition A.1.1 in the Appendix) and depend in a continuous manner both on the realized value of the observed random variable and the parameter θ. The basic fact is then that in any STP_3 family exhibiting these additional continuity properties, an optimal test for equivalence in the sense made precise in (1.1. a,b) [→ p. 5] can be constructed by means of the generalized Fundamental Lemma of Neyman and Pearson (1936). Interestingly, this construction whose mathematical basis is given by Theorem A.1.5 of the Appendix [→ p. 251], leads to tests which are uniformly most powerful (UMP) among *all* tests at level α of the same hypothesis whereas for the dual testing problem $\theta_\circ - \varepsilon_1 \le \theta \le \theta_\circ + \varepsilon_2$ versus $\theta < \theta_\circ - \varepsilon_1$ or $\theta > \theta_\circ + \varepsilon_2$ (sometimes termed the problem of testing for relevant differences by biostatisticians) only a uniformly most powerful unbiased (UMPU) solution exists (see Lehmann, 1986, p .104).

As suggested by intuition, every reasonably structured test for equivalence has a form which is complementary to that of a traditional two-sided test. Thus, optimal solutions to some given problem of equivalence testing have to be sought for in the class of tests whose rejection region can be written as

$$\left\{ \mathbf{x} \,|\, C_1 < T(\mathbf{x}) < C_2 \right\} , \tag{3.7}$$

which means that the null hypothesis H of nonequivalence has to be rejected as long as the observed value of a suitable real-valued statistic remains *within some* sufficiently *short interval.* The limits C_1, C_2 of that critical interval may depend, in addition to the significance level α, on the value observed for some other statistic S, say, which will typically be chosen sufficient for a (maybe multidimensional) nuisance parameter. In order to obtain on optimal test, C_1 and C_2 must be determined in such a way that its (conditional) probability takes on exact value α at both boundaries of the null hypothesis, i.e., under both $\theta = \theta_\circ - \varepsilon_1$ and $\theta = \theta_\circ + \varepsilon_2$. In cases where the distributions of the test statistic $T(\mathbf{X})$ are continuous, this implies that C_1, C_2 must simultaneously satisfy the equations

$$P_{\theta_1}[C_1 < T(\mathbf{X}) < C_2] = \alpha =$$
$$P_{\theta_2}[C_1 < T(\mathbf{X}) < C_2], \quad ,C_1, C_2 \in \mathcal{T}, \;\; C_1 < C_2 \tag{3.8}$$

where $\mathcal{T}$ denotes the range of $T(\cdot)$ and $\theta_1 = \theta_\circ - \varepsilon_1$, $\theta_2 = \theta_\circ + \varepsilon_2$. If the distribution functions of $T(\mathbf{X})$ exhibit jump discontinuities, a solution to (3.8) generally does not exist. Then, one has to deal with the more complicated system

$$P_{\theta_1}\left[C_1 < T(\mathbf{X}) < C_2 \right] + \sum_{\nu=1}^{2} \gamma_\nu \, P_{\theta_1}\left[T(\mathbf{X}) = C_\nu \right] \; = \; \alpha \; =$$

$$P_{\theta_2}\left[C_1 < T(\mathbf{X}) < C_2 \right] + \sum_{\nu=1}^{2} \gamma_\nu \, P_{\theta_2}\left[T(\mathbf{X}) = C_\nu \right],$$
$$C_1, C_2 \in \mathcal{T}, \;\; C_1 \le C_2, \;\; 0 \le \gamma_1, \gamma_2 < 1 \tag{3.9}$$

instead. The existence of a unique solution to (3.9) is guaranteed whenever the family of distributions of $T(\mathbf{X})$ is STP$_3$, and the optimal test entails a randomized decision in favour of equivalence with probability γ_1 or γ_2 if $T(\mathbf{X})$ takes on value C_1 or C_2, respectively. As has been pointed out in the previous chapter in connection with the exact conditional test for one-sided equivalence of two binomial distributions with respect to the odds ratio, in the overwhelming majority of applications of statistical testing procedures to real data randomized decisions between the hypotheses are clearly undesirable. Accordingly, in the noncontinuous case the optimal test for equivalence is usually modified in the following way: The critical interval (C_1, C_2) keeps to be determined by solving (3.9) but at its boundaries, i.e., both for $T(\mathbf{X}) = C_1$ and for $T(\mathbf{X}) = C_2$, the null hypothesis is always accepted (corresponding to the specification $\gamma_1 = 0 = \gamma_2$). In situations where the distributions of $T(\mathbf{X})$ are discrete and at the same time conditional on some other statistic sufficient for the nuisance parameter(s) involved in the underlying model [$\to$ §§5.1, 6.5.1], adopting Boschloo's (1970) technique of raised nominal significance levels [recall §2.3.2] will prove a simple and effective device for reducing the conservatism entailed by accepting nonequivalence whenever we observe that $T(\mathbf{X}) \in \{C_1, C_2\}$.

In the *continuous case*, numerical determination of the optimal critical constants C_1, C_2 is greatly facilitated by the availability of a general result (proved by Lehmann, 1986, as Lemma 2 (iv) of §3.3) on the sign of the difference of the power functions of two tests of the form (3.7) in families with monotone likelihood ratios, which implies the following fact: Let the family of distributions of $T(\mathbf{X})$ be STP$_3$ and (C'_1, C'_2) denote any interval on the real line such that $P_{\theta_1}[C'_1 < T(\mathbf{X}) < C'_2] = \alpha$ but $P_{\theta_2}[C'_1 < T(\mathbf{X}) < C'_2] <$ or $> \alpha$. Then it follows that the optimal critical interval C_1, C_2 whose endpoints satisfy (3.8) lies to the right or left of (C'_1, C'_2), respectively. Clearly, this shows that a simple iteration scheme for approximating the solution of (3.8) to any desired degree of numerical accuracy, consists of the following steps:

(i) Choose some estimate C_1^0, say, of the left-hand limit C_1 of the optimal critical interval.

(ii) Compute the corresponding upper critical bound C_2^0 as $C_2^0 = F_{\theta_1}^{-1}[\alpha + F_{\theta_1}(C_1^0)]$, with F_θ and F_θ^{-1} denoting the distribution and quantile function of $T(\mathbf{X})$, respectively, at an arbitrary point θ in the parameter space.

(iii) Compute the size $\alpha_2^0 = F_{\theta_2}(C_2^0) - F_{\theta_2}(C_1^0)$ of the critical region $\{\mathbf{x} \mid C_1^0 < T(\mathbf{x}) < C_2^0\}$ at $\theta = \theta_2$.

(iv) Update C_1^0 by replacing it with $(\tilde{C}_1 + C_1^0)/2$ or $(C_1^0 + \tilde{\tilde{C}}_1)/2$ depending on whether there holds $\alpha_2^0 > \alpha$ or $\alpha_2^0 < \alpha$ and assuming that $(\tilde{C}_1, \tilde{\tilde{C}}_1)$ has been previously determined as an interval containing both C_1^0 and the exact solution C_1.

(v) Repeat steps (i)-(iv) as many times as required in order to ensure
that $|\alpha_2^0 - \alpha| < \text{TOL}$ with, e.g., $\text{TOL} = 10^{-4}$.

In the *discrete case with integer-valued test statistic* $T(\mathbf{X})$, extensive experience has shown that the following search algorithm (forming the basis of
the programs bi1st, po1st, powsign, bi2st, bi2aeq1 – bi2aeq3) works
very efficiently on finding the solution of (3.9):

(i*) Choose an initial value C_1^0 for the lower critical bound known to be
greater or equal to the correct value C_1.

(ii*) Keeping C_1^0 fixed, find the largest integer $C_2^0 > C_1^0$ such that the
probability of observing $T(\mathbf{X})$ to take on its value in the closed
interval $[C_1^0 + 1, C_2^0 - 1]$ does not exceed α, neither for $\theta = \theta_1$ nor
for $\theta = \theta_2$.

(iii*) Treat (3.9) as a system of linear equations in the two unknowns
γ_1, γ_2 and compute its solution γ_1^0, γ_2^0, say (which of course depends
on C_1^0 and C_2^0).

(iv*) Verify the condition $0 \leq \gamma_1^0, \gamma_2^0 < 1$. If it is satisfied, the solution
of the full system (3.9) is found and given as $(C_1, C_2, \gamma_1, \gamma_2) =
(C_1^0, C_2^0, \gamma_1^0, \gamma_2^0)$; if not, diminish C_1^0 by 1 and repeat steps (ii*) and
(iii*).

Although both of the algorithms outlined in the preceding paragraphs are
logically straightforward, concrete numerical determination of the optimal
critical constants is a much more demanding task for equivalence problems
than for customary one- or two-sided testing problems. This explains why
in the existing literature the number of contributions presenting classical
tests for equivalence as fully explicit decision rules ready for being used
by the working statistician, hardly comes to more than half a dozen (to
our best knowledge, the following list is largely exhaustive: Bondy, 1969;
Wellek and Michaelis, 1991; Wellek, 1993a; Mehring, 1993; Wellek, 1994
[First, German Edition of the present book]; Wang, 1997).

Perhaps, the main fact making optimal tests for equivalence computa-
tionally more complicated than their one- and two-sided analogues, is that
the sampling distributions of customary test statistics are needed in their
noncentral versions in order to determine sizes of rejection regions etc. An
additional complication refers to situations entailing elimination of nuisance
parameters by means of conditioning: The possibility of reducing the conditional tests primarily obtained to equivalent nonconditional procedures,
which is well known (cf. Lehmann, 1986, § 5.1) to lead not infrequently to
considerable simplifications with one- and two-sided problems, generally
does not exist in the equivalence case. Nevertheless, in subsequent chapters the reader will become acquainted with numerous specific equivalence

testing problems for which an optimal procedure can be made available in a form suitable for routine use by anybody having access to standard computational tools.

The computational effort entailed by performing an optimal test for equivalence in practice, reduces to a minimum in all cases where the following bipartite symmetry condition is satisfied:

$$\theta_1 = -\varepsilon, \ \theta_2 = \varepsilon \quad \text{for some} \quad \varepsilon > 0; \tag{3.10a}$$

$$\text{the distribution of } T(\mathbf{X}) \text{ under } \theta = \varepsilon \text{ coincides}$$
$$\text{with that of } -T(\mathbf{X}) \text{ under } \theta = -\varepsilon. \tag{3.10b}$$

In fact, by the result made precise and proved in the Appendix as Lemma A.1.6 [$\to$ p. 252], (3.10) implies that the critical interval for $T(\mathbf{X})$ defining an optimal test for equivalence is symmetric about zero, i.e., of the form $(-C, C)$. In the continuous case, C remains as the only critical constant uniquely determined by the single equation

$$P_\varepsilon[|T(\mathbf{X})| < C] = \alpha, \quad C \in \mathcal{T} \cap (0, \infty). \tag{3.11}$$

An alternative formulation of the same fact is as follows: If, in a situation being symmetric in the sense of (3.10), there exists an optimal test for equivalence, then this can be carried out by means of a p-value defined as the lower tail probability of the absolute value of the test statistic under $\theta = \varepsilon$ or, equivalently, under $\theta = -\varepsilon$. Dropping the continuity assumption, one has $\gamma_1 = \gamma_2 = \gamma$ in addition to $-C_1 = C_2 = C$ where C and γ are defined by

$$C = \max\left\{ t \in \mathcal{T} \cap (0, \infty) \,\middle|\, P_\varepsilon\left[\,|T(\mathbf{X})| < t\,\right] \leq \alpha \right\}, \tag{3.12a}$$

$$\gamma = \left(\alpha - P_\varepsilon\left[\,|T(\mathbf{X})| < C\,\right] \right) \middle/ P_\varepsilon\left[\,|T(\mathbf{X})| = C\,\right]. \tag{3.12b}$$

In particular, an optimal test for equivalence allows this kind of reduction to a one-sided test in terms of the absolute value of the respective test statistic, whenever θ plays the role of a location parameter for the distribution of $T(\mathbf{X})$, provided $\theta = 0$ implies $-T(\mathbf{X}) \overset{d}{=} T(\mathbf{X})$ and we are willing to choose the equivalence range for θ as a symmetric interval. The most important special case of such a location problem occurs if $T(\mathbf{X})$ is normally distributed with unknown expected value $\theta \in \mathbb{R}$ and fixed known variance $\sigma_\circ^2 > 0$ which will be treated in full detail in § 4.1.

The greater part of the equivalence assessment procedures described in the subsequent chapters are tests which maximize the power function uniformly over the class of all valid tests for the same problem, of invariant tests maintaining the prespecified level α, of all unbiased tests at level α, or of all valid tests for an associated asymptotic problem. Although optimal testing procedures generally deserve preference over less powerful tests of the same hypotheses, in providing a sufficiently rich repertoire of equivalence testing procedures unification of the constructional approach seems neither desirable nor promising. In fact, there are many rather elementary equivalence testing problems encountered very frequently in practice which admit no optimal solution. Perhaps, the best known and most important of them refers to location equivalence of two Gaussian distributions $\mathcal{N}(\mu_1, \sigma^2), \mathcal{N}(\mu_2, \sigma^2)$ with common unknown variance. Here, even the construction of an unbiased test for $|\mu_1 - \mu_2| \geq \varepsilon$ vs. $|\mu_1 - \mu_2| < \varepsilon$ proves mathematically quite complicated and leads to rejection regions which in view of several counterintuitive properties seem hardly suitable for practice (for details see Brown, Hwang and Munk, 1997, and § 9.2.1 of the present book). Although the interval inclusion rule with standard equal-tails confidence intervals at two-sided level $(1 - 2\alpha)$ gives a solution to this specific problem which still can be strongly recommended, it would be clearly misleading to suppose that the principle of confidence interval inclusion is generally more easy to implement than the classical approach to constructing equivalence tests. One out of many other important examples showing this not to hold true occurs if, in the setting of the ordinary two-sample t-test, equivalence of $\mathcal{N}(\mu_1, \sigma^2)$ and $\mathcal{N}(\mu_2, \sigma^2)$ is redefined by requiring that we should have $|\mu_1 - \mu_2|/\sigma < \varepsilon$: Computing exact confidence limits for the difference between the standardized means of these distributions is certainly at least as complicated as determining the critical constant of the uniformly most powerful invariant (UMPI) test for the same problem as discussed in § 6.1.

3.4 Construction of asymptotic tests for equivalence

As is true for virtually all areas of statistical inference, the range of equivalence testing problems accessible to exact methods is much too limited for covering even the most basic needs arising in practical data analysis. Problems for which no satisfactory exact solution is available, are by no means predominantly of a kind involving nonparametric or other rather complex models like the proportional hazards model for possibly censored survival times. Even such comparatively simple problems as those of testing for equivalence of binomial proportions with respect to the difference $\delta = p_1 - p_2$ in the analysis of two independent or paired samples of binary data are cases in point. Fortunately, there is an asymptotic approach to the construction of equivalence tests which will enable us to fill a considerable part of the gaps left by exact constructional approaches. It is based on a result which has been established for the two-sample case by Wellek (1996) and can readily be generalized to cover virtually any situation where the equivalence hypothesis to be tested refers to a parameter or (in non- or semiparametric models) to a functional for which an asymptotically normal estimator can be found. In what follows, we give an informal yet exhaustive description of the rationale behind this approach whose rigorous mathematical justification is postponed to the Appendix [→ § A.3].

The notation which was introduced in § 1.2 is interpreted here in its broadest sense covering in particular cases where the target parameter θ depends on more complex characteristics of the distribution functions under comparison than merely their first two moments or selected quantiles. In other words, θ is allowed to have the meaning of an arbitrary functional of the vector of all underlying distribution functions. The dimension of this vector can be any positive integer k which must not vary with the total sample size N. For illustration, let us anticipate a small bit of the material presented in § 6.2 referring to the nonparametric two-sample problem with continuous data $X_1, \ldots, X_m$ and $Y_1 \ldots, Y_n$. In this setting, one wishes to compare $k = 2$ distribution functions usually denoted F and G, and an intuitively appealing choice of a functional which a reasonable measure of distance between them can be based upon, is $\theta = \int G dF = P[X_i > Y_j]$. Returning to the problem of testing for equivalence in its most general formulation, suppose further that for each given value of the total sample size N, there is some real-valued statistic T_N, say, such that the associated sequence $(T_N)_{N \in \mathbb{R}}$ is an asymptotically normal estimator for θ in the sense that we have

$$\sqrt{N}(T_N - \theta)/\sigma \overset{\mathcal{L}}{\to} \mathcal{N}(0,1) \quad \text{as} \quad N \to \infty \qquad (3.13)$$

for a suitable positive functional σ of the vector $(F_1, \ldots, F_k)$ of distribution functions under consideration.

Now, the basic steps leading to an asymptotically valid test of $H : \theta \leq \theta_1$ or $\theta \geq \theta_2$ versus $K : \theta_1 < \theta < \theta_2$ are as follows:

(i) Take (3.13) as if allowing to be strengthened to a statement on the exact sampling distribution of T_N.

(ii) Treat the standard error $\sigma/\sqrt{N}$ of T_N as a known constant τ_N, say, and carry out in terms of T_N the test which is optimal for H vs. K when θ stands for the expected value of a normal distribution with known variance τ_N^2 from which a single observation has been taken.

(iii) Derive an estimator $\hat{\sigma}_N$ which is weakly consistent for σ and plug in $\hat{\tau}_N = \hat{\sigma}_N/\sqrt{N}$ in the expressions obtained in step (ii) at every place where τ_N appears.

The results derived in § 4.1 strongly suggest to use in step (ii) of such a construction the rejection region

$$\left\{ \left| T_N - (\theta_1 + \theta_2)/2 \right| / \tau_N < C_\alpha \left((\theta_2 - \theta_1)/2\tau_N \right) \right\} \qquad (3.14)$$

where for any $\psi > 0$ and $0 < \alpha < 1$, $C_\alpha(\psi)$ has to be taken equal to the square root of the αth quantile of a χ^2-distribution with a single degree of freedom and noncentrality parameter ψ^2. Since the computation of quantiles of noncentral χ^2-distributions is a process perfectly supported by the most widely used statistical software (see the intrinsic function `cinv` of *SAS*, 1999, pp. 288-9), the practical implementation of an asymptotic test for equivalence on the basis of (3.14) is an easy exercise as soon as the test statistic T_N as well as its estimated asymptotic standard error $\hat{\tau}_N$ has been calculated. What remains to be done is to determine the ordinary distance in units of $\hat{\tau}_N$ between T_N and the middle of the equivalence limits specified by the hypothesis, and to compare the result with the number $C_\alpha\big((\theta_2 - \theta_1)/2\hat{\tau}_N\big)$ as a critical upper bound. If the observed value of $\big|T_N - (\theta_1 + \theta_2)/2\big|/\hat{\tau}_N$ is found to be smaller than this bound, nonequivalence can be rejected, and has to be accepted otherwise. Of course, replacing the theoretical standard error τ_N with its consistent estimator $\hat{\tau}_N$ in determining the noncentrality parameter of the χ^2-distribution to be relied upon, makes $C_\alpha\big((\theta_2 - \theta_1)/2\hat{\tau}_N\big)$ a random critical bound rather than a critical constant. Nevertheless, very mild conditions suffice to guarantee that the approach yields a test for equivalence which is asymptotically valid with respect to the significance level.

Usually, the most laborious step to be taken in deriving an asymptotic solution to a concrete equivalence testing problem on the basis of the theory outlined in this section, is to find an explicit expression for the asymptotic standard error of the test statistic as well as for a suitable estimator of it. Except for cases in which the complications entailed in variance calculation prove prohibitive, the approach is very useful. One of its nicest and most important properties stems from the finite-sample behaviour of the corresponding testing procedures which according to the results of extensive simulation studies often turns out to be remarkably good. As one out of not a few noteworthy instances of this, the reader is referred to the log-rank test for equivalence of two survivor functions described in detail in § 6.6. Even if the expected proportion of censored observations contained in the data is about 50% and both sample sizes are as small as 25, the risk of committing a type-I error does not exceed the nominal significance level to a practically relevant extent.

CHAPTER 4

Equivalence tests for selected one-parameter problems

4.1 The one-sample problem with normally distributed observations of known variance

In this section it is assumed throughout that the hypotheses (1.1.a) and (1.1.b) [→ p. 5] refer to the expected value of a single Gaussian distribution whose variance has some fixed known value. In other words we suppose that the data under analysis can be described by a vector $(X_1, \ldots, X_n)$ of mutually independent random variables having all distribution $\mathcal{N}(\theta, \sigma_{\circ}^2)$ where $\sigma_{\circ}^2 > 0$ denotes a fixed positive constant. It is easy to verify that it entails no loss of generality if we set $\sigma_{\circ}^2 = 1$, $\theta_{\circ} - \varepsilon_1 = -\varepsilon$ and $\theta_{\circ} + \varepsilon_2 = \varepsilon$ with arbitrarily fixed $\varepsilon > 0$. In fact, if the variance of the primary observations differs from unity and/or the equivalence interval specified by the alternative hypothesis (1.1.b) fails to exhibit symmetry about zero, both of these properties can be ensured by applying the following simple transformation of the observed variables: $X_i' = (X_i - \theta_{\circ} - (\varepsilon_2 - \varepsilon_1)/2)/\sigma_{\circ}$. In view of the relations $E_{\theta_{\circ} - \varepsilon_1}(X_i') = (\theta_{\circ} - \varepsilon_1 - \theta_{\circ} - (\varepsilon_2 - \varepsilon_1)/2)/\sigma_{\circ} = -(\varepsilon_1 + \varepsilon_2)/2\sigma_{\circ}$, $E_{\theta_{\circ} + \varepsilon_2}(X_i') = (\varepsilon_1 + \varepsilon_2)/2\sigma_{\circ}$, it makes no difference whether we use the original sample to test $\theta \leq \theta_{\circ} - \varepsilon_1$ or $\theta \geq \theta_{\circ} + \varepsilon_2$ versus $\theta_{\circ} - \varepsilon_1 < \theta < \theta_{\circ} + \varepsilon_2$, or base a test of the null hypothesis $\theta' \leq -\varepsilon$ or $\theta' \geq \varepsilon$ versus the alternative $-\varepsilon < \theta' < \varepsilon$ on the transformed sample $(X_1', \ldots, X_n')$, provided we define $\theta' = E(X_i')$ and $\varepsilon = (\varepsilon_1 + \varepsilon_2)/2\sigma_{\circ}$. To simplify notation, we drop the distinction between primed and unprimed symbols and assume that we have

$$X_i \sim \mathcal{N}(\theta, 1), \quad i = 1, \ldots, n \tag{4.1a}$$

and that the equivalence problem referring to these observations reads

$$H : \theta \leq -\varepsilon \text{ or } \theta \geq \varepsilon \quad \text{versus} \quad K : -\varepsilon < \theta < \varepsilon \ . \tag{4.1b}$$

Since (4.1a) implies that the sample mean $\bar{X} = (1/n) \sum_{i=1}^{n} X_i$ and hence also the statistic $\sqrt{n}\bar{X}$ is sufficient for the family of the joint distributions of $(X_1, \ldots, X_n)$, we may argue as follows (using a well-known result to be found, e.g., in Witting, 1985, Theorem 3.30): The distribution of $\sqrt{n}\bar{X}$ differs from that of an individual X_i only by its expected value which is of course given by $\tilde{\theta} = \sqrt{n}\theta$. In terms of $\tilde{\theta}$, the testing problem put forward above reads

$$\tilde{H} : \tilde{\theta} \leq -\tilde{\varepsilon} \text{ or } \tilde{\theta} \geq \tilde{\varepsilon} \quad \text{versus} \quad \tilde{K} : -\tilde{\varepsilon} < \tilde{\theta} < \tilde{\varepsilon}, \tag{4.2}$$

on the understanding that we choose $\tilde{\varepsilon} = \sqrt{n}\varepsilon$. Now, if there is an UMP test, say $\tilde{\psi}$ at level α for (4.2) based on a single random variable Z with

$$Z \sim \mathcal{N}(\tilde{\theta}, 1), \tag{4.3}$$

then a UMP level-α test for the original problem (4.1) is given by $\phi(x_1, \ldots, x_n) = \tilde{\psi}(n^{-1/2} \sum_{i=1}^{n} x_i)$, $(x_1, \ldots, x_n) \in \mathbb{R}^n$.

By (4.3), the possible distributions of Z form a one-parameter exponential family in $\tilde{\theta}$ and Z (cf. Bickel and Doksum, 1977, p. 68), and by Lemma A.1.2 [$\rightarrow$ Appendix, p. 249] this is a specific example of a STP$_3$ family. Moreover, the density functions involved obviously exhibit the continuity properties required in the assumptions of Theorem A.1.5 [$\rightarrow$ Appendix, p. 251], and in view of the symmetry of the standard Gaussian distribution $\mathcal{N}(0, 1)$, the distribution of Z under $\tilde{\theta} = \tilde{\varepsilon}$ is clearly the same as that of $-Z$ under $\tilde{\theta} = -\tilde{\varepsilon}$. Thus, applying Lemma A.1.6 [$\rightarrow$ p. 252] we can conclude that a UMP level-α test for (4.2) is given by

$$\tilde{\psi}(z) = \begin{cases} 1 & \text{for } |z| < C_{\alpha;\tilde{\varepsilon}} \\ 0 & \text{for } |z| \geq C_{\alpha;\tilde{\varepsilon}} \end{cases}, \tag{4.4}$$

where $C_{\alpha;\tilde{\varepsilon}}$ the unique solution of

$$\Phi(C - \tilde{\varepsilon}) - \Phi(-C - \tilde{\varepsilon}) = \alpha, \quad C > 0. \tag{4.5}$$

The expression on the left-hand side of this equation equals to the probability of the event $\{|Z_{\tilde{\varepsilon}}| \leq C\}$ with $Z_{\tilde{\varepsilon}} \sim \mathcal{N}(\tilde{\varepsilon}, 1)$. But $Z_{\tilde{\varepsilon}} \sim \mathcal{N}(\tilde{\varepsilon}, 1)$ implies that $Z_{\tilde{\varepsilon}}^2$ satisfies the definition of a variable whose distribution is noncentral χ^2 with a single degree of freedom (df) and noncentrality parameter $\tilde{\varepsilon}^2$ (cf. Johnson, Kotz and Balakrishnan, 1995, § 29.1). Hence, the solution to equation (4.5) determining the critical constant of a UMP level-α test, admits the explicit representation

$$C_{\alpha;\tilde{\varepsilon}} = \sqrt{\chi^2_{1;\alpha}(\tilde{\varepsilon}^2)}, \tag{4.6}$$

where $\chi^2_{1;\alpha}(\tilde{\varepsilon}^2)$ denotes the αth quantile of a χ^2-distribution with $df = 1$ and noncentrality parameter $\tilde{\varepsilon}^2$. Finally, the desired optimal test for the problem (4.1) we started from, is obtained by applying the decision rule

Reject $H : \theta \leq -\varepsilon$ or $\theta \geq \varepsilon$ in favour of $K : -\varepsilon < \theta < \varepsilon$

if and only if it can be verified that $|\bar{X}| < n^{-1/2} C_{\alpha;\sqrt{n}\varepsilon}$. $\qquad$ (4.7)

In (4.7), the critical constant has to be determined simply by plugging in $\tilde{\varepsilon} = \sqrt{n}\varepsilon$ into (4.5) or (4.6), and constructing a program which computes $C_{\alpha;\tilde{\varepsilon}}$ for any $\tilde{\varepsilon} > 0$ is extremely easy whenever a programming language is used in terms of which the standard normal cdf $\Phi(\cdot)$ is predefined either directly or, like in Fortran, via the so-called error integral

$\mathrm{erf}(z) \equiv (2/\sqrt{\pi}) \int_0^z e^{-y^2} dy$. In fact, as a function of C, $\Phi(C - \tilde{\varepsilon}) - \Phi(-C - \tilde{\varepsilon})$ is continuous and strictly increasing. Hence, as soon as $\Phi(\cdot)$ can be treated as explicitly given, no more than an elementary interval halving algorithm is needed for computing $C_{\alpha;\tilde{\varepsilon}}$ by means of (4.5) to any desired degree of numerical accuracy. Of course, the most convenient way of implementing the optimal test for equivalence of $\mathcal{N}(\theta, 1)$ to $\mathcal{N}(0, 1)$ on the basis of a single sample $(X_1, \ldots, X_n)$ from $\mathcal{N}(\theta, 1)$ is to use a system providing the inverse noncentral χ^2 cdf with $df = 1$ as an intrinsic function (see SAS, 1999, pp. 288-9). For the conventional level $\alpha = .05$ of significance, Table 4.1 gives a tabulation of $C_{\alpha;\tilde{\varepsilon}}$ on the grid $\tilde{\varepsilon} = .1(.1)4.9$.

Table 4.1 *Optimal critical constant $C_{\alpha;\tilde{\varepsilon}}$ [$\to$ (4.5), (4.6)] for equivalence testing at the 5% level in the one-sample case with normally distributed data of known variance*

$\tilde{\varepsilon}$	0.	1.	2.	3.	4.
.0	–	0.10332	0.42519	1.35521	2.35515
.1	0.06302	0.11470	0.49889	1.45517	2.45515
.2	0.06397	0.12859	0.58088	1.55516	2.55515
.3	0.06559	0.14553	0.66944	1.65515	2.65515
.4	0.06793	0.16624	0.76268	1.75515	2.75515
.5	0.07105	0.19157	0.85893	1.85515	2.85515
.6	0.07507	0.22255	0.95696	1.95515	2.95515
.7	0.08011	0.26032	1.05598	2.05515	3.05515
.8	0.08634	0.30608	1.15552	2.15515	3.15515
.9	0.09398	0.36085	1.25530	2.25515	3.25515

Figure 4.1 shows the density functions of the test statistic $\sqrt{n}\bar{X}$ at both boundaries of the hypotheses and the critical interval of the optimal test at level $\alpha = .05$ for the case that the sample consists of $n = 100$ data points and the constant ε defining the width of the equivalence range for the expectation θ of the underlying distribution has been chosen to be $\varepsilon = .25$. As becomes obvious from the graph, the area under both curves over the critical interval $(-C_{\alpha;\sqrt{n}\varepsilon}, C_{\alpha;\sqrt{n}\varepsilon}) = (-.85893, .85893)$ is exactly equal to $.05 = \alpha$. According to Theorem A.1.5, this property characterizes the optimal test.

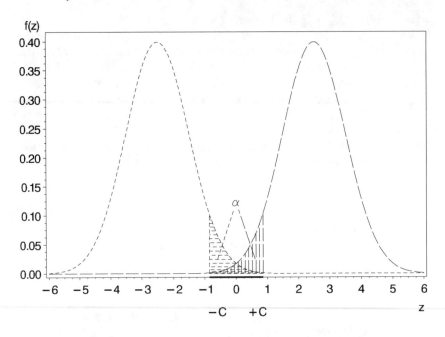

Figure 4.1 *Density of the distributions* $\mathcal{N}(-\sqrt{n}\varepsilon, 1)$ *[left] and* $\mathcal{N}(\sqrt{n}\varepsilon, 1)$ *[right] and critical interval [horizontal bar centred about 0] for* $Z = \sqrt{n}\bar{X}$ *in the UMP test at level* $\alpha = .05$, *with* $\varepsilon = .25$ *and* $n = 100$].

Figure 4.2 shows, for the same values of n, ε and α, the power of the UMP test for (4.1) as a function of the expectation θ of the individual observations $X_1, \ldots, X_n$ [recall (4.1a)]. In accordance with the characterization of the form of the power functions of optimal tests for equivalence in symmetric cases given in general terms in Corollary A.1.7, the curve is strictly unimodal and symmetric about zero. From a practical point of view, perhaps the most striking conclusion to be drawn from this picture is the following: In contrast to tests for traditional one- or two-sided problems, *equivalence tests do not admit the possibility of increasing the power to values arbitrarily close to 100% simply by selecting sufficiently extreme points in the parameter subspace corresponding to the alternative hypothesis under consideration.* The implications of this fact for sample size requirements to be satisfied in equivalence trials are obvious and far-reaching enough.

If we denote for arbitrary values of n, ε and α by $\beta^*_{n,\varepsilon;\,\alpha}$ the ordinate of the peak of the power curve associated to the test (4.7), there holds the simple explicit formula

$$\beta^*_{n,\varepsilon;\,\alpha} = 2\,\Phi(C_{\alpha;\,\sqrt{n}\varepsilon}) - 1 \ . \tag{4.8}$$

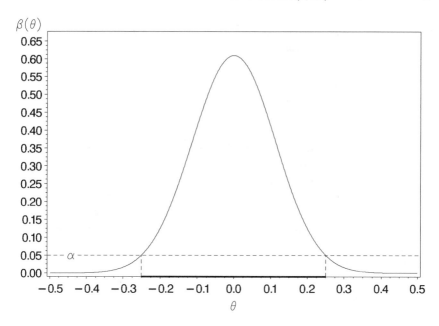

Figure 4.2 *Power function of the UMP test at level* $\alpha = 5\%$ *for* $|\theta| \geq .25$ *vs.* $|\theta| < .25$ *based on* $n = 100$ *observations from* $\mathcal{N}(\theta, 1)$. *[Bold-drawn bar on horizontal coordinate axis* $\leftrightarrow$ *equivalence interval* $(-\varepsilon, \varepsilon) = (-.25, .25)$ *specified by the alternative hypothesis.]*

This implies in particular that the maximum power attainable in any test for the equivalence problem (4.1) likewise depends on n and ε only through $\sqrt{n}\varepsilon = \tilde{\varepsilon}$. Table 4.2 shows, for the same selection of values of $\tilde{\varepsilon}$ covered by the preceding table and again to 5 decimal places, the result of evaluating (4.8). For $\tilde{\varepsilon} = \sqrt{100} \cdot .25 = 2.50$, we read the number .60962 which is the precise value of the maximum ordinate of the curve plotted in Figure 4.2. Conversely, Table 4.2 can be used for obtaining a rough estimate of the sample size required for an equivalence trial to be analyzed in a confirmatory manner by means of (4.7). E.g., the smallest $\tilde{\varepsilon}$ guaranteeing a maximum power of 80% is seen to lie between 2.9 and 3.0. Thus, for a trial in which we aim at establishing equivalence in the sense of $-.25 < \theta < .25$, we need a sample of size $(2.9/.25)^2 = 134.56 < n < 144.00 = (3.0/.25)^2$ in order to detect coincidence of θ with zero with a power of 80%, and so on.

Table 4.2 *Maximum power of the UMP test at level $\alpha = .05$ for the one-sample equivalence problem with Gaussian data of unit variance, for the same grid of values of $\tilde{\varepsilon} = \sqrt{n}\varepsilon$ as covered by Table 4.1*

$\tilde{\varepsilon}$	0.	1.	2.	3.	4.
.0	–	.08229	.32930	.82465	.98148
.1	.05025	.09132	.38214	.85438	.98592
.2	.05101	.10232	.43868	.88009	.98939
.3	.05230	.11571	.49679	.90211	.99207
.4	.05416	.13203	.55434	.92077	.99413
.5	.05665	.15192	.60962	.93642	.99570
.6	.05984	.17611	.66141	.94943	.99687
.7	.06385	.20538	.70902	.96014	.99775
.8	.06880	.24046	.75212	.96885	.99840
.9	.07488	.28179	.79063	.97588	.99887

To be sure, as a testing problem per se, the one-sample problem with normally distributed observations of known variance is of limited practical importance since in real applications precise knowledge of the true value of σ^2 will rarely be available. However, the testing procedure (4.7) which has been shown above to give a UMP solution to this problem, merits due consideration by the fact that it forms the basis of the construction of asymptotically valid tests for equivalence described in general terms in §3.4. Recalling the form of the rejection region of such an asymptotic test [→ (3.14)], it is readily checked that the latter is obtained from the results of the present section by formally treating the test statistic T_N of (3.13) as a single observation from a normal distribution with variance $\hat{\tau}_N^2 = \hat{\sigma}^2/N$ [→ p. 43 (iii)] and expected value $\theta = \theta(F_1, \ldots, F_k)$.

With respect to the existing literature, it is worth noticing that in a paper going back more than 30 years, Bondy (1969) suggested an appropriately modified version of (4.7) as a solution to the problem of testing for equivalence of two Gaussian distributions with known common variance. Bondy's contribution has been almost completely ignored by later authors in the field of equivalence testing (for one of the very few exceptions see Chester, 1986). In particular, although having appeared 3 years earlier than Westlake's seminal paper on the confidence interval inclusion approach, Bondy's idea of having recourse to the classical theory of hypotheses testing has never been referenced by any one of the pioneers of the statistical methodology of bioequivalence assessment. One of the reasons why his paper has been left largely unnoticed in the pertinent literature of the years to come might have been that Bondy gave an unnecessarily complicated representation of the critical constant of his test making it appear hardly suited for applications in routine work. Especially, any hint is missing that the optimal critical constant $C_{\alpha; \tilde{\varepsilon}}$ [$\to$ (4.6)] can be computed by means of the quantile function of a noncentral χ^2-distribution with $df = 1$.

4.2 Test for equivalence of a hazard rate to some given reference value with exponentially distributed survival times

Let X denote a random variable whose density function (with respect to Lebesgue measure on $\mathbb{R}$) is given by

$$f_X(x; \sigma) = (1/\sigma) \exp\{-x/\sigma\}, \quad x > 0. \tag{4.9}$$

As is well known (cf. Johnson, Kotz and Balakrishnan, 1994, § 19.4), under this model the scale parameter $\sigma > 0$ equals the expected value of X. In the sequel, we mostly use the short-hand notation $X \sim \mathcal{E}(\sigma)$ in order to indicate that X is a random variable having density (4.9).

In the present section, it is our purpose to construct an optimal test of $H: \sigma \leq \sigma_1$ or $\sigma \geq \sigma_2$ versus $K: \sigma_1 < \sigma < \sigma_2$ $(0 < \sigma_1 < \sigma_1 < \infty)$ based on a sample $(X_1, \ldots, X_n)$ of mutually independent observations from $\mathcal{E}(\sigma)$. The interval (σ_1, σ_2) specified by that alternative hypothesis K is supposed to contain a point $\sigma_\circ$ serving as the target or reference value of the only parameter appearing in the model under consideration. As is the case in the one-sample problem with normally distributed data of known variance [recall the introductory paragraph of §4.1], it entails no loss of generality to assume that the interval corresponding to K has a normalized form which this time means that we have $\sigma_1 = 1/(1+\varepsilon)$, $\sigma_2 = 1+\varepsilon$ for some $\varepsilon > 0$. In order to induce such a normalization with respect to the form of the equivalence hypothesis, we have simply to apply the following transformation of the individual observations and the parameter, respectively:

$$X_i' = X_i/\sqrt{\sigma_1\sigma_2}, \quad i = 1, \ldots, n; \quad \sigma' = \sigma/\sqrt{\sigma_1\sigma_2}. \tag{4.10}$$

This follows from the obvious fact that for $X_i \sim \mathcal{E}(\sigma)$, the distribution of X_i' is likewise exponential but with scale parameter σ' instead of σ. Moreover, with $\varepsilon = \sqrt{\sigma_2/\sigma_1} - 1$, the condition $\sigma_1 < \sigma < \sigma_2$ is of course logically equivalent to $1/(1 + \varepsilon) < \sigma' < (1 + \varepsilon)$. In view of these relationships, we suppose in analogy to (4.1) that the hypotheses making up our testing problem have been proposed in the form

$$H : \sigma \leq 1/(1 + \varepsilon) \text{ or } \sigma \geq 1 + \varepsilon \text{ versus } K : 1/(1 + \varepsilon) < \sigma < 1 + \varepsilon \tag{4.11a}$$

from the start (with fixed $\varepsilon > 0$), and the data set to be analyzed consists of n mutually independent observations $X_1, \ldots, X_n$ such that

$$X_i \sim \mathcal{E}(\sigma), \quad i = 1, \ldots, n. \tag{4.11b}$$

Now, the distributional assumption (4.11b) is well known to imply that a statistic sufficient for the class of joint distributions of the sample $(X_1, \ldots, X_n)$ is given by $T = \sum_{i=1}^{n} X_i$. The density of the distribution of this T can be shown (see, e.g., Feller, 1971, p. 11) to be:

$$f_\sigma^T(t) = (1/\Gamma(n))\sigma^{-n}t^{n-1}\exp\{-t/\sigma\}, \quad t > 0. \tag{4.12}$$

Since n denotes a known constant whereas σ is allowed to vary over the whole positive half-axis, (4.12) is an element of a one-parameter exponential family in t and $\theta = -1/\sigma$. According to Lemma A.1.2 [$\to$ p. 249], each such family is STP$_\infty$ and thus a fortiori STP$_3$. Furthermore, it is readily verified that the function $(t,\sigma) \mapsto f_\sigma^T(t)$ is continuous in both of its arguments. In view of Theorem A.1.5 [$\to$ p. 251] and the sufficiency of T, we are justified to infer from these facts that the decision rule

$$\text{Reject } H \text{ if and only if } C^1_{\alpha; n, \varepsilon} < \sum_{i=1}^{n} X_i < C^2_{\alpha; n, \varepsilon} \tag{4.13}$$

yields an UMP level-α test for (4.11a), provided the critical bounds $C^1_{\alpha; n, \varepsilon}$, $C^2_{\alpha; n, \varepsilon}$ are determined by solving the system

$$F^T_{1/(1+\varepsilon)}(C_2) - F^T_{1/(1+\varepsilon)}(C_1) = \alpha$$
$$= F^T_{1+\varepsilon}(C_2) - F^T_{1+\varepsilon}(C_1), \quad 0 < C_1 < C_2 < \infty, \tag{4.14}$$

with $F_\sigma^T(\cdot)$ denoting (for any $\sigma > 0$) the cdf corresponding to the density function (4.12).

Unfortunately, notwithstanding the possibility of symmetrizing the hypotheses in the way having lead to (4.11a), the one-sample setting with exponentially distributed data does not satisfy condition (3.10) for symmetrization of the optimal critical interval. In other words, the system (4.14) does not admit reduction to a single equation involving the right-hand critical bound only. Consequently, implementation of (4.13) requires use of the iteration algorithm described in general terms on pp. 39-40. In order to adapt this computational scheme to the specific setting under discussion, using $C_1^\circ = n$ as a starting value of the left-hand critical bound C_1 to T is a sensible choice because T/n is a consistent estimator of σ and the interval of values of σ specified by K contains unity. Generally, if a UMP test for equivalence is based on a statistic which consistently estimates the parameter to be assessed, the critical region will be a proper subset of the interval corresponding to the alternative hypothesis sharing basic formal properties with the latter. Hence, we can take it for granted that the solution (C_1, C_2) to (4.14) gives, after rescaling by the factor $1/n$, an interval covering the point $\sigma = 1$. Thus, we have $C_1 < n < C_2$ so that the initial value $C_1^\circ = n$ is known to lie to the right of the left-hand boundary C_1 of the critical interval to be determined. In accordance with the relationship $C_1 < n$, the *SAS* procedure supplied at http://www.zi-

mannheim.de/wktsheq under the name `exp1st` for computing the solution
to (4.14), runs through a sequence of preliminary steps diminishing C_1° by
$\tau = .05\,n$ each until it occurs that we have $F_{1+\varepsilon}^T(C_2^\circ) - F_{1+\varepsilon}^T(C_1^\circ) \le \alpha$,
with C_2° computed as $C_2^\circ = \left(F_{1/(1+\varepsilon)}^T\right)^{-1}\left[\alpha + F_{1/(1+\varepsilon)}^T(C_1^\circ)\right]$. The point
where this condition is met, is chosen as the value of $\tilde{C}_1$ in the sense of
part (iv) of the general description given on pp. 39-40, and $\tilde{C}_1 + \tau$ as the
corresponding upper bound $\tilde{\tilde{C}}_1$ to C_1. Finally, successive interval halving
is applied to $(\tilde{C}_1, \tilde{\tilde{C}}_1)$ in order to approximate the exact value of C_1 to the
desired degree of accuracy, again as explained on p. 39, (iv).

In addition to the optimal critical constants $C_{\alpha;\,n,\varepsilon}^1$, $C_{\alpha;\,n,\varepsilon}^2$ [to resume
the explicit notation introduced in (4.13)], the *SAS* program `exp1st` also
computes the power of the test established above against the specific alternative $\sigma = 1$. To be sure, this is not the point in the parameter space where
the power function $\beta(\cdot)$, say, of the UMP level-α test for the equivalence
problem made precise in (4.11) takes on its exact maximum. But by the
results to be found in §4.5 we know that the difference between $\beta(1)$ and
$\max_{\sigma>0}\beta(\sigma)$ is asymptotically negligible (as $n \to \infty$). Table 4.3 gives the
critical constants $C_{\alpha;\,n,\varepsilon}^1$, $C_{\alpha;\,n,\varepsilon}^2$ for the level $\alpha = .05$, $\varepsilon \in \{.30, .50\}$, and
sample sizes ≤ 120 being a multiple of 10. The corresponding values of the
power attained at $\sigma = 1$ are displayed in Table 4.4.

Table 4.3 *Critical interval* $(C_{.05;\,n,\varepsilon}^1, C_{.05;\,n,\varepsilon}^2)$ *of the UMP equivalence test at the 5% level for the one-sample setting with exponentially
distributed data, for $\varepsilon = .30, .50$ and $n = 10\,(10)\,120$*

n	$\varepsilon = .30$	$\varepsilon = .50$
10	$(9.610923, 10.167879)$	$(9.302916, 10.179687)$
20	$(19.227987, 20.331723)$	$(18.175346, 20.878033)$
30	$(28.728536, 30.622505)$	$(26.300336, 32.650207)$
40	$(38.059577, 41.104285)$	$(33.955275, 45.339863)$
50	$(47.173320, 51.843905)$	$(41.447117, 58.454257)$
60	$(56.048597, 62.887533)$	$(48.855774, 71.779509)$
70	$(64.711420, 74.228599)$	$(56.204318, 85.244644)$
80	$(73.221500, 85.808680)$	$(63.505485, 98.817061)$
90	$(81.635963, 97.555833)$	$(70.767971, 112.476582)$
100	$(89.991186, 109.414666)$	$(77.998090, 126.208916)$
110	$(98.306216, 121.350753)$	$(85.200605, 140.003340)$
120	$(106.590707, 133.344176)$	$(92.379217, 153.851535)$

Table 4.4 *Power attained at $\sigma = 1$ when using the critical intervals shown in Table 4.3*

n	$\varepsilon = .30$	$\varepsilon = .50$
10	.070340	.111904
20	.098785	.240904
30	.138156	.442380
40	.191426	.635809
50	.260318	.773372
60	.342885	.862271
70	.432381	.917672
80	.520229	.951433
90	.600305	.971657
100	.670069	.983607
110	.729339	.990588
120	.778984	.994629

Example 4.1

In a retrospective study involving $n = 80$ patients, it was one of the aims to rule out the possibility that a particular drug used in the long-term treatment of progressive chronic polyarthritis (PCP) changes the mean lifespan of erythrocytes to a relevant degree. For a reference population, the expected length of the average erythrocytal lifecycle was known to be $3.84 \approx 4$ months.

Let the distribution of the intraindividual mean erythrocytal lifespan be of the form (4.12) and choose the equivalence interval for σ as centred about 4, with length being equal to 2. In the sample recruited for the study a total time of $\sum_{i=1}^{n} X_i = 329.7873$ was obtained. Rescaling the originally measured time values as well as the equivalence limits according to (4.10) yields $T = 329.7873/\sqrt{15} = 85.1507$ and $\varepsilon = \sqrt{5/3} - 1 = 0.2910$. Rounding ε up to .30 we obtain from Table 4.3 $(73.22150, 85.80868)$ as the critical interval to be used in (4.13). Since the observed value of T happens to be an inner point of this interval, we can decide in favour of equivalence between study and reference population with respect to mean erythrocytal lifespan.

Remark on testing for dispersion equivalence of a single sample of normally distributed data. Suppose that the distribution which the random sample $(X_1, \ldots, X_n)$ has been drawn from, is Gaussian with expectation μ and variance σ^2 (with both parameters being unknown) and that our main interest is in establishing dispersion equivalence of this distribution to some reference distribution of the same form whose variance is known to equal σ_o^2. For convenience, let us formulate the equivalence hypothesis in this case as $K : \sigma_1^2 < \sigma^2 < \sigma_2^2$ with (σ_1^2, σ_2^2) as a suitably chosen fixed interval covering the reference value σ_o^2. Applying the same transformation as before [recall (4.10)] and redefining ε as an abbreviation for $\sigma_2/\sigma_1 - 1$ rather than $\sqrt{\sigma_2/\sigma_1} - 1$ leads to the problem of testing

$$H : \sigma^2 \leq 1/(1+\varepsilon) \text{ or } \sigma^2 \geq 1+\varepsilon \text{ versus } K : 1/(1+\varepsilon) < \sigma^2 < 1+\varepsilon \quad (4.15a)$$

with a sample $(X_1, \ldots, X_n)$ of mutually independent observations satisfying

$$X_i \sim \mathcal{N}(\mu, \sigma^2), \quad i = 1, \ldots, n. \quad (4.15b)$$

Now, it is easy to verify that the problem (4.15) remains invariant under arbitrary common translations $X_i \mapsto X_i + c$ of all individual observations contained in the sample. Furthermore, it is well known (see Lehmann, 1986, p. 290) that any test remaining invariant under all transformations of that type, must depend on the data only through the sum of squares $SQ_X = \sum_{i=1}^n (X_i - \bar{X})^2$ or, equivalently, $T = (1/2) \cdot SQ_X$. But under the assumption of (4.15b) the latter statistic has a distribution whose density is precisely $f_{\sigma^2}^T(\cdot)$ as defined in (4.12) with n replaced by $n' = (n-1)/2$ (cf. Stuart and Ord, 1994, p. 385). Hence, in the one-sample setting with normally distributed data, a UMP invariant test for dispersion equivalence in the sense of (4.15a) is obtained simply by comparing the observed value of $T = (1/2) \cdot SQ_X$ with the critical bounds $C_{\alpha; n', \varepsilon}^1, C_{\alpha; n', \varepsilon}^2$ to be computed in exactly the same way as in the case of exponentially distributed survival times. In particular, the critical interval $(73.22150, 85.80868)$ computed in the above example for the sum of $n' = 80$ observations from $\mathcal{E}(\sigma)$ can also be used for testing for dispersion equivalence of $\mathcal{N}(\mu, \sigma^2)$ to $\mathcal{N}(\mu, 1)$ in the sense of $\sqrt{3/5} < \sigma^2 < \sqrt{5/3}$ with a sample of size $n = 2n' + 1 = 161$ and $(1/2) \cdot \sum_{i=1}^n (X_i - \bar{X})^2$ as the test statistic. (Note that the SAS macro exp1st works also for arbitrary noninteger values of the constant n).

4.3 Testing for equivalence of a single binomial proportion to a fixed reference success probability

Both specific equivalence testing problems treated in the preceding sections of this chapter refer to distributions of the absolutely continuous type. In contrast, the present section deals with the most extreme case of a one-sample setting with data following a discrete distribution. More precisely speaking we now assume that each of the n mutually independent observations $X_1, \ldots, X_n$ takes on only two different values, say $0 \,(\leftrightarrow$ "no response") and $1 \,(\leftrightarrow$ "response") with probability p and $1 - p$, respectively.

Once more, the (unweighted) sum of all individual observations turns out to be sufficient for the class of the possible distributions of the vector

$(X_1, \ldots, X_n)$. Of course, the distribution of $T = \sum_{i=1}^{n} X_i$ is now given by the probability mass function

$$b(t; n, p) = \binom{n}{t} p^t (1-p)^{n-t} \quad, \quad t \in \{0, 1, \ldots, n\}. \tag{4.16}$$

Likewise, it is easily seen that the corresponding family $\big(b(\cdot\,; n, p)\big)_{0 < p < 1}$ of densities with respect to the counting measure of the set $\{0, 1, \ldots, n\}$ of possible values of T, is an exponential family in t and $\theta = \log(p/(1-p))$. In view of these facts we can apply essentially the same arguments as were used in §4.2 showing that for

$$H : 0 < p \le p_1 \text{ or } p_2 \le p < 1 \text{ versus } K : p_1 < p < p_2$$

$$(0 < p_1 < p_2 < 1, \text{ fixed}) \tag{4.17}$$

there exists an UMP level-α test defined by the following decision rule:

$$\begin{cases} \text{Rejection of } H \text{ for} \quad C_\alpha^1(n;\, p_1, p_2) < T < C_\alpha^2(n;\, p_1, p_2) \\ \text{Rejection with prob. } \gamma_\alpha^1(n;\, p_1, p_2) \text{ for } T = C_\alpha^1(n;\, p_1, p_2) \\ \text{Rejection with prob. } \gamma_\alpha^2(n;\, p_1, p_2) \text{ for } T = C_\alpha^2(n;\, p_1, p_2) \\ \text{Acceptance for} \quad T < C_\alpha^1(n;\, p_1, p_2) \text{ or } T > C_\alpha^2(n;\, p_1, p_2) \end{cases} \tag{4.18}$$

The optimality property of (4.18) holds on the understanding that the constants $C_\alpha^\nu(n;\, p_1, p_2)$, $\gamma_\alpha^\nu(n;\, p_1, p_2)$, $\nu = 1, 2$, are determined by solving

$$\sum_{t=C_1+1}^{C_2-1} b(t; n, p_1) + \sum_{\nu=1}^{2} \gamma_\nu b(C_\nu; n, p_1) = \alpha = \sum_{t=C_1+1}^{C_2-1} b(t; n, p_2) +$$

$$\sum_{\nu=1}^{2} \gamma_\nu b(C_\nu; n, p_2) \,, \qquad 0 \le C_1 \le C_2 \le n\,, \ 0 \le \gamma_1, \gamma_2 < 1. \tag{4.19}$$

The *SAS* program to be found at http://www.zi-mannheim.de/wktsheq under the name **bi1st** implements the search algorithm described in full generality on p. 40 for this specific case. In addition, the program computes the power of the test (4.18) against the special alternative that the true value of the response probability p coincides with the midpoint $(p_1 + p_2)/2$ of the interval corresponding to K. In view of the undesirability of using external chance mechanisms in real applications of statistical inference, the program also calculates the power against $p = (p_1 + p_2)/2$ of the nonrandomized version of the test as obtained by adding both boundary points of the rejection interval to the acceptance region.

The sufficient condition (3.10) for symmetrizing the optimal critical interval is satisfied here whenever we are willing to choose $p_1 = 1/2 - \varepsilon$, $p_2 = 1/2 + \varepsilon$ which seems especially natural in those applications of the test where the X_i are in fact indicators of the sign of intra-subject differences between paired continuous observations [for details see §5.1]. Trivially, the distribution of $\sum_{i=1}^{n} X_i - n/2$ under $p = 1/2 + \varepsilon$ is the same as that of

$n/2 - \sum_{i=1}^{n} X_i$ under $p = 1/2 - \varepsilon$. Since, as a test statistic, $\sum_{i=1}^{n} X_i - n/2$ is equivalent to $T = \sum_{i=1}^{n} X_i$ and, for $p_1 = 1/2 - \varepsilon$, $p_2 = 1/2 + \varepsilon$, (4.17) can equivalently be written $H : |\theta| \geq \varepsilon$ vs. $K : |\theta| < \varepsilon$ with $\theta = p - 1/2$, we may conclude from (3.12) that in the symmetric case, the optimal critical interval for T is given by

$$\left(C_\alpha^1(n; 1/2 - \varepsilon, 1/2 + \varepsilon), C_\alpha^2(n; 1/2 - \varepsilon, 1/2 + \varepsilon) \right) =$$
$$\left(n - C_\alpha^*(n; \varepsilon), C_\alpha^*(n; \varepsilon) \right) \qquad (4.20a)$$

where

$$C_\alpha^*(n; \varepsilon) = n/2 + \max \left\{ c \left| \sum_{n/2-c+1}^{n/2+c-1} b(t; n, 1/2 + \varepsilon) \leq \alpha, \right. \right.$$
$$\left. 0 < c \leq n/2 + 1, (c + n/2) \in \mathbb{Z} \right\}. \qquad (4.20b)$$

Furthermore, specializing (3.12) to the case $T(\mathbf{X}) = \sum_{i=1}^{n} X_i - n/2$, it is easy to check that the nonrandomized version of the test (4.18) can also be based on a p-value in the usual sense. For that purpose, one has to define the significance probability of the observed value $t \in \{0, 1, \ldots, n\}$ of T by

$$p_{obs}(t) = \sum_{j=n-\tilde{t}}^{\tilde{t}} b(j; n, 1/2 + \varepsilon) \qquad (4.21a)$$

with

$$\tilde{t} = \max\{t, n - t\}. \qquad (4.21b)$$

Table 4.5 shows the critical interval $\left(C_{.05}^1(n; p_1, p_2), C_{.05}^1(n; p_1, p_2) \right)$ to be used in (4.18) at the 5% level for various choices of the equivalence interval (p_1, p_2) and a selection of sample sizes ranging from 25 to 125. The power of the corresponding tests (with and without randomization) against the alternative $p = (p_1 + p_2)/2$ is given in Table 4.6. It should be noticed that these tables cover, for the same values of n, also the cases $(p_1, p_2) \in \{(.10, .30), (.20, .40), (.30, .50), (.05, .35)\}$. Generally, it is not hard to establish the relationships

$$C_\alpha^\nu(n; 1 - p_2, 1 - p_1) = n - C_\alpha^{3-\nu}(n; p_1, p_2), \quad \nu = 1, 2 ; \qquad (4.22a)$$

$$\beta_{n,\alpha}^{1-p_2, 1-p_1}(1 - p) = \beta_{n,\alpha}^{p_1, p_2}(p) , \quad \tilde{\beta}_{n,\alpha}^{1-p_2, 1-p_1}(1 - p) = \tilde{\beta}_{n,\alpha}^{p_1, p_2}(p) , \qquad (4.22b)$$

of which the latter refer to the power function of the UMP test (4.18) $[\rightarrow \beta_{n,\alpha}^{q_1, q_2}(\cdot)]$ and its nonrandomized version $[\rightarrow \tilde{\beta}_{n,\alpha}^{q_1, q_2}(\cdot)]$, respectively.

Table 4.5 *Critical interval* $(C^1_{.05}(n; p_1, p_2), C^2_{.05}(n; p_1, p_2))$ *for the test (4.18) at the 5% level, for various specifications of* (p_1, p_2) *and* $n = 25(25)125$

				$(p_1, p_2) =$		
n	$(.40, .60)$	$(.50, .70)$	$(.60, .80)$	$(.70, .90)$	$(.35, .65)$	$(.65, .95)$
25	$(12, 13)$	$(15, 16)$	$(17, 18)$	$(20, 21)$	$(12, 13)$	$(20, 22)$
50	$(24, 26)$	$(29, 31)$	$(35, 36)$	$(40, 42)$	$(23, 27)$	$(38, 45)$
75	$(36, 39)$	$(44, 47)$	$(51, 54)$	$(59, 63)$	$(33, 42)$	$(55, 68)$
100	$(48, 52)$	$(58, 63)$	$(68, 73)$	$(77, 85)$	$(43, 57)$	$(73, 91)$
125	$(59, 66)$	$(72, 79)$	$(84, 93)$	$(96, 107)$	$(53, 72)$	$(90, 115)$

Table 4.6 *Power of the UMP tests with critical intervals shown in Table 4.5 against the alternative* $p = (p_1 + p_2)/2$ *[italicized values* $\leftrightarrow$ *nonrandomized version of the tests]*

				$(p_1, p_2) =$		
n	$(.40, .60)$	$(.50, .70)$	$(.60, .80)$	$(.70, .90)$	$(.35, .65)$	$(.65, .95)$
25	.0816	.0847	.0900	.1093	.1551	.3167
	.0000	*.0000*	*.0000*	*.0000*	*.0000*	*.1867*
50	.1367	.1428	.1663	.2451	.4124	.7193
	.1123	*.1146*	*.0000*	*.1364*	*.3282*	*.6626*
75	.2201	.2347	.2918	.4419	.6815	.8940
	.1824	*.1854*	*.1987*	*.3288*	*.6443*	*.8899*
100	.3368	.3602	.4429	.6319	.8392	.9583
	.2356	*.3157*	*.3367*	*.6104*	*.8067*	*.9418*
125	.4685	.4980	.5924	.7611	.9231	.9844
	.4083	*.4149*	*.5590*	*.7166*	*.8930*	*.9801*

Figure 4.3 shows the complete power function of the UMP test for $K: .70 < p < .90$ at level $\alpha = .05$ based on a sample of size $n = 82$, along with its counterpart referring to the nonrandomized version of (4.18). An obvious feature evident in both curves is the lack of symmetry about the midpoint of the equivalence interval specified by the alternative hypothesis. Furthermore, a comparison of both graphs discloses that even in applica-

tions with rather large samples the gain in power attained by exhausting the significance level through randomized decisions on the boundaries of the critical interval, is by no means negligible.

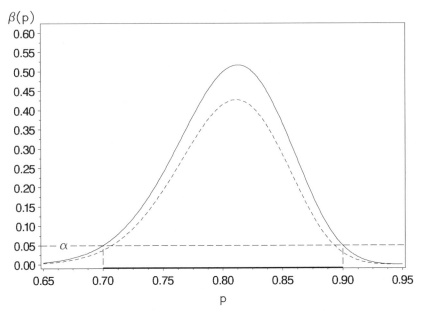

Figure 4.3 *Power function of the UMP level-α test of p ≤ .70 or p ≥ .90 vs. .70 < p < .90 [solid line] and its nonrandomized counterpart [broken line] for n = 82 and α = .05.*

Example 4.2

In an observational study of an improved combination regime for the adjuvant chemotherapy of a particular tumour entity, the investigators aimed at showing that a highly toxic drug which had been used in the past as one of the components could be replaced with a much better tolerable substance without inducing a relevant change in patients' prognosis. The sample comprised $n = 273$ patients suffering from the respective tumour. Each patient had been under follow-up for at least 24 months. From extensive clinical experience the traditionally administered combination containing the toxic ingredient was known to provide a 2-year progression-free survival rate of 73%. The interval of acceptable deviations from this reference value was specified to be $(p_1, p_2) = (.65, .75)$. In the current study a number of $t = 191$ patients survived the first 24 months since initiation of treatment without exhibiting signs of a progression. The limits of the critical interval of the test (4.18) at level $\alpha = .05$ are computed (by means of the *SAS* macro mentioned above) to be $C^1_{.05}(273; .65, .75) = 189$, $C^2_{.05}(273; .65, .75) = 194$ leading to a rejection of the null hypothesis of nonequivalence. Power calculation shows the probability of detecting exact coincidence of the parameter p with the reference value .73 in the nonrandomized test to be .1216. When randomized decisions are admitted for $T = 189$ and $T = 194$, this value is slightly increased to .1435. If the true value of p coincides with the midpoint of the equivalence interval instead, the rejection probability amounts to .2082 (nonrandomized version of the test) and .2431 (UMP test at exact level .05), respectively.

4.4 Confidence-interval inclusion rules as asymptotically UMP tests for equivalence

At first glance the principle of confidence interval inclusion and the classical approach to the construction of equivalence tests seem to have nothing in common except for yielding procedures which are valid in the sense of maintaining the significance level. Nevertheless, it can be shown that an interval inclusion test based on a pair of confidence bounds at one-sided level $1 - \alpha$ [recall § 3.1] approximates, under suitable conditions, the optimal test for the same problem with arbitrarily high precision if the sample size is chosen sufficiently large. A rigorous mathematical proof of this result is technically rather complicated and will not be given here (readers interested in the details may be referred to Wellek, 1994, pp. 96-103, despite the difference in language). However, in the one-sample setting with normally distributed observations of unit variance and symmetrically chosen equivalence interval for the parameter θ [$\rightarrow$ (4.1)], it admits a simple heuristic derivation which will be presented on the following pages.

If the values realized in a sample of size n from $\mathcal{N}(\theta, 1)$ are $x_1, \ldots, x_n$ with $\bar{x}_n$ as their ordinary arithmetic mean, the standard method of interval estimation yields the number $\bar{x}_n - u_{1-\alpha}/\sqrt{n}$ and $\bar{x}_n + u_{1-\alpha}/\sqrt{n}$ as a lower and upper $(1 - \alpha)$−confidence bound for θ, respectively. Hence, rejection of the null hypothesis $|\theta| \geq \varepsilon$ in the interval inclusion test requires in this case that both of the inequalities $\bar{x}_n - u_{1-\alpha}/\sqrt{n} > -\varepsilon$ and $\bar{x}_n + u_{1-\alpha}/\sqrt{n} < \varepsilon$ must be satisfied. Clearly, this holds true if and only if $\sqrt{n}\bar{x}_n$ is a point in the open interval with limits $\mp(\sqrt{n}\varepsilon - u_{1-\alpha})$. In other words, the interval inclusion test rejects if and only if we have $\sqrt{n}|\bar{x}_n| < \sqrt{n}\varepsilon - u_{1-\alpha}$. Accordingly, its rejection region is exactly of the same form as that of the optimal level-α test [$\rightarrow$ (4.7)], with the sole difference that the critical constant $C_{\alpha; \sqrt{n}\varepsilon}$ as defined by (4.6) is replaced by $\sqrt{n}\varepsilon - u_{1-\alpha}$.

Trivially, the equation determining $C_{\alpha; \sqrt{n}\varepsilon}$ according to (4.5) can be rewritten as

$$\Phi(c - \sqrt{n}\varepsilon) + \Phi(c + \sqrt{n}\varepsilon) = 1 + \alpha \ , \quad 0 < c < \infty. \qquad (4.23)$$

Since ε stands for a positive number, one has of course $\sqrt{n}\varepsilon \to +\infty$ (as $n \to \infty$) and consequently $c - \sqrt{n}\varepsilon \to -\infty$, $c + \sqrt{n}\varepsilon \to +\infty$. In view of $\Phi(-\infty) = 0$, $\Phi(+\infty) = 1$ this implies $\Phi(c - \sqrt{n}\varepsilon) \to 0$, $\Phi(c + \sqrt{n}\varepsilon) \to 1$. Furthermore, like every reasonable testing procedure, the UMP level-α test for (4.1b) is consistent (Wellek, 1994, Lemma A.3.3). But convergence of the rejection probability to 1 under any $\theta \in (-\varepsilon, \varepsilon)$ implies [recall (4.5)] that the area under the density curve of a Gaussian variable with unit variance over the critical interval $(-C_{\alpha; \sqrt{n}\varepsilon}, C_{\alpha; \sqrt{n}\varepsilon})$ tends to 1 which can only be true if the length of that interval and hence $C_{\alpha; \sqrt{n}\varepsilon}$ itself increases to ∞ as $n \to \infty$. In view of this, the values of c to be taken into consideration when solving equation (4.23) are very large positive numbers if n is large, and for fixed $c \gg 0$, $\Phi(c + \sqrt{n}\varepsilon)$ will come very close to its limit, i.e., to 1, already for values of n which are still too small for carrying $\Phi(c - \sqrt{n}\varepsilon)$ into a small neighbourhood of zero. According to this intuitive notion the solution to (4.23), i.e., the optimal critical constant $C_{\alpha; \sqrt{n}\varepsilon}$ satisfies the approximate equation

$$\Phi(C_{\alpha; \sqrt{n}\varepsilon} - \sqrt{n}\varepsilon) \approx \alpha \ . \qquad (4.24)$$

On the other hand, in view of the definition of u_γ and the symmetry of the standard normal distribution we clearly have $\alpha = \Phi(-u_{1-\alpha})$. Hence, (4.24) holds if and only if

$$\Phi(C_{\alpha; \sqrt{n}\varepsilon} - \sqrt{n}\varepsilon) \approx \Phi(-u_{1-\alpha}). \qquad (4.25)$$

Since the standard normal cdf has a continuous inverse we are justified to drop $\Phi(\cdot)$ on both sides of (4.25) and write for "sufficiently large" sample sizes n

$$C_{\alpha; \sqrt{n}\varepsilon} \approx \sqrt{n}\varepsilon - u_{1-\alpha} \ . \qquad (4.26)$$

Finally, each of the two tests under comparison is uniquely determined by one of the critical bounds $C_{\alpha; \sqrt{n}\varepsilon}$ and $\sqrt{n}\varepsilon - u_{1-\alpha}$ being approximately equal according to (4.26). In view of this, we have given a heuristic proof of the assertion that approximate identity holds between both tests with respect to all probabilistic properties, in particular the power against any specific alternative $\theta \in (-\varepsilon, \varepsilon)$. In fact, according to the result proved as Theorem A.3.5 in Wellek (1994), still more can be said: *Asymptotically, the interval inclusion test is uniformly most powerful for the equivalence problem* (4.1) even if tests are admitted which maintain the nominal level only in the limit and/or the arbitrarily selected alternative $\theta \in K$ is allowed to converge to one of the boundary points of the equivalence interval rather than kept fixed for all values of n.

To be sure, demonstration of asymptotic optimality of a test per se is mainly of theoretical interest. The actual relevance of such a result can only be assessed if detailed numerical investigations have been performed providing in particular precise information on the order of magnitude of the sample sizes required to ensure that the loss of power entailed by replacing the optimal finite-sample test with the asymptotic procedure under consideration be practically negligible. Since both the UMP level-α test and the test based on the principle of confidence interval inclusion depends on n and ε only through $\tilde{\varepsilon} = \sqrt{n}\varepsilon$, it suffices to compare the procedures for various values of this latter quantity.

Tables 4.7 and 4.8 are the direct counterparts of Tables 4.1 and 4.2 for the interval inclusion test at the same level $\alpha = .05$. Inspecting the entries in Table 4.8 as compared to the corresponding values shown in Table 4.2 leads to the following major conclusions:

(i) As long as $\tilde{\varepsilon} = \sqrt{n}\varepsilon$ fails to exceed the value 1.7 the interval inclusion test is very unsatisfactory since its maximum power falls below the significance level. In contrast, for $\tilde{\varepsilon} = 1.7$ the power of the UMP test against $\theta = 0$ amounts to 21% and is thus more than four times larger than α.

(ii) The cases where the interval inclusion test does better than the trivial procedure rejecting H with constant probability α (independently of the data), but is still markedly inferior to the UMP test at the same level are characterized by the condition $1.7 < \tilde{\varepsilon} \leq 2.3$.

(iii) If $\tilde{\varepsilon}$ is increased beyond the right-hand limit of this interval (by weakening the equivalence condition under the hypothesis and/or increasing the sample size), the difference between both tests disappears very quickly (except of course for some remainder being negligible for all practical purposes).

Table 4.7 *Critical constant $\tilde{\varepsilon} - u_{.95}$ for the interval inclusion test at level $\alpha = .05$ in the one-sample setting with data from $\mathcal{N}(\theta, 1)$*

$\tilde{\varepsilon}$	0.	1.	2.	3.	4.
.0	–	-.64485	0.35515	1.35515	2.35515
.1	-1.5449	-.54485	0.45515	1.45515	2.45515
.2	-1.4449	-.44485	0.55515	1.55515	2.55515
.3	-1.3449	-.34485	0.65515	1.65515	2.65515
.4	-1.2449	-.24485	0.75515	1.75515	2.75515
.5	-1.1449	-.14485	0.85515	1.85515	2.85515
.6	-1.0449	-.04485	0.95515	1.95515	2.95515
.7	-.94485	0.05515	1.05515	2.05515	3.05515
.8	-.84485	0.15515	1.15515	2.15515	3.15515
.9	-.74485	0.25515	1.25515	2.25515	3.25515

Table 4.8 *Power of the test with critical region* $\left\{\sqrt{n}\,|\bar{X}_n| < \tilde{\varepsilon} - u_{.95}\right\}$ *against* $\theta = 0$ *for the same grid of values of* $\tilde{\varepsilon} = \sqrt{n}\varepsilon$ *as covered by Table 4.7*

$\tilde{\varepsilon}$	0.	1.	2.	3.	4.
.0	–	.00000	.27752	.82463	.98148
.1	.00000	.00000	.35100	.85437	.98592
.2	.00000	.00000	.42121	.88009	.98939
.3	.00000	.00000	.48763	.90211	.99207
.4	.00000	.00000	.54984	.92077	.99413
.5	.00000	.00000	.60753	.93642	.99570
.6	.00000	.00000	.66050	.94943	.99687
.7	.00000	.04398	.70864	.96014	.99775
.8	.00000	.12329	.75197	.96885	.99840
.9	.00000	.20139	.79057	.97588	.99887

Numerical power comparisons for various other one-sample problems whose results are not reported in detail here, fully confirm these findings. Summarily speaking, the gain from applying the UMP instead of the corresponding interval inclusion test is very modest whenever the power attained in the former has the order of magnitude usually required in a study to be analyzed by means of a conventional one- or two-sided test. However, in equivalence testing power values exceeding 50% can only be obtained if either the equivalence range specified by the alternative hypothesis is chosen extremely wide or the sample size requirements are beyond the scope of feasibility for most if not all applications.

Clearly, the intuitive notion of equivalence suggests to tolerate only small deviations of the parameter θ from its target value θ_o. If we adopt this point of view there is no choice but to either refrain from launching a suitable study at all, or to be content with power values falling distinctly below 50%. The latter case is the one where replacing an interval inclusion procedure with an optimal test typically yields the most marked gains in power which can amount to up to 30% in these instances. In addition to such considerations concerning power and efficiency, there is another major reason (which has been alluded to already in §3.3) why there is a real need for carrying out classical optimal constructions of tests for equivalence in spite of the option of solving testing problems of that kind by means of the interval inclusion principle: The range of settings for which well-established interval estimation procedures exist, is by far too narrow to provide a clinical or experimental investigator with a sufficiently rich arsenal of specific equivalence testing methods.

CHAPTER 5

Equivalence tests for designs with paired observations

5.1 Sign test for equivalence

The assumptions which must be satisfied in order to ensure that the sign test for equivalence be an exactly valid procedure exhibiting some basic optimality property are as weak as in the case of its traditional one- and two-sided analogue. This means that the data have to be given by n mutually independent pairs $(X_1, Y_1), \ldots, (X_n, Y_n)$ of random variables following all the same bivariate distribution which may be of arbitrary form. In particular, the distribution of the (X_i, Y_i) is allowed to be discrete. Within each such random pair, the first and second component gives the result of applying the two treatments, say A and B, under comparison to the respective observational unit. Except for treatment, the observations X_i and Y_i are taken under completely homogeneous conditions so that each intraindividual difference $D_i \equiv X_i - Y_i$ can be interpreted as an observed treatment effect. For definiteness, we assume further that large values of the X's and Y's are favourable which implies that A has been more efficient than B in the ith individual if and only if the value taken on by D_i turns out to be positive.

Now, let us agree on defining equivalence of both treatments by means of the condition that, except for practically irrelevant differences, the probability $p_+ \equiv P[D_i > 0]$ of observing A to turn out superior to B in a randomly selected individual, coincides with the probability $p_- \equiv P[D_i < 0]$ of observing A to yield a weaker effect than B. In view of our aim to construct an optimal testing procedure, it proves advisable that we relate this condition to the logarithmic scale which leads to considering the statement $-\varepsilon_1 < \log p_+ - \log p_- < \varepsilon_2$ (with sufficiently small positive real numbers $\varepsilon_1, \varepsilon_2$) as the equivalence hypothesis of interest.

In fact, the mathematically natural choice of a target parameter for the inferential problem in mind is given by

$$\theta = \log(p_+/p_-) \ . \tag{5.1}$$

This is readily seen by examining the joint distribution of the usual counting statistics $N_+ = \#\{i \mid D_i > 0\}$, $N_0 = \#\{i \mid D_i = 0\}$, $N_- = \#\{i \mid D_i < 0\}$

whose probability mass function admits the representation

$$f(n_+, n_0, n_-; n, \theta, \zeta) = \frac{n!}{n_+! n_0! n_-!} \exp\{n_+\theta + n_0\zeta\}\, (1 + e^\theta + e^\zeta)^{-n}\,, \quad (5.2)$$

where

$$\theta = \log(p_+/p_-)\,, \quad \zeta = \log(p_0/p_-)\,. \quad (5.3)$$

Furthermore, the argument made explicit in Lehmann (1986, pp. 168-9) shows that a test which is uniformly most powerful unbiased (UMPU) in the class of those level-α tests of

$$H : \theta \le -\varepsilon_1 \vee \theta \ge \varepsilon_2 \text{ versus } K : -\varepsilon_1 < \theta < \varepsilon_2 \quad (5.4)$$

which depend on the data only through (N_+, N_0, N_-), uniformly maximizes the power also within the class of *all* unbiased tests at the same level for (5.4).

By (5.2), the class of all possible joint distributions of (N_+, N_0, N_-), i.e., of all trinomial distributions based on a sample of size n, is a two-parameter exponential family in (θ, ζ) and (N_+, N_0). Hence, we can apply Theorem A.2.2 [$\rightarrow$ Appendix, p. 255] with $k = 1$, $T = N_+$, $S = N_0$ which implies that a UMPU level-α test for the problem (5.4) exists and is of the following form: Given the observed number of ties between A and B, i.e., of zeroes contained in the sample $(D_1, \ldots, D_n)$, is $n_0 \in \{0, 1, \ldots, n\}$, the null hypothesis H of nonequivalence has to be rejected if the number N_+ of positive signs satisfies the double inequality $C^1_{\alpha|n_0} + 1 \le N_+ \le C^2_{\alpha|n_0} - 1$. On the boundaries of the corresponding critical interval, i.e., for $N_+ = C^\nu_{\alpha|n_0}$, a randomized decision in favour of K has to be taken with probability $\gamma^\nu_{\alpha|n_0}$ ($\nu = 1, 2$). The complete set $C^\nu_{\alpha|n_0}$, $\gamma^\nu_{\alpha|n_0}$, $\nu = 1, 2$, of (conditional) critical constants has to be determined by solving the equations

$$\sum_{n_+ = C^1_{\alpha|n_0} + 1}^{C^2_{\alpha|n_0} - 1} P_{-\varepsilon_1}[N_+ = n_+ | N_0 = n_0] \quad +$$

$$\sum_{\nu=1}^{2} \gamma^\nu_{\alpha|n_0} P_{-\varepsilon_1}\left[N_+ = C^\nu_{\alpha|n_0} \mid N_0 = n_0\right] = \alpha\,, \quad (5.5a)$$

$$\sum_{n_+ = C^1_{\alpha|n_0} + 1}^{C^2_{\alpha|n_0} - 1} P_{\varepsilon_2}[N_+ = n_+ | N_0 = n_0] \quad +$$

$$\sum_{\nu=1}^{2} \gamma^\nu_{\alpha|n_0} P_{\varepsilon_2}\left[N_+ = C^\nu_{\alpha|n_0} \mid N_0 = n_0\right] = \alpha\,. \quad (5.5b)$$

Since the conditional distribution of N_+ given $N_0 = n_0$ is well known (cf.

Johnson, Kotz and Balakrishnan, 1997, p. 35) to be binomial with parameters $n - n_0$ and $p_+/(p_+ + p_-) = e^\theta/(1 + e^\theta)$ for each $n_0 \in \{0, 1, \ldots, n\}$ and $\theta \in \mathbb{R}$, the system (5.5) differs from (4.19) only by changes in notation. More precisely speaking, (5.5) turns into the system of equations to be solved in testing for equivalence of a single binomial proportion to $1/2$ simply by making the substitution $n \leftrightarrow n - n_0$, $p_1 \leftrightarrow e^{-\varepsilon_1}/(1 + e^{-\varepsilon_1})$, $p_2 \leftrightarrow e^{\varepsilon_2}/(1 + e^{\varepsilon_2})$.

Thus, it eventually follows that an UMPU level-α test for the nonparametric equivalence problem proposed at the beginning of this section is obtained by treating the observed number n_0 of pairs with tied components as a fixed quantity and carrying out the test derived in § 4.3 with $n - n_0$ as nominal sample size and $\left(e^{-\varepsilon_1}/(1 + e^{-\varepsilon_1}), e^{\varepsilon_2}/(1 + e^{\varepsilon_2})\right)$ as the equivalence range for the binomial parameter. Accordingly, the practical implementation of the decision rule to be used in the sign test for equivalence entails no new computational steps. In particular, in the symmetric case $\varepsilon_1 = \varepsilon_2 = \varepsilon$, the nonrandomized version of the test can be carried out by means of the p-value as defined in (4.21) (with ε and n replaced with $e^\varepsilon/(1 + e^\varepsilon) - 1/2$ and $n - n_0$, respectively), and even the table of critical bounds to the test statistic presented before for the binomial one-sample problem can be used for some values of $n - n_0$ and some specifications of ε. The only true extension brought into play when using the binomial one-sample test of § 4.3 as a conditional procedure for testing the hypotheses (5.4) concerns the computation of power values and minimum sample sizes required for guaranteeing specified lower bounds to the power. As is generally the case with conditional testing procedures, the power function of the sign test for equivalence is of practical interest only in its nonconditional form, which implies that the respective computations involve averaging with respect to the distribution of the conditioning statistic N_0. Obviously, irrespective of the form of the hypotheses under consideration, the nonconditional power function of any test based on the statistics N_+ and N_0 is a function of two arguments, viz. p_+ and p_0. A *SAS* macro which enables to compute the rejection probability of both the exact and the nonrandomized version of the UMPU level-α test for (5.4) against the specific alternative $\theta = 0$ (or, equivalently, $p_+ = p_-$ which in turn is equivalent to $p_+ = (1 - p_0)/2$ for arbitrary rates p_0 of zeroes among the intra-subject differences D_i), can be found at http://www.zi-mannheim.de/wktsheq under the program name powsign.

Clearly, the problem of inducing considerable conservatism by not allowing randomized decisions in favour of the alternative hypothesis which has been discussed in detail in connection with the Fisher type exact test for one-sided equivalence of two binomial distributions in § 2.3.2, affects the sign test for (two-sided) equivalence as well. Again, mitigating this conservatism by increasing the nominal significance level as far as possible without increasing the nonconditional rejection probability under any null parameter constellation above the target level, provides a very satisfactory compromise between maximization of power and suitability of the resulting testing procedure for real applications. For sample sizes up to 150 being multiples of 25 and cases where the equivalence limits to the target parameter θ are chosen in accordance with Table 1.1 (note that in presence of ties, $p_+/(1 - p_0) = p_+/(p_+ + p_-)$ is the analogue to p_+ as to be considered in the continuous case), Table 5.1 shows maximally increased nominal levels α^* for use in the nonrandomized sign test for equivalence at target level $\alpha = .05$.

Table 5.1 *Nominal significance levels and sizes of improved nonrandomized sign tests for equivalence at target level 5% for $\varepsilon_1 = \varepsilon_2 = \varepsilon = log\,(6/4),\ log\,(7/3)$ and $n = 25(25)150$ [Number in ( ): size of the nonrandomized test at nominal level $\alpha = .05$; p_0^* = value of the nuisance parameter maximizing the rejection probability of H]*

ε	n	α^*	p_0^*	Size	
.405465	25	.11714	.0675	.04746	(.00000)
"	50	.08429	.0000	.04046	(.04046)
"	75	.06699	.0113	.04832	(.04014)
"	100	.05802	.0671	.04413	(.03935)
"	125	.05750	.0296	.04743	(.04018)
"	150	.05709	.0408	.04899	(.04366)
.847298	25	.07060	.0000	.03825	(.03825)
"	50	.06580	.2214	.04831	(.04771)
"	75	.06000	.0206	.04928	(.04133)
"	100	.05305	.0494	.04545	(.04101)
"	125	.06000	.3580	.04983	(.04157)
"	150	.05963	.4851	.04888	(.04704)

Example 5.1

In a study based on a sample of size $n = 50$, the number of patients doing better under treatment A as compared to B was observed to be $n_+ = 17$. In $n_0 = 13$ patients, no difference between the responses to A and B could be detected. The equivalence interval for $\theta = \log(p_+/p_-)$ was chosen symmetric about 0 specifying $\varepsilon_1 = \varepsilon_2 = \varepsilon = \log(7/3) = .847298$ which is the same as requiring of the parameter of the conditional binomial distribution of N_+ given $N_0 = n_0$ to fall in the interval $(3/10,\ 7/10)$. With these data and specifications of constants, the sign test for equivalence has to be carried out as a binomial test for equivalence of $p = e^\theta/(1+e^\theta)$ to $1/2$ in a sample of size $n' = n - n_0 = 37$ and equivalence limits $.5 \mp .2$ to p. At the 5% level, the rejection region of this test is computed (by means of the *SAS* program `bilst` introduced in § 4.3) to be the set $\{\, 16 < N_+ < 21 \,\}$. Since the observed value of the test statistic N_+ is an element of this set, we are justified to reject nonequivalence in the sense of $|\log(p_+/p_-)| \geq .847298$.

For assessing the power of the test let us assume that the true proportion p_0 of patients responding equally well to both treatments coincides with the observed relative frequency $13/50 = .26$ of ties and that in the subpopulation of patients providing nonindifferent responses, superiority of A to B is exactly as frequent as inferiority. Running the enclosed *SAS* program `powsign` we find the power against this specific alternative to be 61.53% (UMPU test) and 54.19% (nonrandomized version), respectively. Replacing the target significance level .05 with the raised nominal level α^* = .0658 as displayed in the pertinent line of the above table, the power of the nonrandomized test increases to 60.91%. Thus, under the present circumstances, the loss of efficiency entailed by discarding randomization can be compensated almost completely without changing the basic structure of the test.

5.2 Equivalence tests for the McNemar setting

The test commonly named after McNemar (1947) deals with a setting which is just a special case of that underlying the previous section. Specialization results from the fact that all primary observations X_i and Y_i are now assumed to be binary response-status indicators taking on values 1 ($\leftrightarrow$ success) and 0 ($\leftrightarrow$ failure), respectively. (Of course, any other way of coding the two alternative elementary outcomes leads to the same inferences.) This obviously implies that the set $(X_1, Y_1), \ldots, (X_n, Y_n)$ of bivariate data points make up a sample of size n from a quadrinomial distribution with parameters $p_{00}, \ldots, p_{11}$, say, given by $p_{00} = P[X_i = 0, Y_i = 0]$, $p_{01} = P[X_i = 0, Y_i = 1]$, $p_{10} = P[X_i = 1, Y_i = 0]$, $p_{11} = P[X_i = 1, Y_i = 1]$. In view of the sufficiency of the respective frequencies for the corresponding family of joint distributions of all n random pairs, there is no loss of efficiency in reducing the full data set as directly observed, to the entries in a 2×2 contingency table of the form displayed in Table 5.2.

As is the case in the "classical" McNemar test concerning an ordinary one- or two-sided problem, in constructing a test for equivalence of the two treatments A and B based on a contingency table of that structure, the difference rather than the ratio of the probabilities p_{10}, p_{01} of the two possible kinds of discordant pairs of primary observations will be regarded as the target parameter. Evidently, establishing equivalence with respect

Table 5.2 *Outline of a 2×2 contingency table for use in the analysis of a trial yielding paired binary data*

Treat- ment A	Treatment B		
	0	1	Σ
0	N_{00} (p_{00})	N_{01} (p_{01})	$N_{0 \cdot}$ $(p_{0 \cdot})$
1	N_{10} (p_{10})	N_{11} (p_{11})	$N_{1 \cdot}$ $(p_{1 \cdot})$
Σ	$N_{\cdot 0}$ $(p_{\cdot 0})$	$N_{\cdot 1}$ $(p_{\cdot 1})$	n (1.00)

to p_{10}/p_{01} leads not to a new testing problem but can be done simply by applying the test obtained in § 5.1 with $N_{+} = N_{10}$, $N_{-} = N_{01}$ and the analogous replacements among the p's. Hence, the testing problem to which we want to derive a solution in the present section is given by

$$H : \delta \le -\delta_1 \text{ or } \delta \ge \delta_2 \text{ versus } K : -\delta_1 < \delta < \delta_2 \qquad (5.6)$$

where

$$\delta = p_{10} - p_{01} \; , \qquad \delta_1, \delta_2 \in (0, 1) \, . \qquad (5.7)$$

For notational convenience, let us further agree to denote the probability of observing in a randomly selected experimental unit a constellation belonging to the off-diagonal cells of Table 5.2 by some extra symbol, say η defining

$$\eta = p_{10} + p_{01} \; . \qquad (5.8)$$

5.2.1 Large-sample solution

A large-sample solution to the testing problem (5.6) is obtained by applying the theory outlined in § 3.4. In fact, standard results on the limiting distribution of arbitrary linear functions of the absolute frequencies appearing as entries in a contingency table with random marginal sums (see, e.g., Rao, 1973, p. 383, 6a.1(i)) imply that the statistic $\sqrt{n}(\hat{\delta}_n - \delta)/\sqrt{\eta - \delta^2}$, with $\hat{\delta}_n = (N_{10} - N_{01})/n$, is asymptotically a standard normal variate. Furthermore, $\sqrt{\eta - \delta^2}$ is obviously a continuous function of the basic multinomial parameters $p_{00}, \ldots, p_{11}$ so that plugging in the natural estimators $\hat{\eta}_n = (N_{10} + N_{01})/n$, $\hat{\delta}_n = (N_{10} - N_{01})/n$ yields a consistent estimator of the standard error of the numerator of that statistic (as follows from another well-known result – see Rao, loc. cit., p. 345 – on the asymptotic properties of the multinomial family). Hence, on the understanding that both extreme constellations $\eta = 0$ and $|\delta| = 1$ under which the variance of $\sqrt{n}(\hat{\delta}_n - \delta)$ vanishes can be ruled out, the testing problem (5.6) satisfies all conditions of using the approach of §3.4 with the following specifications: $N = n$, $T_N = \hat{\delta}_n$, $\theta = \delta$, and $\hat{\tau}_N = [(\hat{\eta}_n - \hat{\delta}_n^2)/n]^{1/2}$. In terms of the off-diagonal frequencies N_{10} and N_{01}, the decision rule of the corresponding asymptotically valid test for the problem (5.6) admits the following representation:

$$\text{Reject nonequivalence iff } \frac{n^{1/2}|(N_{10} - N_{01}) - n(\delta_2 - \delta_1)/2|}{[n\,(N_{10} + N_{01}) - (N_{10} - N_{01})^2]^{1/2}} <$$

$$C_\alpha \left(\frac{n^{3/2}(\delta_1 + \delta_2)/2}{[n\,(N_{10} + N_{01}) - (N_{10} - N_{01})^2]^{1/2}} \right). \qquad (5.9)$$

For definiteness, let us recall that the critical upper bound appearing in the above rule has to be determined as the square root of the lower $100\,\alpha$ percentage point of a χ^2-distribution with a single degree of freedom and a (random) noncentrality parameter which equals the square of the expression in the argument to the functional symbol C_α, i.e., $n^3(\delta_1 + \delta_2)^2/4[n\,(N_{10} + N_{01}) - (N_{10} - N_{01})^2]$.

Example 5.2

We illustrate the asymptotic testing procedure given by (5.9), by analyzing a contingency table compiled from data contained in the reference database of the CSE (**C**ommon **S**tandards for Quantitative **E**lectrocardiography) project launched in the early 1980's. One of the major objectives of this project was the establishment of tools for a comparative assessment of the diagnostic accuracy of various computer programs for the automatic classification of electrocardiograms (ECGs). For that purpose, a diagnostic "gold standard" was set up by classifying many hundred subjects with well-documented ECG recordings into clear-cut diagnostic categories by means of carefully validated clinical criteria irrespective of the ECG. In the version underlying the report of Willems et al. (1990), the database contained $n = 72$ ECGs recorded from patients suffering from left ventricular hypertrophy (LVH), a pathological condition of the heart notoriously difficult to recognize by means of noninvasive methods. Table 5.3 summarizes the results of the assessment of these ECGs by a panel of human experts (CR [*"Combined Referee"*]) on the one hand, and one specific computer program denoted by F on the other. In this table, 0 stands for classification into a wrong category (different from LVH) whereas 1 indicates that the LVH was recognized from the patient's ECG. For the general purposes of the CSE project, it was in particular of interest to assess the equivalence of the computer program to the human experts with respect to the capability of diagnosing LVH. Since the difference between the respective probabilities of detecting an existing hypertrophy of the left ventricle equals to δ as defined in (5.7), this amounts to raising a testing problem of the form (5.6). Finally, let us choose the equivalence interval once more in a symmetric manner setting $\delta_1 = \delta_2 = .20$, and use the conventional value $\alpha = .05$ for the nominal significance level.

Table 5.3 *Comparison between the computer program F and the "Combined Referee" (CR) in the diagnostic classification of the ECGs of 72 patients with clinically proven hypertrophy of the left ventricle of the heart [data from Willems et al. (1990, p. 113)]*

		F		
C				
R	0	1	Σ	
0	47	5	52	
	(.6528)	(.0694)	(.7222)	
1	4	16	20	
	(.0556)	(.2222)	(.2778)	
Σ	51	21	72	
	(.7083)	(.2917)	(1.000)	

With $\delta_1 = \delta_2$ and the observed frequencies displayed in the above table, the expression on the left-hand side of the critical inequality (5.9) becomes

$$\frac{n^{1/2}|(N_{10} - N_{01}) - n(\delta_2 - \delta_1)/2|}{[n\,(N_{10} + N_{01}) - (N_{10} - N_{01})^2]^{1/2}}$$

$$= \frac{\sqrt{72}|4 - 5|}{\sqrt{72\,(4 + 5) - (4 - 5)^2}} = \sqrt{\frac{72}{647}} = \sqrt{.111283} = .3336\,.$$

On the other hand, we get for the noncentrality parameter of the χ^2-squared distribution providing an upper critical bound to our test statistic:

$$\hat{\psi}^2 = \left[\frac{n^{3/2}(\delta_1 + \delta_1)/2}{[n\,(N_{10} + N_{01}) - (N_{10} - N_{01})^2]^{1/2}}\right]^2$$

$$= \frac{72^3 \cdot .20^2}{72 \cdot 9 - (-1)^2} = 23.075611\,.$$

But the .05-quantile of a χ^2-distribution with a single degree of freedom and that noncentrality parameter is computed (by means of the *SAS* intrinsic function cinv) to be 9.978361. Consequently, as the critical upper bound we obtain

$$C_\alpha \left(\frac{n^{3/2}(\delta_1 + \delta_2)/2}{[n\,(N_{10} + N_{01}) - (N_{10} - N_{01})^2]^{1/2}} \right) = \sqrt{9.978361} = 3.1589\,.$$

Since the latter is much larger than the observed value of the test statistic $n^{1/2}|(N_{10} - N_{01}) - n(\delta_2 - \delta_1)/2|/[n\,(N_{10} + N_{01}) - (N_{10} - N_{01})^2]^{1/2}$, it follows that at the 5% level, the data of Table 5.3 allow a decision in favour of equivalence of F and CR in the sense of $-.20 < \delta < .20$.

5.2.2 Corrected finite-sample version of the large-sample test

In view of the purely asymptotic nature of the approach leading to (5.9), the validity of the procedure in finite samples can obviously not be taken for granted without further study. The clearest and most reliable answer to the question of possible discrepancies between actual and nominal level of an asymptotic testing procedure is obtained by determining the rejection probability under arbitrary null parameter constellations by means of exact computational methods. For that purpose, it is convenient to introduce the following transformation of variables and parameters, respectively:

$$U = N_{10}\,, \quad V = N_{10} + N_{01}\,; \quad \pi = p_{10}/\eta\,, \tag{5.10}$$

with η defined as in (5.8). In terms of (U, V), the critical region of the test (5.9) can be rewritten

$$\left\{ (u, v) \in \mathbb{N}_0^2 \,\middle|\, 0 \le u \le v \le n,\ T_n^{\delta_1, \delta_2}(u, v) < c_{\alpha;\,n}^{\delta_1, \delta_2}(u, v) \right\} \tag{5.11}$$

where

$$T_n^{\delta_1, \delta_2}(u, v) = \frac{\sqrt{n}\,|(2u - v) - n(\delta_2 - \delta_1)/2|}{[nv - (2u - v)^2]^{1/2}}\,,$$

$$c_{\alpha;\,n}^{\delta_1, \delta_2}(u, v) = C_\alpha \left(\frac{n^{3/2}(\delta_1 + \delta_2)/2}{[nv - (2u - v)^2]^{1/2}} \right).$$

The advantage of representing the critical region in this form stems from the fact that the conditional distribution of U given $\{V = v\}$ is binomial with parameters (v, π) for any $v = 0, 1, \ldots n$, and the marginal distribution of V is likewise binomial, with parameters (n, η). Hence, the rejection probability of the test (5.9) under any (π, η) admits the representation

$$Q_{\alpha, n}^{\delta_1, \delta_2}(\pi, \eta) = \sum_{v=0}^{n} \left\{ \sum_{u \in \mathcal{U}_{\alpha, n}^{\delta_1, \delta_2}(v)} b(u;\, v, \pi) \right\} b(v;\, n, \eta)\,, \tag{5.12}$$

where $\mathcal{U}_{\alpha, n}^{\delta_1, \delta_2}(v)$ denotes the v-section of the set (5.11) given by

$$\mathcal{U}_{\alpha, n}^{\delta_1, \delta_2}(v) = \left\{ u \in \mathbb{N}_0 \,\middle|\, u \le v,\ T_n^{\delta_1, \delta_2}(u, v) < c_{\alpha;\,n}^{\delta_1, \delta_2}(u, v) \right\}, \tag{5.13}$$

which is typically an (maybe empty) interval of nonnegative integer numbers $\leq v$.* Furthermore, in (5.12), both symbols of the type $b(k\,;m,p)$ stand for the respective binomial point masses.

Now, in order to determine the actual size of the asymptotic McNemar test for equivalence, we have to maximize $Q_{\alpha,n}^{\delta_1,\delta_2}(\pi,\eta)$ over the set of all $(\pi,\eta)\in(0,1)^2$ satisfying the above $[\to(5.6)]$ null hypothesis H of nonequivalence. As an immediate consequence of the definition of the parametric functions π, δ and η, one has $\pi=(\delta+\eta)/2\eta$ so that for any fixed $\eta>0$ the η-section of H equals the complement of the interval $(1/2-\delta_1/2\eta,\,1/2+\delta_2/2\eta)$. Hence, for the size of the test we obtain the formula

$$SIZE_\alpha(\delta_1,\delta_2;\,n)=\sup\left\{Q_{\alpha,n}^{\delta_1,\delta_2}(\pi,\eta)\,\Big|\,0<\eta<1,\right.$$

$$\left.0<\pi\leq 1/2-\delta_1/2\eta \text{ or } 1/2+\delta_2/2\eta\leq\pi<1\right\}. \qquad (5.14)$$

Qualitatively speaking, the results to be obtained by evaluating the right-hand side of (5.14) numerically admit the conclusion that the finite-sample behaviour of the asymptotic test given by (5.9) is surprisingly poor (in the subsequent sections and chapters, the reader will find numerous applications of the theory of §3.4 to much more complex models yielding very satisfactory solutions to the respective equivalence testing problem). In fact, the convergence of the exact size of the test to its limiting value, i.e., the target significance level α, turns out to be extremely slow, with a general tendency towards anticonservatism. For instance, in the specific case of Example 5.2, the exact size of the critical region is seen to be as large as .0721 although the size of the sample distinctly exceeds that available for many equivalence studies conducted in practice. Even if the number of observations in the sample is raised to 150 and thus more than doubled, the smallest significance level maintained by the asymptotic test is still .0638 rather than .05.

Clearly, these results together with many other examples pointing in the same direction, strongly suggest replacing the asymptotic solution to the problem of testing for equivalence in McNemar's setting by a finite-sample version corrected with respect to the significance level. Provided repeated evaluation of (5.14) with sufficiently high numerical precision causes no serious problem with respect to computing time, such a correction is easily carried out: All that remains is to determine by means

---

* By "typically", we mean in the present context that in constructing the respective sets explicitly by direct computation, we never found an exception but no mathematical proof of the corresponding general assertion is available. In view of this, both computer programs implementing evaluations of (5.12) (mcnemasc, mcnempow), although working on the understanding that it is a generally valid fact, check upon it during each individual run. In case of finding an exception, either program would stop and produce an error message.

of an iteration process the largest nominal significance level α^* such that $SIZE_{\alpha^*}(\delta_1, \delta_2; n) \leq \alpha$. Of course, it is tempting to speed up this procedure by restricting at each step the search for the maximum probability of an incorrect decision in favour of equivalence to the boundary of the null hypothesis H of (5.6). Since, in terms of (π, η), the latter is given as the set $\{(1/2 - \delta_1/2\eta, \eta) \,|\, \delta_1 < \eta < 1\} \cup \{(1/2 + \delta_2/2\eta, \eta) \,|\, \delta_2 < \eta < 1\}$, this leads to determining for varied values of α

$$SIZE_\alpha^B(\delta_1, \delta_2; n) = \max\Big\{ \sup_{\eta > \delta_1} Q_{\alpha,n}^{\delta_1,\delta_2}(1/2 - \delta_1/2\eta, \eta),$$

$$\sup_{\eta > \delta_2} Q_{\alpha,n}^{\delta_1,\delta_2}(1/2 + \delta_2/2\eta, \eta) \Big\} \qquad (5.15)$$

instead of $SIZE_\alpha(\delta_1, \delta_2; n)$ as obtained by searching through the whole set of parameter values compatible with H. Although, in general we can only state that there holds the inequality $SIZE_\alpha^B(\delta_1, \delta_2; n) \leq SIZE_\alpha(\delta_1, \delta_2; n)$, taking for granted that the sets $\mathcal{U}_{\alpha,n}^{\delta_1,\delta_2}(v)$ [$\to$ (5.13)] are intervals allows to restrict the search for the maximum probability of a type-I error to the common boundary of the hypotheses (5.6) whenever the equivalence range for δ is chosen as a symmetric interval. In fact, $\delta_1 = \delta_2$ clearly implies that each such interval in the sample space of $U|\{V = v\}$ must be symmetric about $v/2$ from which it can be concluded by means of elementary arguments (starting from the well-known relationship between the binomial cdf and the incomplete beta integral – see, e.g., Feller, 1968, p. 173) that, as a function of π, the vth inner sum of (5.12) is nondecreasing on $(0, 1/2]$ and nonincreasing on $[1/2, 1)$. The SAS macro mcnemasc which for cases with $\delta_1 = \delta_2 = \delta_\circ$ serves the purpose of determining a nominal significance level α^* such that the exact size of the respective test for (5.6) approaches the target level from below as closely as possible, exploits this possibility of simplifying the search for the maximum of the rejection probability (5.12) over the null hypothesis.

For two symmetric choices of the equivalence range $(-\delta_1, \delta_2)$ for $\delta = p_{10} - p_{01}$ and selected sample sizes ranging from 50 to 200, corrected nominal levels computed in this way are shown in Table 5.4, together with the exact size of the corrected test and that of the original large-sample procedure. All results presented in this table have been obtained by means of mcnemasc setting the fineness of the grid of η-values searched through for the maximum rejection probability under nonequivalence [recall (5.14)] equal to .0005 throughout. Strikingly, neither the difference between the target significance level α and the nominal level to be used in the corrected test, nor between α and the size attainable under the correction decreases monotonically with n, and even with samples comprising several hundred observations it happens that the nominal level has to be halved.

Table 5.4 *Nominal significance level and exact size for the corrected McNemar test for equivalence maintaining the 5% level in finite samples of size $n = 50(25)200$, for $\delta_1 = \delta_2 = \delta_o = .2, .4$ [Number in ( ): size of the noncorrected test at nominal level $\alpha = .05$]*

δ_o	n	α^*	$SIZE_{\alpha^*}(\delta_o, \delta_o; n)$	
.20	50	.024902	.0480	(.1034)
"	75	.016406	.0267	(.0928)
"	100	.036718	.0488	(.0844)
"	125	.037207	.0477	(.0747)
"	150	.032324	.0414	(.0638)
"	175	.027832	.0358	(.0750)
"	200	.025000	.0430	(.0640)
.40	50	.029296	.0353	(.0565)
"	75	.039746	.0420	(.0626)
"	100	.043164	.0474	(.0615)
"	125	.043164	.0460	(.0598)
"	150	.041601	.0436	(.0561)
"	175	.039257	.0408	(.0536)
"	200	.037500	.0475	(.0533)

Table 5.5 *Exact power of the corrected version of (5.9) against the alternative $\delta = 0$ [$\Leftrightarrow \pi = 1/2$] for $n = 50$, $\delta_1 = \delta_2 = .20$, $\alpha^* = .024902$ and various values of the nuisance parameter η*

η	.0002	.002	.005	.01	..02
$Q^{.20,.20}_{\alpha^*,50}(1/2, \eta)$	.00995	.09525	.22169	.39499	.63581
	.20	.40	.60	.80	1.00
	.73720	.29702	.11515	.06281	.11228

Once the corrected nominal level has been determined, computing the exact power of the corresponding finite-sample test for the equivalence problem (5.6) against arbitrary specific alternatives $\delta \in (-\delta_1, \delta_2)$ is comparatively easy since it requires only a single evaluation of the double sum on the right-hand side of (5.12). However, given the alternative of interest in terms of δ, the power depends in a rather complicated way on the nuisance parameter η. As becomes obvious from the numerical example shown in Table 5.5, the power is in particular neither monotonic nor concave in η. Generally, the *SAS* macro mcnempow allows the computation of the exact rejection probability of the test (5.9) at any nominal significance level $\tilde{\alpha}$ under arbitrary parameter constellations (p_{10}, p_{01}).

Example 5.2 (continued)

For $n = 72$ and $\delta_1 = \delta_2 = .20$, the smallest nominal level α^* to be used in (5.9) in order to maintain the target significance level $\alpha = .05$, is obtained (by running the program mcnemasc) to be $\alpha^* = .027148$. Since the noncentrality parameter of the χ^2-distribution through which the critical upper bound to the test statistic $n^{1/2}|(N_{10} - N_{01})|/[n(N_{10} + N_{01}) - (N_{10} - N_{01})^2]^{1/2}$ has to be determined, has been estimated by means of the data of the present example to be $\hat{\psi}^2 = 23.075611$, recomputing the critical bound with α^* instead of α gives: $C_{\alpha^*}(\hat{\psi}) = \sqrt{\texttt{cinv}(.027148, 1, 23.075611)}$ $= \sqrt{8.290026} = 2.8792$, after another application of the *SAS* intrinsic function cinv. This bound is still much larger than the value which has been observed for the test statistic so that the decision keeps the same as if the nominal level was set equal to the target significance level. Finally, let us assume that the true rates of discordant pairs of both kinds in the underlying population coincide with the corresponding relative frequencies of the observed 2×2 table so that we have $p_{10} = 4/9$, $p_{01} = 5/9$. Running program mcnempow, the power of the corrected test against this "observed alternative" is found to be only slightly larger than the target significance level, namely .0599, as compared to .1794 which turns out to be the power of the noncorrected asymptotic test (5.9) against the same alternative.

5.3 Paired t-test for equivalence

In this section, we assume throughout that the setting described in §5.1 has to be considered in the special version that the distribution of the intraindividual differences D_i between the measurements taken under both treatments is Gaussian with (unknown) parameters $\delta = E(D_i)$ and $\sigma_D^2 = \text{Var}(D_i)$. In the special case

$$D_i \sim \mathcal{N}(\delta, \sigma_D^2) \quad \forall i = 1, \ldots, n, \qquad (5.16)$$

the hypothesis of equivalence with respect to the probability of a positive sign [cf. (5.1), (5.4)] reduces to a statement about the *standardized* expected value δ/σ_D. In fact, under the parametric model (5.16), we have $p_0 = 0$ and hence $p_- = 1 - p_+$. Consequently, we may write: $-\varepsilon_1 < \log(p_+/p_-) < \varepsilon_2$ $\Leftrightarrow -\varepsilon_1 < \log(p_+/(1 - p_+)) < \varepsilon_2 \Leftrightarrow e^{-\varepsilon_1} < p_+/(1 - p_+) < e^{\varepsilon_2} \Leftrightarrow e^{-\varepsilon_1}/(1 + e^{-\varepsilon_1}) < p_+ < e^{\varepsilon_2}/(1 + e^{\varepsilon_2})$. On the other hand, under (5.16), p_+ admits the representation $p_+ = P[D_i > 0] = 1 - P[(D_i - \delta)/\sigma_D < -\delta/\sigma_D] = 1 - \Phi(-\delta/\sigma_D) = \Phi(\delta/\sigma_D)$. Since the standard normal distribution function Φ is strictly increasing and continuous, we eventually see that under (5.16), the hypothesis $-\varepsilon_1 < \log(p_+/p_-) < \varepsilon_2$ to be established by means of the sign test for equivalence is logically equivalent to $\Phi^{-1}(e^{-\varepsilon_1}/(1+e^{-\varepsilon_1})) < \delta/\sigma_D < \Phi^{-1}(e^{\varepsilon_2}/(1 + e^{\varepsilon_2}))$. Hence, setting for brevity $\Phi^{-1}(e^{-\varepsilon_1}/(1 + e^{-\varepsilon_1})) = \theta_1$, $\Phi^{-1}(e^{\varepsilon_2}/(1 + e^{\varepsilon_2})) = \theta_2$, the testing problem which in its nonparametric form was dealt with in § 5.1, can now be written

$$H : \delta/\sigma_D \le \theta_1 \vee \delta/\sigma_D \ge \theta_2 \quad \text{vs.} \quad K : \theta_1 < \delta/\sigma_D < \theta_2 \ . \tag{5.17}$$

Evidently, this problem does not change if the observations D_i are re-scaled by multiplying each of them by the same positive constant c. Put in more technical terms, this means that the parametric equivalence testing problem (5.17) remains invariant under all transformations of the sample space $\mathbb{R}^n$ of $(D_1, \ldots, D_n)$ taking the form of $(d_1, \ldots, d_n) \mapsto (cd_1, \ldots, cd_n)$, with arbitrary $c > 0$. As is shown in Lehmann (1986, § 6.4), the construction of a test of the ordinary one-sided null hypothesis about δ/σ_D which is uniformly most powerful among all tests being invariant against all transformations of that type, conveniently starts from reducing the data $(D_1, \ldots, D_n)$ to the sufficient statistics $(\bar{D}, S_D)$ before applying the principle of invariance. The same two-step reduction can be carried out in the present context which implies that a uniformly most powerful invariant (UMPI) level α test for (5.17) is obtained in the following way: After reducing the primary data set $(D_1, \ldots, D_n)$ to the usual one-sample t-statistic

$$T = \sqrt{n}\bar{D}/S_D , \tag{5.18}$$

a UMP level-α test based on T is carried out for

$$\tilde{H} : \tilde{\theta} \le \sqrt{n}\theta_1 \vee \tilde{\theta} \ge \sqrt{n}\theta_2 \quad \text{vs.} \quad \tilde{K} : \sqrt{n}\theta_1 < \tilde{\theta} < \sqrt{n}\theta_2 , \tag{$\widetilde{5.17}$}$$

where $\tilde{\theta}$ denotes the parameter of a noncentral t-distribution with $n - 1$ degrees of freedom.

Denoting the density function of that distribution by $g_{\tilde{\theta}}(\cdot)$, we know from a result derived in Karlin (1968, §4(iii)) [cf. also Lemma A.1.3 of Appendix A to this book] that the family $(g_{\tilde{\theta}})_{\tilde{\theta} \in \mathbb{R}}$ is strictly positive of any order and hence a fortiori STP_3. Furthermore, for arbitrary $(\tilde{\theta}, t)$, $g_{\tilde{\theta}}(t)$ admits the representation

$$g_{\tilde{\theta}}(t) = e^{-\tilde{\theta}^2/2}(n - 1 + t^2)^{-n/2} \sum_{j=0}^{\infty} c_j [h(t, \tilde{\theta})]^j , \tag{5.19}$$

where

$$h(t, \tilde{\theta}) = t\tilde{\theta}\sqrt{2}/\sqrt{n - 1 + t^2} \tag{5.20}$$

and the power series $\sum_{j=0}^{\infty} c_j x^j$ converges for any $x \in \mathbb{R}$ (see Johnson, Kotz and Balakrishnan, 1995, p. 516). This ensures continuity of $g_{\tilde{\theta}}(t)$ in both of its arguments so that the family $(g_{\tilde\theta})_{\tilde\theta\in\mathbb{R}}$ of noncentral t-densities with an arbitrary number $(n-1)$ of degrees of freedom satisfies all the conditions of Theorem A.1.5 [$\rightarrow$ Appendix, p. 251]. Hence, we may conclude that an UMP level-α test for $\widetilde{(5.17)}$ exists and is given by the critical region

$$\left\{ \tilde{C}^1_{\alpha;\,n-1}(\theta_1,\theta_2) < T < \tilde{C}^2_{\alpha;\,n-1}(\theta_1,\theta_2) \right\} , \qquad (5.21)$$

where the bounds $\tilde{C}^\nu_{\alpha;\,n-1}(\theta_1,\theta_2)$ are uniquely determined by the equations

$$G_{\tilde\theta_1}(C_2) - G_{\tilde\theta_1}(C_1) = \alpha = G_{\tilde\theta_2}(C_2) - G_{\tilde\theta_2}(C_1),$$
$$-\infty < C_1 < C_2 < \infty. \qquad (5.22)$$

In (5.22), $G_{\tilde\theta}(\cdot)$ denotes for any $\tilde\theta\in\mathbb{R}$ the cumulative distribution function associated to $g_{\tilde\theta}(\cdot)$, and $\tilde\theta_\nu$ has to be set equal to $\sqrt{n}\theta_\nu$ both for $\nu = 1$ and $\nu = 2$. Both in view of the form of the statistic T and the distribution which the computation of the critical constants has to be based upon, the term paired t-test seems fully appropriate for the testing procedure given by (5.21).

A glance at (5.19) and (5.20) shows that we have $g_{-\tilde\theta}(-t) = g_{\tilde\theta}(t) \; \forall(\tilde\theta, t) \in \mathbb{R}^2$. Hence, for any $\tilde\theta > 0$, the distribution of $-T$ under $-\tilde\theta$ coincides with that of T under $\tilde\theta$ so that for a *symmetric choice of the equivalence interval*, i.e., for $\theta_1 = -\varepsilon, \theta_2 = \varepsilon$ and correspondingly for $\tilde\theta_1 = -\tilde\varepsilon, \tilde\theta_2 = \tilde\varepsilon$ with $\varepsilon > 0$, $\tilde\varepsilon = \sqrt{n}\varepsilon$, the conditions of Lemma A.1.6 are satisfied as well. Applying this result we see that in the symmetric case, (5.21) and (5.22) can be simplified to

$$\left\{ |T| < \tilde{C}_{\alpha;\,n-1}(\varepsilon) \right\} \qquad (5.23)$$

and

$$G_{\tilde\varepsilon}(C) - G_{\tilde\varepsilon}(-C) = \alpha, \;\; 0 < C < \infty, \qquad (5.24)$$

respectively, where $\tilde{C}_{\alpha;\,n-1}(\varepsilon)$ stands for the solution of the latter equation. Furthermore, it is seen at once that the expression on the left-hand side of (5.24) is equal to the probability of the event $\{|T| < C\} = \{T^2 < C^2\}$ under $\tilde\theta = \tilde\varepsilon$. Since it is a well known fact (cf. Johnson, Kotz and Balakrishnan, loc. cit.) that squaring a random variable following a t-distribution with $n-1$ degrees of freedom and noncentrality parameter $\tilde\varepsilon$ yields a variable which is noncentral F with $1, n-1$ degrees of freedom and $\tilde\varepsilon^2$ as the noncentrality parameter, it follows that the solution to (5.24) admits the explicit representation

$$\tilde{C}_{\alpha;\,n-1}(\varepsilon) = \left[F_{1,n-1;\,\alpha}(\tilde\varepsilon^2) \right]^{1/2} , \qquad (5.24')$$

where $F_{1,n-1;\,.}(\tilde\varepsilon^2)$ denotes the quantile function of that F-distribution.

Due to the relationship (5.24′), when the equivalence hypothesis is formulated symmetrically setting $-\theta_1 = \theta_2 = \varepsilon > 0$, the practical implementation of the paired t-test for equivalence providing an UMPI solution to

(5.17), involves only slightly more effort than that of the ordinary one- or two-sided t-test for paired observations. In fact, from the viewpoint of any user having access to up-to-date statistical software, the noncentral versions of the basic sampling distribution functions as well as their inverses,

Table 5.6 *Critical constant $\tilde{C}_{.05;\,n-1}(\varepsilon)$ of the one-sample t-test for equivalence at level $\alpha = 5\%$ in the symmetric case $(\theta_1, \theta_2) = (-\varepsilon, \varepsilon)$, for $\varepsilon = .25(.25)1.00$ and $n = 10(10)100$*

| | | $\varepsilon\,=$ | | |
n	.25	.50	.75	1.00
10	0.08811	0.22188	0.73424	1.46265
20	0.11855	0.61357	1.67161	2.70944
30	0.16079	1.08722	2.40334	3.68005
40	0.21752	1.50339	3.02359	4.50470
50	0.29164	1.87104	3.57213	5.23475
60	0.38432	2.20387	4.06944	5.89697
70	0.49319	2.51030	4.52773	6.50742
80	0.61250	2.79581	4.95499	7.07666
90	0.73573	3.06421	5.35682	7.61210
100	0.85817	3.31826	5.73729	8.11913

Table 5.7 *Power attained at $\theta = \delta/\sigma_D = 0$ when using the critical constants shown in Table 5.6 for the one-sample t-statistic*

| | | $\varepsilon\,=$ | | |
n	.25	.50	.75	1.00
10	.06828	.17064	.51851	.82241
20	.09313	.45323	.88901	.98610
30	.12662	.71411	.97713	.99905
40	.17106	.85921	.99560	.99994
50	.22821	.93268	.99919	1.0000
60	.29787	.96855	.99986	1.0000
70	.37656	.98559	.99998	1.0000
80	.45803	.99350	1.0000	1.0000
90	.53617	.99711	1.0000	1.0000
100	.60713	.99873	1.0000	1.0000

can be considered as explicitly given. In particular, the *SAS* system provides an intrinsic function named finv returning specific quantiles of F-distributions with arbitrary numbers of degrees of freedom and values of the noncentrality parameter with very high numerical accuracy (for details about the syntax to be used in calling this routine and the underlying algorithm see *SAS*, 1999, pp. 278, 362-4). The above Table 5.6 enables the reader to perform the test in the symmetric case without any computational tools at the 5% level, for sample sizes up to 100 being multiples of 10 and right-hand equivalence limit $\varepsilon = .25(.25)1.00$. The corresponding maximum rejection probabilities $\tilde{\beta}_{\alpha;\,n-1}(\varepsilon)$ attained at $\delta = 0$ ($\Leftrightarrow P[D_i > 0] = 1/2$) are shown in Table 5.7. The latter are readily computed by means of the central t-distribution function $G_0(\cdot)$, say, using the formula

$$\tilde{\beta}_{\alpha;\,n-1}(\varepsilon) = 2\,G_0(\tilde{C}_{\alpha;\,n-1}(\varepsilon)) - 1\,. \tag{5.25}$$

Example 5.3

In an experimental study of the effects of increased intracranial pressure on the cortical microflow of rabbits, a preliminary test had to be done to ensure that the measurements exhibit sufficient stability during a pre-treatment period of 15 minutes' duration. In a sample of $n = 23$ animals, at the beginning and the end of that period the mean flow [ml/min/100g body mass] was observed to be $\bar{X} = 52.65$ and $\bar{Y} = 52.49$, respectively, corresponding to a mean change of $\bar{D} = 0.16$; the standard deviation of the intraindividual changes was computed to be $S_D = 3.99$ (data from Ungersböck and Kempski, 1992). The equivalence limits for the standardized expected change of the microflow were chosen to be $\mp\varepsilon$ with $\varepsilon = .50$.

For the values of n and ε applying to the present example, the noncentrality parameter of the F-distribution to be referred to for computing the critical upper bound to the absolute value of the t-statistic, is $\psi^2 = 23\cdot 0.50^2 = 5.75$. In order to compute the critical bound using *SAS*, one has to write in a data step just the single statement csquare=finv(.05,1,22,5.75) which yields the output: csquare=.576779. From this, the critical constant itself is $\tilde{C}_{.05;22}(.50) = \sqrt{.576779} = .7595$.

On the other hand, for a sample of size $n = 23$, the t-value corresponding to the observed point $(0.16, 3.99)$ in the space of the sufficient statistic $(\bar{D}, S_D)$, is .1923. Thus, we have $|T| < \tilde{C}_{.05;22}(.50)$ indeed which implies that the observed value of $(\bar{D}, S_D)$ belongs to the rejection region of our test. Accordingly, we can conclude that at the 5% level, the experimental data of the present example contain sufficient evidence in support of the hypothesis that the cortical microflow of rabbits does not change to a relevant extent over a time interval of 15 minutes during which no active treatment is administered. The power of the UMPI test at level $\alpha = .05$

for (5.17) with $\theta_1 = -.50$, $\theta_2 = .50$ and sample size $n = 23$ is computed by means of formula (5.25) at 54.44%.

If the equivalence hypothesis K of (5.17) is formulated in a nonsymmetric way, computation of the critical constants $\tilde{C}^\nu_{\alpha;\,n-1}(\theta_1, \theta_2)$, $\nu = 1, 2$ of the one-sample t-test for equivalence becomes considerably more complicated. It requires an iterative algorithm, then, for solving the system (5.22) of equations numerically. An iteration procedure for accomplishing this task can be obtained by suitable modifications to the algorithm described in §4.2 for the one-sample equivalence testing problem with exponentially distributed data. It suffices to replace the gamma distribution function $F^T_{\sigma_\nu}(\cdot)$ being the basic building block there, by the noncentral t-distribution function $G_{\tilde{\theta}_\nu}(\cdot)$ (for $\nu = 1, 2$) and redefine the initial value C°_1 of C_1. Extensive experience has shown that $C^\circ_1 = (\tilde{\theta}_1 + \tilde{\theta}_2)/2 = \sqrt{n}(\theta_1 + \theta_2)/2$ is a sensible choice. The SAS macro `tt1st` to be found at http://www.zi-mannheim.de/wktsheq implements this computational procedure for determining the critical constants of the one-sample t-test for equivalence in cases of an arbitrary choice of the equivalence range for δ/σ_D.

In concluding this section, a remark on the possible role of the test discussed on the preceding pages in bioequivalence assessment seems in place: Under a set of conditions satisfied by the majority of comparative bioavailability trials conducted in practice (lognormality of the intraindividual bioavailability ratios; negligibility of period effects), the procedure has much to recommend it as an alternative to the conventional interval inclusion approach to so-called average bioequivalence [a more elaborate argument for this view will be given in Ch. 9].

5.4 Signed rank test for equivalence

The testing procedure to be derived in the present section is a natural nonparametric competitor to the paired t-test for equivalence as discussed in §5.3. It will be obtained by modifying the most frequently applied nonparametric test for paired data in such a way that the resulting test for equivalence is both interpretable in terms of a sensible measure of distance between distribution functions on $\mathbb{R}$ and fairly easy to implement in practice. The assumptions which the construction to be described on the pages to follow starts from, are as weak as those underlying the sign test for equivalence with continuously distributed intraindividual differences D_i. This means that, in contrast to the "classical" signed rank test of the hypothesis of symmetry of the distribution of the D_i, the distribution function F of the D_i is not assumed symmetric, neither under the null nor the alternative hypothesis. Basically, this possibility of enlarging the class of admissible distributions is a consequence of the fact that the procedure we propose to term signed rank for equivalence, is asymptotic in nature.

However, we will be able to show by means of the results of suitable simulation experiments that under surprisingly mild restrictions on the order of magnitude of the sample size n, the discrepancies between the nominal level of significance and the actual size of the test are practically negligible even if the distribution of the D_i exhibits gross asymmetry.

As is well known from textbooks on nonparametric statistics (see, e.g., Lehmann, 1975, p. 129, (3.16)), for continuously distributed D_i, the test statistic V, say, of the ordinary signed rank test admits the representation

$$V = \sum_{i=1}^{n} I_{(0,\infty)}(D_i) + \sum_{i=1}^{n-1} \sum_{j=i+1}^{n} I_{(0,\infty)}(D_i + D_j) \; , \qquad (5.26)$$

with $I_{(0,\infty)}(\cdot)$ as the indicator of a positive sign of any real number defined formally by

$$I_{(0,\infty)}(x) = \begin{cases} 1 & \text{for } x > 0 \\ 0 & \text{for } x \le 0 \end{cases} \; . \qquad (5.27)$$

From (5.26) it is obvious that the finite-sample expectation of the signed rank statistic is a weighted sum of the two parameters (functionals) $p_+ = P[D_i > 0]$ and

$$q_+ = P[D_i + D_j > 0] \; . \qquad (5.28)$$

On the other hand, it seems reasonable to formulate the equivalence hypothesis to be established by means of the test to be constructed in the present section, in terms of the mean of the asymptotic distribution of the customary signed rank statistic. In view of this, it is preferable to drop the first term on the right-hand side of (5.26) and base the construction on the statistic

$$U_+ = \binom{n}{2}^{-1} \sum_{i=1}^{n-1} \sum_{j=i+1}^{n} I_{(0,\infty)}(D_i + D_j) \qquad (5.29)$$

instead of V. In fact, U_+ is an unbiased estimator of the probability q_+ of getting a positive sign of the so-called Walsh-average within any pair of D's and is asymptotically equivalent to V, in the sense that the difference between the standardized versions of both statistics vanishes in probability for $n \to \infty$ under any specification of the true distribution of D_i (cf. Randles and Wolfe, 1979, pp. 84-5).

Therefore, as an asymptotic procedure, the conventional signed rank test is a test of a hypothesis on q_+ and accordingly, we refer throughout this section to the following equivalence testing problem:

$$H : 0 < q_+ \le q'_+ \vee q''_+ \le q_+ < 1 \text{ versus } K : q'_+ < q_+ < q''_+ \; , \qquad (5.30)$$

where the limits q'_+, q''_+ of the equivalence range can be chosen as arbitrary fixed numbers satisfying $0 < q'_+ < q''_+ < 1$. The exact finite-sample variance of U_+ admits the representation

$$\text{Var}[U_+] = \binom{n}{2}^{-1} \{ 2(n-2)[q^+_{1(2,3)} - q_+^2] + q_+(1 - q_+) \} \; , \qquad (5.31)$$

with

$$q_{1(2,3)}^{+} = P[D_i + D_j > 0, D_i + D_k > 0] \qquad (5.32)$$

(cf. Randles and Wolfe, 1979, (3.1.21)). For $q_{1(2,3)}^{+}$, there exists a natural estimator as well which exhibits the form of a U-statistic and is given by

$$\hat{q}_{1(2,3)}^{+} = \binom{n}{3}^{-1} \sum_{i=1}^{n-2} \sum_{j=i+1}^{n-1} \sum_{k=j+1}^{n} (1/3) \Big[I_{(0,\infty)}(D_i + D_j) \cdot$$
$$I_{(0,\infty)}(D_i + D_k) + I_{(0,\infty)}(D_i + D_j)I_{(0,\infty)}(D_j + D_k) +$$
$$I_{(0,\infty)}(D_i + D_k)I_{(0,\infty)}(D_j + D_k) \Big]. \qquad (5.33)$$

From the general theory of U-statistic estimators, it is in particular known that $\hat{q}_{1(2,3)}^{+}$ as defined by (5.33) is consistent for $q_{1(2,3)}^{+}$ (see once more Randles and Wolfe, loc. cit., Corollary 3.2.5), which implies that the variance of U_{+} can in turn be estimated consistently by

$$\hat{\sigma}^2[U_+] = \binom{n}{2}^{-1}\{2(n-2)[\hat{q}_{1(2,3)}^{+} - U_+^2] + U_+(1 - U_+)\} . \qquad (5.34)$$

Since $(U_+ - q_+)/\sqrt{\text{Var}[U_+]}$ is asymptotically standard normal for any distribution of the D_i under which $\text{Var}[U_+]$ does not vanish, we may apply the result presented in §3.4 yielding the decision rule

Reject nonequivalence $\Leftrightarrow$

$$\Big|U_+ - (1/2)(q_+' + q_+'')\Big|/\hat{\sigma}[U_+] < C_{\pm R}(\alpha; q_+', q_+''), \qquad (5.35)$$

with

$$C_{\pm R}(\alpha; q_+', q_+'') = \Big\{ 100\alpha-\text{percentage point of the } \chi^2 - \text{distri-}$$
$$\text{bution with } df = 1 \text{ and } \lambda_{nc}^2 = (q_+'' - q_+')^2/4\hat{\sigma}^2[U_+]\Big\}^{1/2}. \qquad (5.36)$$

Although the quantile function of any noncentral χ^2-distribution is predefined in well-known software packages for use in statistics, the practical implementation of the signed rank test for equivalence based on (5.35) entails considerably more effort as that of the conventional one- and two-sided Wilcoxon test for paired observations. The reason is that in addition to U_+ or V, the quantity $\hat{q}_{1(2,3)}^{+}$ not appearing in the "ordinary" signed rank test, is needed. Hence, at the URL associated with this book, the reader may find another *SAS* macro [program name: **sgnrk**] designed for carrying out all computational steps to be taken in an application of (5.36). As input data, it requires in addition to the size n of the sample, the nominal level α of significance and the limits q_+', q_+'' of the equivalence range for the target parameter q_+, only the name of a raw-data file containing just the observed values of the D_i.

Example 5.4

In a pilot study preceding a large-scale multicenter trial of the antihypertensive efficacy of various drugs, the aim was to establish comparability of the measurements of blood pressure (BP) taken with two different automatic devices (denoted by A and B in the sequel). In each of a total of 20 volunteers participating in the pilot study, 12 repeated BP measurements were taken during the same session, 6 using each of the two devices. The temporal spacing of all individual measurements was strictly uniform, with an interval of 2 minutes between consecutive readings and altering between A and B. The 6 values produced by each device within one such series were collapsed to a single one by simple averaging.

For the analysis of the data of this pilot study, the comparison of both measurement devices with respect to the diastolic BP (DBP) was of primary interest. Correspondingly, Table 5.8 shows for each subject the averages of 6 DBP values obtained by the first device (A) as compared to B. The limits of the equivalence range for q_+ were set equal to $q'_+ = .2398$,

Table 5.8 *Results of a pilot study on the comparability of two different devices A ($\leftrightarrow X_i$) and B ($\leftrightarrow Y_i$) for measuring diastolic blood pressure*

i	X_i	Y_i	D_i	i	X_i	Y_i	D_i
1	62.167	62.667	-0.500	11	74.500	76.667	-2.167
2	85.667	85.333	0.333	12	91.667	93.500	-1.833
3	80.667	80.000	0.667	13	73.667	69.167	4.500
4	55.167	53.833	1.333	14	63.833	71.333	-7.500
5	92.000	93.500	1.500	15	80.333	77.667	2.667
6	91.000	93.000	-2.000	16	61.167	57.833	3.333
7	107.833	108.833	-1.000	17	63.167	67.333	-4.167
8	93.667	93.833	-0.167	18	73.167	67.500	5.667
9	101.167	100.000	1.667	19	103.333	101.000	2.333
10	80.500	79.667	0.833	20	87.333	89.833	-2.500

$q''_+ = .7602$, which can be motivated as follows: In the specific case that the D_i are normal with expectation δ and variance σ_D^2, it is easily verified that there holds the relationship $q_+ = \Phi(\sqrt{2}\,\delta/\sigma_D)$, and this suggests to transform the interval $(-.5, .5)$ making up a reasonable equivalence range in terms of δ/σ_D [recall Tab. 1.1 (iv)], to the set $\{q_+ \mid \Phi(-\sqrt{2}\,\delta/\sigma_D) < q_+ < \Phi(\sqrt{2}\,\delta/\sigma_D)\} = (.2398, .7602)$.

Now, in order to test for equivalence of the measuring devices A and B, we apply the above decision rule (5.35) with these value of q'_+ and q''_+, $\alpha = .05$, and the $n = 20$ intra-subject differences shown in the above table as the observations eventually to be analyzed. Running the program `sgnrk` we find $U_+ = .55263$, $\hat{\sigma}[U_+] = .12071$, $C_{\pm R}(.05; .2398, .7602) = 0.54351$, and it follows that $|U_+ - (1/2)(q'_+ + q''_+)|/\hat{\sigma}[U_+] = |.55263 - .50000|/.12071 = .43600 < C_{\pm R}(.05; .2398, .7602)$. Hence, we can reject the null hypothesis of nonequivalence of the two measuring devices under comparison.

For the remaining part of this section, we restrict consideration to the well-known semiparametric shift model assuming that the density and cumulative distribution function of the intraindividual differences D_i is given by $z \mapsto f_o(z - \vartheta)$ and $z \mapsto F_o(z - \vartheta)$ with fixed (though unspecified) baseline $f_o : \mathbb{R} \to [0, \infty)$ and $F_o : \mathbb{R} \to [0, 1]$, respectively. Even under this comparatively simple submodel, exact computation of rejection probabilities of the test (5.35) is unfeasible so that for purposes of investigating the finite-sample power function of the signed rank test for equivalence we have recourse to simulation methods. A question of particular interest to be answered by this way concerns the possible dependence of the power against some specific alternative in terms of the target functional q_+, on the form of the baseline distribution function F_o.

Let us denote by $\beta(F_o; q_+)$ the probability that the test rejects its null hypothesis if it is performed with data $D_1, \ldots, D_n$ from a distribution which belongs to the location parameter family generated by baseline cdf F_o such that the true value of $P[D_i + D_j > 0]$ is q_+. Clearly, in a simulation experiment carried out in order to determine $\beta(F_o; q_+)$, we have to generate sets of values of random variables of the form $D_i = D_i^\circ + \vartheta(q_+)$ where D_i° has distribution function F_o for all $i = 1, \ldots, n$, and $\vartheta(q_+)$ is the unique solution of the equation

$$\int_{-\infty}^{\infty} [1 - F_o(-2\vartheta - z)]dF_o(z) = q_+ , \quad \vartheta \in \mathbb{R} . \qquad (5.37)$$

Given some specific baseline cdf F_o, the expression on the left-hand side of (5.37) is a function, say $w_+(\vartheta)$, of the location parameter which admits an explicit representation only for some of the most common location families. Table 5.9 gives a summary of the pertinent formulae. Making use of these relationships, for the models covered by the table, the solution $\vartheta(q_+)$ to (5.37) can either be written down explicitly (Gaussian, Cauchy, uniform, exponential distribution) or computed numerically by means of a simple interval halving algorithm (Laplace, logistic distribution). Furthermore, it follows immediately from a general result of advanced mathematical analysis (see Pratt, 1960, Corollary 3) that $w_+(\vartheta)$ is a continuous function of ϑ in each location parameter family generated by a continuously differentiable baseline cdf $F_o(\cdot)$. Hence, to each specification of the equivalence range

Table 5.9 *Explicit representation of* $w_+(\vartheta) = P[\,(D_i^\circ + \vartheta) + (D_j^\circ + \vartheta) > 0\,]$
for independent random variables D_i°, D_j° *with common density* $f_\circ(\cdot)$

Location Family	$f_\circ(z)$	$w_+(\vartheta) = \int_{-\infty}^{\infty}[1 - F_\circ(-2\vartheta - z)]\,dF_\circ(z)$
Gaussian	$(2\pi)^{-1/2}e^{-z^2/2}$	$\Phi(\sqrt{2}\vartheta)$
Cauchy	$\pi^{-1}(1 + z^2)^{-1}$	$1/2 + \pi^{-1}\arctan(\vartheta)$
Uniform*	$I_{(-1/2,\,1/2)}(z)$	$1/2 + 2\vartheta(1 - \vartheta)$ for $0 \le \vartheta < 1/2$; 1 for $\vartheta \ge 1/2$
Exponential†	$e^{-z}I_{(0,\infty)}(z)$	$1 - G_{4;\,0}((-4\vartheta) \vee 0)$
Laplace*	$e^{-|z-\vartheta|}$	$1 - (1/2)e^{-2\vartheta}(1 + \vartheta)$ for $\vartheta \ge 0$
Logistic	$e^{-z}(1 + e^{-z})^{-2}$	$e^{2\vartheta}(e^{2\vartheta} - 1 - 2\vartheta)(e^{2\vartheta} - 1)^{-2}$

* For $\vartheta < 0$, the relationship $w_+(-\vartheta) = 1 - w_+(\vartheta)$ can be made use of being valid for arbitrary location families with symmetric baseline density $f_\circ(\cdot)$.

† In the formula given for $w_+(\vartheta)$, $G_{4;\,0}(\cdot)$ is to denote the cdf of a central χ^2-distribution with $df = 4$. Furthermore, $(-4\vartheta) \vee 0$ stands for $\max\{-4\vartheta, 0\}$.

Table 5.10 *Equivalence range for* ϑ *corresponding to* $(q_+', q_+'') = (.3618,.6382)$ *and* $(q_+', q_+'') = (.2398,.7602)$, *respectively, in the location parameter families covered by Table 5.9*

Family of distribution	Equivalence Range $(\vartheta_1, \vartheta_2)$ corresponding to $(q_+', q_+'') =$	
	$(0.3618,\ 0.6382)$	$(0.2398,\ 0.7602)$
Gaussian	$(-0.2500,\ 0.2500)$	$(-0.5000,\ 0.5000)$
Cauchy	$(-0.4637,\ 0.4637)$	$(-1.0662,\ 1.0662)$
Uniform	$(-0.0747,\ 0.0747)$	$(-0.1537,\ 0.1537)$
Exponential	$(-1.0853,-0.6340)$	$(-1.3748,-0.4668)$
Laplace	$(-0.2885,\ 0.2885)$	$(-0.6035,\ 0.6035)$
Logistic	$(-0.4245,\ 0.4245)$	$(-0.8563,\ 0.8563)$

(q'_+, q''_+) for the target functional q_+, there corresponds a unique interval $(\vartheta_1, \vartheta_2)$, say, of values of the parameter indexing the specific location model in mind. In Table 5.10, one finds the thus associated equivalence interval for ϑ for both specifications of (q'_+, q''_+) used in the simulation study and all location families appearing in Table 5.9.

The simulation study whose results are presented below in Table 5.11, was performed to provide sufficiently complete data both on the level properties and the maximum power of the signed rank test for equivalence. Therefore, for each specification of $F_\circ$ and $(\vartheta_1, \vartheta_2)$ appearing in Table 5.10, 100,000 samples of the respective size $n \in \{20, 30, 50\}$ were drawn from the distributions given by $F_\circ(\cdot - \vartheta_1)$, $F_\circ(\cdot - \vartheta_2)$ and $F_\circ(\cdot - \vartheta_\circ)$ where $\vartheta_\circ$ denotes that point in the parameter space which satisfies $w_+(\vartheta_\circ) = 1/2$. The case that ϑ coincides with $\vartheta_\circ$ or, equivalently, q_+ with $1/2$, occurs in particular if for each $i = 1, \ldots, n$, the random pair (X_i, Y_i) giving rise to the intraindividual difference D_i is continuous and exchangeable in the sense of having the same distribution as (Y_i, X_i). Of course, exchangeability is a natural assumption whenever both treatments under comparison are actually identical and assessed by means of an endpoint criterion admitting numerically precise measurement. To be sure, exchangeability of an continuously distributed random pair (X_i, Y_i) implies still more than the validity of $P[D_i + D_j > 0] = 1/2$, namely symmetry about zero of the distribution of the associated intrapair difference $D_i = X_i - Y_i$.

Going through the rejection probabilities shown in Table 5.11, one notices in particular (see the entries in line 4) that in the setting of the above Example 5.4 with normally distributed intra-subject differences, the nominal level of significance is strictly maintained. Furthermore, it can be seen that the power attained against the alternative of no difference between both measuring devices comes out as low as 37.5%. On the one hand, this value is exceeded by that of the optimal parametric test for the same setting by about 8%. On the other, the power of the sign test for equivalence with limits $\Phi(\mp.5) = .5 \mp .1915$ to p_+, against $p_+ = 1/2$ falls short of that of the signed rank test by almost 15% even if the former is performed in its randomized version.

From a more general perspective, the simulation results shown in Table 5.11 admit the following conclusions:

Table 5.11 *Simulated rejection probability of the signed rank test for equivalence at level $\alpha = .05$ at both boundaries of the null hypothesis (columns 4 and 5) and at $q_+ = 1/2$ (rightmost column) for the distributional shapes and equivalence ranges covered by Table 5.10 [Italicized values: power of the paired t-test for equivalence against the alternative $q_+ = 1/2$]*

Location Family	$\left(q'_+, q''_+\right)$	n	$\beta(F_\circ; q'_+)$	$\beta(F_\circ; q''_+)$	$\beta(F_\circ; 1/2)$	
Gaussian	(.3618, .6382)	20	.04398	.04299	.07982	*.09313*
"		30	.04869	.04912	.11893	*.12662*
"		50	.04982	.04895	.20635	*.22821*
	(.2398, .7602)	20	.04287	.04145	.37516	*.45323*
"		30	.04133	.03977	.63069	*.71411*
"		50	.03785	.03858	.89987	*.93268*
Cauchy	(.3618, .6382)	20	.04441	.04460	.07785	
"		30	.05150	.05041	.11613	
"		50	.04952	.04970	.20805	
	(.2398, .7602)	20	.04578	.04647	.37366	
"		30	.04215	.04195	.63091	
"		50	.04126	.03885	.89866	
Uniform	(.3618, .6382)	20	.04058	.04293	.07828	
"		30	.04713	.04750	.11698	
"		50	.04761	.04822	.21146	
	(.2398, .7602)	20	.03996	.03980	.37255	
"		30	.03822	.03901	.63042	
"		50	.03871	.03804	.89656	
Exponential	(.3618, .6382)	20	.04587	.04048	.07311	
"		30	.05315	.04661	.11383	
"		50	.05135	.04580	.19046	
	(.2398, .7602)	20	.04589	.03932	.34001	
"		30	.04129	.03656	.59280	
"		50	.03919	.03602	.87640	
Laplace	(.3618, .6382)	20	.04543	.04338	.07807	
"		30	.05004	.04990	.12144	
"		50	.04990	.04850	.20773	
	(.2398, .7602)	20	.04302	.04435	.37238	
"		30	.04070	.04035	.63089	
"		50	.03959	.03941	.89908	
Logistic	(.3618, .6382)	20	.04497	.04314	.07831	
"		30	.05021	.05028	.11682	
"		50	.05037	.04954	.20822	
	(.2398, .7602)	20	.04322	.04284	.37418	
"		30	.04010	.03995	.63520	
"		50	.03900	.03829	.89718	

(i) Even for sample sizes as small as 20 and highly skewed distributions ($\to$ exponential location parameter family), there is no reason to suspect that the nominal significance level could be exceeded to a practically relevant extent.

(ii) Both the effective size and the power of the signed rank test for equivalence seems rather robust even against gross changes in the form of the underlying distribution.

(iii) If the distribution of the intra-subject differences D_i is Gaussian, the loss in efficiency of the signed rank as compared to the t-statistic seems to be considerably more marked in the equivalence case than in testing problems with conventional form of the hypotheses (cf. Randles and Wolfe, 1979, Tab. 4.1.7).

Remark. Except for the case that the underlying distribution is exponential, the corresponding entries in column 4 and 5 of the above Table 5.11 are strikingly similar suggesting that each such pair actually gives two repeated estimates of the same quantity. This impression is far from misleading since it is not hard to derive analytically the following general result: Whenever the equivalence limits q'_+, q''_+ are chosen symmetricly about $1/2$ and the location family under consideration is generated by a baseline distribution function symmetric about 0, the power function $q_+ \mapsto \beta(F_\circ; q_+)$ of the signed rank test for equivalence is symmetric for its own part.

5.5 A generalization of the signed rank test for equivalence for noncontinuous data

In the previous section, the construction of an equivalence version of the signed rank test was carried out under the basic assumption that the distribution of the intraindividual differences $D_1, \ldots, D_n$ is of the continuous type. For a considerable proportion of possible applications of the procedure to concrete data sets, this restriction is prohibitive since in practice the occurrence of ties between the D_i is quite common. Lack of continuity of the distribution of the D_i implies in particular that the probability

$$q_0 = P[D_i + D_j = 0] \tag{5.38}$$

of observing a pair of intra-subject differences of equal absolute value but opposite sign, does not necessarily vanish but might take on any value in the unit interval. Obviously, for $q_0 > 0$, it no longer makes sense to compare the true value of the functional q_+ to $1/2$ and consider $|q_+ - 1/2|$ as a reasonable measure of distance between the actual distribution of the D_i and a distribution exhibiting the same form but being centred about 0. Hence, what we primarily need for purposes of adapting the signed rank test for equivalence to settings with noncontinuous data, is a meaningful generalization of the basic distance measure $|q_+ - 1/2|$.

In the continuous case, we obviously have $q_+ = 1 - q_-$ with

$$q_- = P[D_i + D_j < 0] \tag{5.39}$$

so that $|q_+ - 1/2| = 0$ is satisfied if and only if there holds $q_+ = q_-$. Irrespective of the type of the distributions involved, marked discrepancies between q_+ and q_- are always at variance with equivalence of the treatments behind the primary observations X_i and Y_i from which the ith intra-subject difference is computed. In fact, even if the joint distribution of (X_i, Y_i) is discrete, it must be exchangeable whenever there exists no treatment difference at all, and exchangeability of (X_i, Y_i) clearly implies $D_i = X_i - Y_i \overset{d}{=} Y_i - X_i = -D_i$ and hence $q_+ = P[(-D_i) + (-D_j) > 0] = q_-$. Now, in view of the basic restriction $q_+ + q_0 + q_- = 1$, q_+ and q_- coincide if and only if there holds the equation $2q_+ + q_0 = 1$, or equivalently, $q_+/(1 - q_0) = 1/2$. The latter fact suggests to replace q_+ by its conditional counterpart $q_+/(1 - q_0)$ throughout, where conditioning is on absence of any pair (i, j) of sampling units such that the Walsh average $(D_i + D_j)/2$ of the associated intra-subject differences vanishes. This leads to use $|q_+/(1 - q_0) - 1/2|$ as a basic measure of distance suitable for any type of distribution of the D_i. Defining, as usual, equivalence by the requirement that the value taken on by the selected measure of distance between the distributions under comparison be sufficiently small, the nonparametric testing problem to be dealt with in this section reads

$$H : \frac{q_+}{1 - q_0} \leq 1/2 - \varepsilon_1 \text{ or } \frac{q_+}{1 - q_0} \geq 1/2 + \varepsilon_2$$

$$\text{versus} \quad K : 1/2 - \varepsilon_1 < \frac{q_+}{1 - q_0} < 1/2 + \varepsilon_2 . \tag{5.40}$$

As before, the construction of an asymptotically valid testing procedure will be based on a natural estimator of the target functional in terms of which the hypotheses have been formulated. This estimator is given by

$$U_+^* = U_+/(1 - U_0) \tag{5.41}$$

where U_+ is as in (5.29) and U_0 denotes the U-statistic estimator of q_0 to be computed analogously, namely as

$$U_0 = \binom{n}{2}^{-1} \sum_{i=1}^{n-1} \sum_{j=i+1}^{n} I_{\{0\}}(D_i + D_j) \tag{5.42}$$

with

$$I_{\{0\}}(z) = \begin{cases} 1 & \text{for } z = 0 \\ 0 & \text{for } z \in \mathbb{R} \setminus \{0\} \end{cases} . \tag{5.43}$$

In order to determine the large-sample distribution of U_+^* and in particular its asymptotic variance, we first consider the joint large-sample distribution of (U_+, U_0). From the general asymptotic distribution theory for U-statistics (see ,e.g., RANDLES and WOLFE, 1979, Sec. 3.6), it follows that $\sqrt{n}(U_+ - q_+, U_0 - q_0)$ is asymptotically bivariate normal with expectation $\mathbf{0}$. The covariance matrix $\mathbf{\Sigma}_n = \begin{pmatrix} \sigma_{+n}^2 & \sigma_{0+;n} \\ \sigma_{+0;n} & \sigma_{0n}^2 \end{pmatrix}$, say, of this distribution can be computed exactly, and with a view to using the testing procedure under derivation in finite samples, we prefer to keep the terms of order $O(1/n)$ in the following formulae:

$$\sigma_{+n}^2 = \frac{4(n-2)}{n-1}\left(q_{1(2,3)}^+ - q_+^2\right) + \frac{2}{n-1}q_+(1-q_+), \tag{5.44a}$$

$$\sigma_{0n}^2 = \frac{4(n-2)}{n-1}\left(q_{1(2,3)}^0 - q_0^2\right) + \frac{2}{n-1}q_0(1-q_0), \tag{5.44b}$$

$$\sigma_{+0;n} = \frac{4(n-2)}{n-1}\left(q_{1(2,3)}^{+0} - q_+q_0\right) + \frac{2}{n-1}q_+q_0. \tag{5.44c}$$

In these expressions, the symbol $q_{1(2,3)}^+$ has the same meaning as before [recall (5.32)] whereas $q_{1(2,3)}^0$ and $q_{1(2,3)}^{+0}$ have to be defined by

$$q_{1(2,3)}^0 = P[D_i + D_j = 0, D_i + D_k = 0] \tag{5.45}$$

and

$$q_{1(2,3)}^{+0} = P[D_i + D_j > 0, D_i + D_k = 0], \tag{5.46}$$

respectively. Now, we can proceed by applying the so-called δ-method (cf. Bishop, Fienberg and Holland, 1975, §14.6) which allows us to infer that $\sqrt{n}(U_+^* - q_+/(1-q_0))$ is asymptotically univariate normal with mean 0 and variance $\sigma_{*n}^2 = \nabla g(q_+, q_0)\, \mathbf{\Sigma}_n\, (\nabla g(q_+, q_0))'$ where $\nabla g(q_+, q_0)$ stands for the gradient (row) vector of the transformation $(q_+, q_0) \mapsto q_+/(1-q_0)$. Writing down $\nabla g(q_+, q_0)$ explicitly and expanding the quadratic form yields after some straightforward algebraic simplifications the expression:

$$\sigma_{*n}^2 = \frac{\sigma_{+n}^2}{(1-q_0)^2} + \frac{q_+^2\sigma_{0n}^2}{(1-q_0)^4} + \frac{2q_+\sigma_{+0;n}}{(1-q_0)^3}. \tag{5.47}$$

The natural way of estimating the asymptotic variance σ_{*n}^2 of $\sqrt{n}U_+^*$ consists in plugging in U-statistic estimators of all functionals of the distribution of the D_i appearing on the right-hand side of equations (5.44a) – (5.44c). Since the U-statistics for q_+, $q_{1(2,3)}^+$ and q_0 have already been defined [recall (5.29), (5.33) and (5.42), respectively], all what remains to be done is to provide explicit formulae for the analogous estimators of $q_{1(2,3)}^0$ and $q_{1(2,3)}^{+0}$:

$$\hat{q}^0_{1(2,3)} = \binom{n}{3}^{-1} \sum_{i=1}^{n-2} \sum_{j=i+1}^{n-1} \sum_{k=j+1}^{n} (1/3) \Big[I_{\{0\}}(D_i + D_j) \cdot$$

$$I_{\{0\}}(D_i + D_k) + I_{\{0\}}(D_i + D_j) I_{\{0\}}(D_j + D_k)$$

$$+ I_{\{0\}}(D_i + D_k) I_{\{0\}}(D_j + D_k) \Big], \quad (5.48)$$

$$\hat{q}^{+0}_{1(2,3)} = \binom{n}{3}^{-1} \sum_{i=1}^{n-2} \sum_{j=i+1}^{n-1} \sum_{k=j+1}^{n} (1/6) \Big[I_{(0,\infty)}(D_i + D_j) \cdot$$

$$I_{\{0\}}(D_i + D_k) + I_{(0,\infty)}(D_i + D_j) I_{\{0\}}(D_j + D_k)$$

$$+ I_{(0,\infty)}(D_i + D_k) I_{\{0\}}(D_j + D_k) + I_{(0,\infty)}(D_i + D_k) \cdot$$

$$I_{\{0\}}(D_i + D_j) + I_{(0,\infty)}(D_j + D_k) I_{\{0\}}(D_i + D_j)$$

$$+ I_{(0,\infty)}(D_j + D_k) I_{\{0\}}(D_i + D_k) \Big]. \quad (5.49)$$

Additional results from the asymptotic theory of U-statistics (see, e.g., Lee, 1990, §3.4.2) ensure the (strong) consistency of all these estimators for their expectations. This implies that the plug-in estimator $\hat{\sigma}^2_{+n}$ obtained from (5.44a) by replacing q_+ and $q^+_{1(2,3)}$ with U_+ and $\hat{q}^+_{1(2,3)}$, respectively, is consistent for σ^2_{+n}, and so on for $\hat{\sigma}^2_{0n}$ and $\hat{\sigma}_{+0;n}$. Finally, consistency of U_+, U_0, $\hat{\sigma}^2_{+n}$, $\hat{\sigma}^2_{0n}$ and $\hat{\sigma}_{+0;n}$ ensures that the asymptotic variance σ^2_{*n} of $\sqrt{n} U^*_+ = \sqrt{n} U_+/(1 - U_0)$ can be consistently estimated by

$$\hat{\sigma}^2_{*n} = \frac{\hat{\sigma}^2_{+n}}{(1 - U_0)^2} + \frac{U^2_+ \hat{\sigma}^2_{0n}}{(1 - U_0)^4} + \frac{2U_+ \hat{\sigma}_{+0;n}}{(1 - U_0)^3}. \quad (5.50)$$

Now, in order to complete the derivation of a signed rank test for equivalence being asymptotically valid for arbitrary noncontinuous distributions of the D_i, it suffices to invoke for another time the general result stated in §3.4, with the following specifications: $N = n$, $T_N = U_+/(1 - U_0)$, $\theta = q_+/(1 - q_0)$, $\sigma = \lim_{n \to \infty} \sigma_{*n}$, $k = 1$, and $\tau_N = \sigma_{*n}/\sqrt{n}$. This verifies that the decision rule

Reject $H : \dfrac{q_+}{1 - q_0} \leq 1/2 - \varepsilon_1$ or $\dfrac{q_+}{1 - q_0} \geq 1/2 + \varepsilon_2$ iff

$$\sqrt{n} \Big| U_+/(1 - U_0) - (1 - \varepsilon_1 + \varepsilon_2)/2) \Big| / \hat{\sigma}_{*n} < C^*_{\pm R}(\alpha; \varepsilon_1, \varepsilon_2), \quad (5.51)$$

with

$$C^*_{\pm R}(\alpha; \varepsilon_1, \varepsilon_2) = \Big\{ 100\alpha - \text{percentage point of the } \chi^2 - \text{distri-}$$

$$\text{bution with } df = 1 \text{ and } \lambda^2_{nc} = n(\varepsilon_1 + \varepsilon_2)^2/4\hat{\sigma}^2_{*n} \Big\}^{1/2} \quad (5.52)$$

defines an asymptotically valid test for the nonparametric equivalence problem (5.40), provided the limit σ_*^2, say, of (5.47) is a positive number.

An *SAS* macro which allows to carry out the generalized signed rank test for equivalence with arbitrary sets $\{D_1, \ldots, D_n\}$ of observed intra-subject differences, is provided at http://www.zi-mannheim.de/wktsheq under the program name `srktie_d`.

5.5.1 Simplifying computations by reducing raw data to counts

Often computation of the U-statistics required for carrying out the generalized signed rank test for equivalence can largely be simplified by determining in a preliminary step the configuration of ties which occurred in the observed vector $(D_1, \ldots, D_n)$ of intra-subject differences. This is the case whenever the D_i take on their values in a finite lattice of known span $w > 0$, say. Without loss of generality, this lattice can be assumed symmetric about 0, i.e., as a set of the form $\{ -rw, -(r-1)w, \ldots, -w, 0, w, \ldots, (r-1)w, rw \}$ where $r \in \mathbb{N}$ denotes the number of points lying on both sides of the origin. Of course, a particularly frequent specific case of that kind occurs when the D_i are integer-valued random variables with finite support. Given a lattice containing the set of possible values of each D_i in the sample of intra-subject differences, let us define

$$M_k = \# \{ i \mid D_i = kw \}, \quad k = -r, \ldots r \qquad (5.53)$$

so that for any $k \in \{-r, \ldots, r\}$, M_k counts the number of sample points tied at the respective point of the lattice. (Note that some of the frequencies M_k may and typically will be equal to zero.)

In terms of the frequencies M_k, the formulae for the U-statistic estimators to be considered in connection with the generalized signed rank test for equivalence can be rewritten as follows:

$$U_+ = \frac{1}{n(n-1)} \left[2 \sum_{k=1}^{r} \sum_{l=-k+1}^{k-1} M_k M_l + \sum_{k=1}^{r} M_k^2 - \sum_{k=1}^{r} M_k \right], \qquad (5.29^*)$$

$$\hat{q}_{1(2,3)}^{+} = \frac{1}{n(n-1)(n-2)} \left[\sum_{k=-r+1}^{r} M_k \left(\sum_{l=-k+1}^{r} M_l \right)^2 - \sum_{k=1}^{r} M_k^2 \right.$$
$$\left. - 2 \sum_{k=1}^{r} \sum_{l=-k+1}^{k-1} M_k M_l + 2 \sum_{k=1}^{r} M_k - 2 \sum_{k=1}^{r} \sum_{l=-k+1}^{r} M_k M_l \right], \qquad (5.33^*)$$

$$U_0 = \frac{1}{n(n-1)} \left[2 \sum_{k=1}^{r} M_k M_{-k} + M_0(M_0 - 1) \right], \qquad (5.42^*)$$

$$\hat{q}^0_{1(2,3)} = \frac{1}{n(n-1)(n-2)} \left[\sum_{k=-r}^{r} M_k M_{-k}^2 - 2 \sum_{k=1}^{r} M_k M_{-k} \right.$$

$$\left. -3M_0^2 + 2M_0 \right], \qquad (5.48^*)$$

$$\hat{q}^{+0}_{1(2,3)} = \frac{1}{n(n-1)(n-2)} \left[\sum_{k=-r+1}^{r} \left(M_k M_{-k} \sum_{l=-k+1}^{r} M_l \right) \right.$$

$$\left. - \sum_{k=1}^{r} M_k (M_{-k} + M_0) \right]. \qquad (5.49^*)$$

These identities (formally proved in Firle, 1998, pp. 86-88) underlie the *SAS* macro named `srktie_m` which allows its user to compute both the test statistic and its critical upper bound at any desired significance level α. Of course, in every setting such that the D_i are lattice variables, the macro `srktie_d` can be used instead, and the results will necessarily coincide with those obtained by means of `srktie_m`. The only difference is that the algorithm underlying the M-version of the program enables to dispense with triple loops and typically needs much shorter execution time.

Example 5.5

In a comparative trial of the efficacy of two mydriatic agents [compounds administered for the purpose of dilating the eye pupils] A and B, each of $n = 24$ patients got dropped substance A to the one eye and B to the other. The outcome was measured as the increase of the pupil diameter [mm] attained after 30 minutes since administration of the tinctures. The individual results obtained in this way are shown in Table 5.12. Due to limited accuracy of measurements, all X_i and Y_i observed in this trial are multiples of $w = 0.1$, and so are the associated intra-subject differences $D_i = X_i - Y_i$. In order to test for equivalence in efficacy of both mydriatic drugs, decision rule (5.52) is clearly appropriate. Using the same equivalence limits as have been proposed in Example 5.4 for q_+, i.e., setting $\varepsilon_1 = \varepsilon_2 = .2602$ and $\alpha = .05$, the macro `srktie_m` yields with the entries in column 4 of the table as raw data the following results: $U_+^* = .57769$, $\hat{\sigma}_{*n} = .59819$, $C^*_{\pm R}(\alpha; \varepsilon_1, \varepsilon_2) = .52345$. But with $n = 24$ and $\varepsilon_1 = \varepsilon_2 = .2602$, these values do not lead to a rejection of the null hypothesis $H : q_+/(1 - q_0) \le 1/2 - \varepsilon_1$ or $q_+/(1 - q_0) \ge 1/2 + \varepsilon_2$ since we have $\sqrt{24} |.57769 - 1/2|/.59819 = .63626 > C^*_{\pm R}(\alpha; \varepsilon_1, \varepsilon_2)$.

Table 5.12 *Results of a comparative trial of two mydriatic agents, with*
X_i *and* Y_i *as the increase of the pupil diameter [mm] attained in the ith*
patient 30 minutes after administration of drug A and B, respectively

i	X_i	Y_i	D_i	i	X_i	Y_i	D_i
1	2.4	1.6	0.8	13	3.8	4.1	-0.3
2	2.6	2.4	0.2	14	4.2	4.2	0.0
3	3.3	3.3	0.0	15	3.5	3.4	0.1
4	3.9	4.0	0.1	16	3.6	3.3	0.3
5	3.6	3.9	-0.3	17	4.0	4.3	-0.3
6	2.7	2.4	0.3	18	3.6	3.5	0.1
7	4.4	4.5	-0.1	19	3.8	4.0	-0.2
8	3.7	3.3	0.4	20	3.3	3.8	-0.5
9	3.6	3.0	0.6	21	2.7	2.5	0.2
10	3.4	3.2	0.2	22	4.0	4.1	-0.1
11	2.6	2.6	0.0	23	3.7	3.5	0.2
12	3.9	4.1	-0.2	24	3.3	3.4	-0.1

Table 5.13 is to give an impression of the multiformity of discrete distributions concentrated on the specific lattice $\{-2, -1, 0, 1, 2\}$ leading to the
same selected value of the target functional $q_+/(1-q_0)$. From the entries in

Table 5.13 *Examples of distributions on a five-point lattice belonging to*
the left [(a),(d)], the right [(c),(g)] boundary and the centre [(b), (e), (f)]
of the equivalence hypothesis K of (5.41) with $\varepsilon_1 = \varepsilon_2 = .2602$

	$P[D_i = -2]$	$P[D_i = -1]$	$P[D_i = 0]$	$P[D_i = 1]$	$P[D_i = 2]$
(a)	.313300	.249480	.229700	.086820	.120700
(b)	.091300	.346251	.229700	.116049	.216700
(c)	.120700	.086820	.229700	.249480	.313300
(d)	.300000	.366789	.000000	.233211	.100000
(e)	.200000	.400000	.000000	.100000	.300000
(f)	.369855	.130145	.000000	.130145	.369855
(g)	.299300	.052384	.000000	.048016	.600300

Table 5.14 *Simulated rejection probabilities[†] of the tie-corrected version of the signed rank test for equivalence under the distributions shown in Table 5.13, for sample sizes varying over $\{20, 30, 50, 100\}$ [The values obtained under (a), (d) and (c), (g) allow to estimate the actual type-I error risk in finite samples; the entries into lines (b), (e) and (f) are values of the power against $q_+/(1-q_0) = 1/2$]*

	$n = 20$	$n = 30$	$n = 50$	$n = 100$
(a)	.03910	.03657	.03606	.03619
(d)	.03695	.03738	.03422	.03622
(c)	.03834	.03485	.03263	.03537
(g)	.03348	.03790	.03445	.03564
(b)	.19518	.36714	.70671	.97368
(e)	.17185	.33191	.67104	.96635
(f)	.12228	.24260	.53774	.92583

[†] 100,000 replications of each Monte Carlo experiment

lines (b), (e) and (f), it becomes in particular obvious that symmetry of the distribution of the D_i is sufficient but by no means necessary for minimizing the distance measure $|q_+/(1 - q_0) - 1/2|$ underlying hypotheses formulation (5.40). The rejection probabilities of the generalized signed rank test for equivalence under all specific distributions covered by Table 5.13 have been determined by means of Monte Carlo simulation. The results of this simulation study which are shown in Table 5.14 allow the conclusion that correcting the equivalence version of the signed rank test for ties in the way established in this section, is another instance of an asymptotic construction along the lines of § 3.4 yielding an equivalence testing procedure which tends to mild conservatism in finite samples. Furthermore, by comparison with Table 5.11, it can be seen that the maximum power attainable with a given sample size n, is markedly lower in the discrete than in the continuous case, as to be expected according to intuition.

Discussion

In order to gain better insight into the meaning of the distance measure $|q_+/(1-q_0)-1/2|$ we chose as a basis for formulating a nonparametric equivalence hypothesis for settings with noncontinuous paired observations, it is helpful to analyze the extreme case that the D_i can take on only three different values, namely -1, 0 and $+1$. Denoting the probabilities of these values by p_-, p_0 and p_+, respectively, it is easily verified that we can write

$q_+ = 2p_0 p_+ + p_+^2$, $q_0 = 2(1 - p_0 - p_+)p_+ + p_0^2$. Hence, in the trinomial case, the alternative hypothesis to be established by means of the tie-corrected signed rank test for equivalence corresponds to the following subset of the parameter space:

$$
\widetilde{K}^{\pm R}_{\varepsilon_1, \varepsilon_2} = \left\{ (p_0, p_+) \in (0,1)^2 \,\middle|\, p_0 + p_+ \leq 1, 1/2 - \varepsilon_1 < \right.
$$
$$
\left. \frac{2p_0 p_+ + p_+^2}{1 - 2(1 - p_0 - p_+)p_+ - p_0^2} < 1/2 + \varepsilon_2 \right\}. \quad (5.54)
$$

In contrast, in the sign test for equivalence which, after the appropriate sufficiency reduction, refers to exactly the same family of distributions, the alternative hypothesis [cf. p. 66, (5.4)] is easily seen to admit the representation

$$
\widetilde{K}^{S}_{\varepsilon_1', \varepsilon_2'} = \left\{ (p_0, p_+) \in (0,1)^2 \,\middle|\, p_0 + p_+ \leq 1, \ 1/2 - \varepsilon_1' < \right.
$$
$$
\left. \frac{p_+}{1 - p_0} < 1/2 + \varepsilon_2' \right\} \quad (5.55)
$$

where the ε_ν', like the ε_ν ($\nu = 1,2$) of (5.54) can be arbitrarily chosen in the interval $(0, 1/2)$.

The graphs presented in Figure 5.1 and 5.2 visualize the differences in geometrical shape of the subspaces $\widetilde{K}^{\pm R}_{\varepsilon_1, \varepsilon_2}$ and $\widetilde{K}^{S}_{\varepsilon_1', \varepsilon_2'}$: Whereas the boundaries of the latter are simply straight lines, those of $\widetilde{K}^{\pm R}_{\varepsilon_1, \varepsilon_2}$ are slightly curved. If, as done in the first couple of graphs, the tolerances ε_ν and ε_ν' are set equal to each other (both for $\nu = 1$ and $\nu = 2$), the alternative hypothesis of the sign test for equivalence is much larger than that of the generalized signed rank test. On the other hand, if the ε_ν and ε_ν' are chosen in a way ensuring that the vertical section at $p_0 = 0$ of both parameter subspaces coincide, then $\widetilde{K}^{\pm R}_{\varepsilon_1, \varepsilon_2}$ covers $\widetilde{K}^{S}_{\varepsilon_1', \varepsilon_2'}$, as illustrated by Figure 5.2. All in all it is clear that we have no possibility to make the two versions of an alternative hypothesis about (p_0, p_+) perfectly coincident by a suitable adjustment of the respective tolerances ε_ν and ε_ν'. Admittedly, it would be desirable to base a nonparametric equivalence test for paired noncontinuous observations on a functional which reduces in the case of trinomially distributed D_i to the parametric function underlying the sign test for equivalence. However, there seems to exist no possibility to implement this idea without discarding all other information provided by the observations except that contained in the counting statistic (N_0, N_+) to which the data are reduced in the sign test.

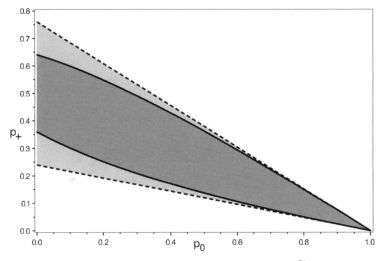

Figure 5.1 *Boundaries of the equivalence hypotheses* $\widetilde{K}^{\pm R}_{\varepsilon_1,\varepsilon_2}$ *(——) and* $\widetilde{K}^{S}_{\varepsilon'_1,\varepsilon'_2}$ *(- - - -) for* $\varepsilon_1 = \varepsilon'_1 = \varepsilon'_2 = \varepsilon_2 = .2602$

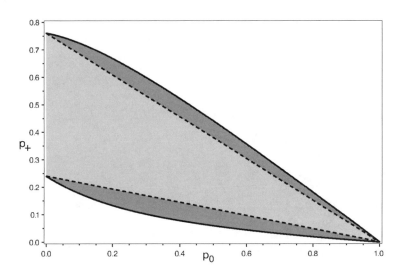

Figure 5.2 *Boundaries of the equivalence hypotheses* $\widetilde{K}^{\pm R}_{\varepsilon_1,\varepsilon_2}$ *(——) and* $\widetilde{K}^{S}_{\varepsilon'_1,\varepsilon'_2}$ *(- - - -) for* $\varepsilon_1 = \varepsilon_2 = .2602$, $\varepsilon'_1 = \varepsilon'_2 = .4095$

CHAPTER 6

Equivalence tests for two unrelated samples

6.1 Two-sample t-test for equivalence

If the trial run in order to compare the two treatments A and B follows an ordinary two-arm design, the data set to be analyzed consists of $m + n$ mutually independent observations $X_1, \ldots, X_m, Y_1, \ldots, Y_n$. For definiteness, we keep assigning the X's to treatment group A, whereas the Y's are assumed to belong to the group of subjects or patients given treatment B. The statistical model which is assumed to hold for these variables is the same as in the ordinary two-sample t-test for conventional one- and two-sided hypotheses. Accordingly, we suppose throughout this section that both the X_i and the Y_j follow a normal distribution with some common variance and possibly different expected values where all three parameters are unknown constants allowed to vary unrestrictedly over the respective part of the parameter space. Formally speaking, this means that the observations are assumed to satisfy the basic parametric model

$$X_i \sim \mathcal{N}(\xi, \sigma^2) \ \forall \, i = 1, \ldots, m, \quad Y_j \sim \mathcal{N}(\eta, \sigma^2) \ \forall \, j = 1, \ldots, n, \quad (6.1)$$

with $\xi, \eta \in \mathbb{R}$, $\sigma^2 \in \mathbb{R}_+$.

In § 1.4, we have argued that the most natural measure of dissimilarity of two homoskedastic Gaussian distributions is the standardized difference of their means. Accordingly, under the present parametric model, we define equivalence of treatments A and B through the condition that the true value of this measure falls into a sufficiently narrow interval $(-\varepsilon_1, \varepsilon_2)$ around zero. In other words, we formulate the testing problem as

$$H : (\xi - \eta)/\sigma \leq -\varepsilon_1 \text{ or } (\xi - \eta)/\sigma \geq \varepsilon_2$$
$$\text{versus } K : -\varepsilon_1 < (\xi - \eta)/\sigma < \varepsilon_2 \quad (\varepsilon_1, \varepsilon_2 > 0), \quad (6.2)$$

in direct analogy to the setting of the paired t-test for equivalence [recall (5.16), (5.17)].

The construction of an optimal solution to this problem exploits essentially the same ideas as underlie the derivation of the paired t-test for equivalence. In the unpaired case, both hypotheses remain invariant under any transformation of the form $(x_1, \ldots, x_m, y_1, \ldots, y_n) \mapsto (a + bx_1, \ldots, a + bx_m, a + by_1, \ldots, a + by_n)$ with $(a, b) \in \mathbb{R} \times \mathbb{R}_+$, applying to each coordinate of a point in the joint sample space $\mathbb{R}^N$ (with $N = m + n$) the same scale change and the same translation. Denoting the group of all transformations of this form by $\mathcal{G}$, it is easy to show that the construction of a test which is uniformly most powerful among all level-α tests for (6.2) remaining invariant under $\mathcal{G}$ has been accomplished as soon as a test has been found which is UMP at the same level for the reduced problem

$$\tilde{H} : \tilde{\theta} \le -\tilde{\varepsilon}_1 \text{ or } \tilde{\theta} \ge \tilde{\varepsilon}_2 \quad \text{versus} \quad \tilde{K} : -\tilde{\varepsilon}_1 < \tilde{\theta} < \tilde{\varepsilon}_2 \ . \tag{$\widetilde{6.2}$}$$

In the two-sample case, $\tilde{\theta}$ has to be interpreted as the parameter of a noncentral t-distribution with $m + n - 2 = N - 2$ degrees of freedom, and $(-\tilde{\varepsilon}_1, \tilde{\varepsilon}_2)$ denotes the equivalence interval of (6.2) rescaled by multiplication with $\sqrt{mn/N}$.

Except for differences in notation for the number of degrees of freedom and the limits of the equivalence range, $(\widetilde{6.2})$ is the same as the testing problem $(\widetilde{5.17})$ which has been considered in § 5.3 in connection with the paired t-test for equivalence. Hence, it follows [cf. (5.21), (5.22)] that in order to obtain a UMP level-α test for $(\widetilde{6.2})$, we have to use a critical region of the form

$$\left\{ \tilde{C}^1_{\alpha; m,n}(-\varepsilon_1, \varepsilon_2) < T < \tilde{C}^2_{\alpha; m,n}(-\varepsilon_1, \varepsilon_2) \right\} , \tag{6.3}$$

where the critical constants $\tilde{C}^k_{\alpha; m,n}(-\varepsilon_1, \varepsilon_2)$, $k = 1, 2$, have to be determined by solving the equation system

$$G^*_{-\tilde{\varepsilon}_1}(C_2) - G^*_{-\tilde{\varepsilon}_1}(C_1) = \alpha =$$
$$G^*_{\tilde{\varepsilon}_2}(C_2) - G^*_{\tilde{\varepsilon}_2}(C_1), \quad -\infty < C_1 < C_2 < \infty. \tag{6.4}$$

In (6.4), the superscript $*$ is added to the symbol $G_{\tilde{\varepsilon}}(\cdot)$ which has been used in § 5.3 for noncentral t-distribution functions, in order to make conspicuous the change in the way the number of degrees of freedom has to be determined. In the two-sample case, the latter must be set equal to $N - 2$ instead of $n - 1$. The desired UMPI (uniformly most powerful invariant) test for the primary problem (6.2) is obtained by applying (6.3) with T as the ordinary two-sample t-statistic to be computed from the individual observations by means of the well known formula

$$T = \sqrt{mn(N-2)/N}\,(\bar{X} - \bar{Y})/\left\{ \sum_{i=1}^{m}(X_i - \bar{X})^2 + \sum_{j=1}^{n}(Y_j - \bar{Y})^2 \right\}^{1/2}. \tag{6.5}$$

The simplified computational scheme for determining the critical bounds to the t-statistic derived in § 5.3 for symmetrically chosen equivalence limits to the standardized population mean, has likewise its direct counterpart in the two-sample case. More precisely speaking, it follows by Lemma A.1.6 that whenever both tolerances ε_1 and ε_2 are set equal to some common value $\varepsilon > 0$, say, the critical region (6.3) admits the representation

$$\left\{ |T| < \tilde{C}_{\alpha;\,m,n}(\varepsilon) \right\} , \tag{6.6}$$

where $\tilde{C}_{\alpha;\,m,n}(\varepsilon)$ is explicitly given as the square root of the lower $100\,\alpha$ percentage point of an F-distribution with $1, N-2$ degrees of freedom and noncentrality parameter $\lambda_{nc}^2 = mn\varepsilon^2/N$. In view of this, the practical implementation of the two-sample t-test for equivalence in a symmetric sense is extremely easy in any programming environment providing an intrinsic function for the computation of quantiles of noncentral F-distributions (like finv in SAS). Moreover, making use of Table 6.1, no extra computational tools are needed at all to carry out the test in cases of balanced designs with common sample sizes being multiples of 5 between 10 and 75, pro-

Table 6.1 *Critical constant* $\tilde{C}_{.05;\,n,n}(\varepsilon)$ *of the two-sample t-test for equivalence at level* $\alpha = 5\%$ *with common size* n *of both samples in the symmetric case* $(\varepsilon_1, \varepsilon_2) = (-\varepsilon, \varepsilon)$, *for* $\varepsilon = .25(.25)1.00$ *and* $n = 10(5)75$

		ε =		
n	.25	.50	.75	1.00
10	0.07434	0.11864	0.25412	0.61365
15	0.07997	0.16083	0.46595	1.08697
20	0.08626	0.21755	0.73546	1.50303
25	0.09313	0.29167	1.00477	1.87065
30	0.10058	0.38434	1.25435	2.20346
35	0.10866	0.49320	1.48481	2.50990
40	0.11738	0.61250	1.69952	2.79542
45	0.12681	0.73572	1.90128	3.06383
50	0.13698	0.85816	2.09219	3.31790
55	0.14795	0.97741	2.27384	3.55971
60	0.15977	1.09257	2.44747	3.79090
65	0.17248	1.20355	2.61406	4.01275
70	0.18615	1.31055	2.77441	4.22631
75	0.20082	1.41389	2.92917	4.43246

vided one chooses $\varepsilon_1 = \varepsilon_2 = \varepsilon \in \{.25, .50, .75, 1.00\}$. The maxima of the power functions of the tests determined by these critical constants are shown in Table 6.2. Denoting, for $\varepsilon_1 = \varepsilon_2 = \varepsilon$ and $m = n$, the rejection probability of the test with critical region (6.3) against the specific alternative $\theta = (\xi - \eta)/\sigma = 0$ $[\leftrightarrow \xi = \eta]$ by $\tilde{\beta}_{\alpha;n,n}(\varepsilon)$, this maximal power is readily computed by means of the simple formula

$$\tilde{\beta}_{\alpha;n,n}(\varepsilon) = 2\,G_0^*(\tilde{C}_{\alpha;\,n,n}(\varepsilon)) - 1\,, \tag{6.7}$$

with $G_0^*(\cdot)$ as the central version of the t-distribution function with $N-2$ degrees of freedom.

Table 6.2 *Power attained at* $\theta = (\xi - \eta)/\sigma = 0$ *when using the critical constants shown in Table 6.1 for the two-sample t-statistic*

	$\varepsilon =$			
n	.25	.50	.75	1.00
10	.05844	.09312	.19772	.45288
15	.06317	.12662	.35514	.71368
20	.06829	.17106	.53343	.85890
25	.07381	.22820	.67995	.93250
30	.07977	.29786	.78525	.96845
35	.08620	.37654	.85779	.98554
40	.09314	.45801	.90679	.99348
45	.10062	.53614	.93946	.99710
50	.10867	.60710	.96099	.99873
55	.11734	.66945	.97505	.99945
60	.12666	.72319	.98414	.99976
65	.13667	.76901	.98998	.99990
70	.14740	.80781	.99370	.99996
75	.15888	.84051	.99606	.99998

    Even if the restriction of a symmetric choice of the equivalence limits to the target parameter $\theta = (\xi - \eta)/\sigma$ has to be abandoned, the practical implementation of the two-sample t-test for equivalence continues to be a quick and easy matter, provided one makes use of an appropriate computer program. A *SAS* macro which does all necessary computations determining in particular both critical bounds to the test statistic, is to be found at http://www.zi-mannheim.de/wktsheq under the program name tt2st. The basic algorithm is the same as that underlying its analogue for the one-sample case [$\rightarrow$ tt1st]. In addition to solving the pair of equations (6.4) for arbitrary choices of ε_1 and $\varepsilon_2 > 0$, it outputs the power of the test against the alternative of coincident expected values.

Example 6.1

Table 6.3 shows the raw data obtained from a comparative trial of moxonodin [an alpha receptor blocking agent] and captopril [an inhibitor of
the angiotensin converting enzyme] in the antihypertensive treatment of
patients suffering from major depression. Since moxonodin was known to

Table 6.3 *Reduction of diastolic blood pressure [mm Hg] observed in patients suffering from major depression after 4 weeks of daily treatment
with 0.2 – 0.4 mg moxonodin (a) and 25 – 50 mg captopril (b), respectively*

(a) Moxonidin   *(b) Captopril*

i	X_i	j	Y_j
1	10.3	1	3.3
2	11.3	2	17.7
3	2.0	3	6.7
4	-6.1	4	11.1
5	6.2	5	-5.8
6	6.8	6	6.9
7	3.7	7	5.8
8	-3.3	8	3.0
9	-3.6	9	6.0
10	-3.5	10	3.5
11	13.7	11	18.7
12	12.6	12	9.6
$\bar{X} = 4.175, S_X = 7.050$		$\bar{Y} = 7.208, S_Y = 6.625$	

have not only antihypertensive but also neuroregulative effects alleviating
some of the key symptoms making up a major depression, the aim of the
trial was to establish equivalence of this drug to the ACE inhibitor with
respect to antihypertensive efficacy. Furthermore, only rather extreme increases in the reduction of blood pressure induced by captopril were considered undesirable, on the ground that the latter drug was known to produce
comparatively weak effects. On the other hand, only comparatively small
losses in antihypertensive effectiveness were considered compatible with
equivalence. Making allowance for both of these aspects, a nonsymmetric
choice of the equivalence range for the standardized difference of means
was considered appropriate specifying $(-\varepsilon_1, \varepsilon_2) = (-0.50, 1.00)$.

With the data given in the above table, the test statistic (6.5) is com-

puted to be $T = \sqrt{12^2 \cdot 22/24} \cdot (4.175 - 7.208)/\sqrt{11 \cdot 7.050^2 + 11 \cdot 6.625^2}$
$= -1.086$. On the other hand, with $\alpha = .05$, $m = n = 12$, $\varepsilon_1 = 0.50$ and
$\varepsilon_2 = 1.00$, the *SAS* macro tt2st yields $(0.27977, 0.93088)$ as the critical
interval for T. Since the observed value of T falls clearly outside this interval, the data do not allow to reject the null hypothesis of nonequivalence
of moxonodin to captopril with respect to antihypertensive efficacy. Furthermore, the power against the alternative that the underlying Gaussian
distributions coincide, is computed to be .21013. Thus, even under the most
extreme alternative, the chance of establishing equivalence was rather low
in the present study. In view of the small size of both samples, this is hardly
surprising.

6.2 Mann-Whitney test for equivalence

The equivalence testing problem treated in the previous section can easily
be embedded in a purely nonparametric framework. To see this, it suffices
to recall the elementary fact that under the specific parametric assumption that both the X_i and the Y_j are normally distributed with common
variance σ^2 and arbitrary expectation ξ and η, respectively, the probability π_+, say, of obtaining an observation from the first distribution which
exceeds some single observation drawn from the second, can be written
$\pi_+ = \Phi((\xi - \eta)/\sqrt{2}\sigma)$. Since the standard normal cdf Φ is well known to
be both continuous and strictly increasing, this identity implies that the
testing problem (6.2) is equivalent to

$$H : \pi_+ \leq (1/2) - \varepsilon_1' \text{ or } \pi_+ \geq (1/2) + \varepsilon_2'$$
$$\text{versus} \quad K' : (1/2) - \varepsilon_1' < \pi_+ < (1/2) + \varepsilon_2' , \qquad (6.8)$$

provided π_+ and the ε_ν' are defined by

$$\pi_+ = P[X_i > Y_j]; \ \varepsilon_1' = -(1/2) + \Phi\left(\frac{\varepsilon_1}{\sqrt{2}}\right), \ \varepsilon_2' = \Phi\left(\frac{\varepsilon_2}{\sqrt{2}}\right) - (1/2). \ (6.9)$$

Since the Mann-Whitney functional π_+ is well defined for any pair (F, G)
of *continuous* distribution functions on $\mathbb{R}^1$ such that

$$X_i \sim F \ \forall i = 1, \ldots, m , \qquad Y_j \sim G \ \forall j = 1, \ldots, n , \qquad (6.10)$$

it is natural to treat (6.8) as a nonparametric formulation of the problem of
testing for equivalence of two continuous distributions of arbitrary shape.
On the following pages, we will show how an asymptotically distribution-
free solution to that testing problem can be based on the large-sample
distribution of the U-statistic estimator W_+, say, of π_+. As is well known
(see, e.g., Lehmann, 1975, p. 335), this estimator is simply given as the
Wilcoxon two-sample statistic in its Mann-Whitney form divided by mn

so that we have

$$W_+ = (1/mn) \sum_{i=1}^{m} \sum_{j=1}^{n} I_{(0,\infty)}(X_i - Y_j) \ . \tag{6.11}$$

Not surprisingly, the role played here by the statistic W_+ and the functional π_+ will be analogous to that of the quantities U_+ [$\to$ p. 83, (5.29)] and q_+ [$\to$ (5.28)] in the derivation of a nonparametric equivalence test for paired observations.

Irrespective of the shape of the underlying cdf's F and G, the exact variance of W_+ is given as

$$\text{Var}[W_+] = (1/mn) \cdot$$
$$\left(\pi_+ - (m + n - 1)\pi_+^2 + (m - 1)\Pi_{XXY} + (n - 1)\Pi_{XYY} \right), \tag{6.12}$$

where

$$\Pi_{XXY} = P[X_{i_1} > Y_j, X_{i_2} > Y_j],$$
$$\Pi_{XYY} = P[X_i > Y_{j_1}, X_i > Y_{j_2}] \tag{6.13}$$

(see, e.g., Lehmann, 1975, (2.20)). Natural estimators of the functionals Π_{XXY} and Π_{XYY} are given by the U-statistics

$$\widehat{\Pi}_{XXY} = \frac{2}{m(m-1)\,n} \times$$
$$\sum_{i_1=1}^{m-1} \sum_{i_2=i_1+1}^{m} \sum_{j=1}^{n} I_{(0,\infty)}(X_{i_1} - Y_j) \cdot I_{(0,\infty)}(X_{i_2} - Y_j), \tag{6.14a}$$

$$\widehat{\Pi}_{XYY} = \frac{2}{m\,n(n-1)} \times$$
$$\sum_{i=1}^{m} \sum_{j_1=1}^{n-1} \sum_{j_2=j_1+1}^{n} I_{(0,\infty)}(X_i - Y_{j_1}) \cdot I_{(0,\infty)}(X_i - Y_{j_2}). \tag{6.14b}$$

As is true for any two-sample U-statistic estimator with square integrable kernel (cf. Randles and Wolfe, 1979, Corollary 3.4.9), W_+, $\widehat{\Pi}_{XXY}$ and $\widehat{\Pi}_{XYY}$ are consistent for the respective estimands π_+, Π_{XXY} and Π_{XYY}. Hence, a consistent estimator of $\text{Var}[W_+]$ is given by

$$\hat{\sigma}^2[W_+] = \frac{1}{mn} \left(W_+ - (m + n - 1)W_+^2 + \right.$$
$$\left. (m - 1)\widehat{\Pi}_{XXY} + (n - 1)\widehat{\Pi}_{XYY} \right). \tag{6.15}$$

In view of the asymptotic normality of the Mann-Whitney statistic (see, e.g., Lehmann, 1975, p. 69), consistency of $\hat{\sigma}^2[W_+]$ implies that the statistic $(W_+ - \pi_+)/\hat{\sigma}[W_+]$ converges in law to a standard Gaussian variable whenever we have $0 < \pi_+ < 1$, $m, n \to \infty$ and $m/n \to \lambda$ (with λ denoting some positive real number). Hence, we can apply once more the general theory outlined in § 3.4 leading to the conclusion that an asymptotically valid testing procedure for the equivalence problem (6.8) is obtained by using the decision rule

Reject nonequivalence if and only if

$$\left|W_+ - (1/2) - (\varepsilon_2' - \varepsilon_1')/2)\right| / \hat{\sigma}[W_+] < C_{MW}(\alpha; \varepsilon_1', \varepsilon_2'), \quad (6.16)$$

with

$$C_{MW}(\alpha; \varepsilon_1', \varepsilon_2') = \Big\{ 100\alpha - \text{percentage point of the } \chi^2 - \text{distri-}$$

$$\text{bution with } df = 1 \text{ and } \lambda_{nc}^2 = (\varepsilon_1' + \varepsilon_2')^2 / 4\hat{\sigma}^2[W_+] \Big\}^{1/2}. \quad (6.17)$$

At the URL associated with this book, one finds also a tool for the quick and easy implementation of the testing procedure (6.16), appropriately termed Mann-Whitney test for equivalence in the research paper where its basic properties have first been rigorously established (Wellek, 1996). The program which has been once more written in *SAS* as a macro, is named mawi and requires as input data the actual values of the significance level α, the sample sizes m, n and the tolerances ε_1', ε_2', as well as the name of a file containing the raw data under analysis. In the output, the user finds in addition to the input data, the values computed for the Mann-Whitney statistic W_+, its estimated standard deviation $\hat{\sigma}[W_+]$, the critical bound $C_{MW}^a(\alpha; \varepsilon_1', \varepsilon_2')$ and an indicator which is set equal to 1 if and only if the data fall into the rejection region corresponding to (6.16).

Example 6.1 (continued)

In order to illustrate the use of the testing procedure (6.16), we reanalyze the blood pressure reduction data of Table 6.3 by means of the Mann-Whitney statistic. According to (6.9), the equivalence hypothesis $-.50 < (\xi - \eta)/\sigma < 1.00$ on two Gaussian distributions with means ξ, η and common variance σ^2 can be rewritten as $.3618 < \pi_+ < .7602$. The corresponding specification of the ε_ν' in (6.8), (6.16), (6.17) is $\varepsilon_1' = .1382$, $\varepsilon_2' = .2602$. With these values and the raw data displayed in Table 6.3, the *SAS* macro mawi yields $W_+ = .41667$, $\hat{\sigma}[W_+] = .10807$, $C_{MW}(.05; \varepsilon_1', \varepsilon_2') = .32861$. Since we have $|.41667 - 1/2 - (.2602 - .1382)/2| / .10807 = 1.3355$, the observed value of the test statistic clearly exceeds its critical upper bound. Thus it follows that the Mann-Whitney test for equivalence leads to the same decision as the parametric test derived in the previous subsection, namely acceptance of the null hypothesis of nonequivalence of both drugs with respect to their antihypertensive efficacy.

In order to investigate the level and power of the Mann-Whitney test for equivalence in real applications with samples of finite or even small size, one has to rely on Monte Carlo simulation once more. The fact that the ordinary Mann-Whitney test is well known (see Hájek and Šidák, 1967, p. 87) to be optimal against logistic shift alternatives suggests to restrict such an investigation to constellations where the cdf and the density of the Y_j has one of the standard forms listed in Table 5.9 and the distribution of the X_i is the result of shifting that of the Y_j by a real constant ϑ. Accordingly, in the majority of simulation experiments run to study the finite sample behaviour of the testing procedure (6.16), random numbers of the form $X_i = X_i^\circ + \vartheta, Y_j = Y_j^\circ$ were generated with $(X_1^\circ, \ldots, X_m^\circ, Y_1^\circ, \ldots, Y_n^\circ)$ as a sample of size $m + n$ from a standardized Gaussian, Cauchy, uniform, exponential, Laplace and logistic distribution, respectively. In addition, one constellation was investigated where both distributions under comparison differ in form. The rationale behind the procedure of generating pairs of samples from distributions of this latter kind was the same as for the location models: The distribution from which the Y_j were taken, was fixed (at $\mathcal{N}(0, 1)$, i.e., the standard Gaussian), and the centre ϑ of the distribution of the X_i (belonging to the Gaussian family as well but with threefold standard deviation) was successively shifted from zero to the point at which the functional π_+ [recall (6.9)] reaches $1/2 - \varepsilon_1', 1/2 + \varepsilon_2'$, and $1/2$, respectively.

For $X_i = X_i^\circ + \vartheta, Y_j = Y_j^\circ$ with X_i° and Y_j° following the (continuous) cdf $F_\circ$ and $G_\circ$, respectively, the functional π_+ with respect to which equivalence of the underlying distributions is asserted under the alternative hypothesis of (6.8), admits the representation

$$\pi_+ = \int_{-\infty}^{\infty} [1 - F_\circ(y - \vartheta)] dG_\circ(y) \; . \tag{6.18}$$

It is easy to verify that in any setting with $F_\circ = G_\circ$ and $F_\circ(-x) = 1 - F_\circ(x) \, \forall x \in \mathbb{R}$, i.e., in any ordinary shift model with a symmetric common baseline cdf, the integral on the right-hand side of (6.18) coincides with the expression on the left of equation (5.37), provided, ϑ is replaced with $\vartheta/2$ in the latter. Hence except for the exponential distribution, for all baseline cdf's considered in § 5.4, the limits $-\varepsilon_1, \varepsilon_2$, say, of the equivalence range for the location parameter ϑ which corresponds to some given equivalence range $(1/2 - \varepsilon_1', 1/2 + \varepsilon_2')$ for π_+ under the two-sample shift-model generated by $F_\circ$, can be determined by means of the formulae shown in the third column of Table 5.9. In the two-sample shift-model obtained by setting $F_\circ(x) = \Phi(x/3), G_\circ(y) = \Phi(y)$ such that the distributions under comparison differ in dispersion for any value of the location parameter, π_+ admits a simple representation through the normal distribution function as well. It reads $\pi_+ = \Phi(\vartheta/\sqrt{10})$, in close analogy to the ordinary Gaussian shift model given by $F_\circ = G_\circ = \Phi$. Making use of these relationships one

obtains the values displayed in Table 6.4 which is a direct two-sample counterpart to Table 5.10. Specifying the equivalence limits to π_+ by choosing
$\varepsilon_1' = \varepsilon_2' = .20$ can be motivated as explained in §1.5 [cf. Table 1.1, (ii)].
The other specification of $\varepsilon_1', \varepsilon_2'$ referred to in Table 6.4 corresponds to the
equivalence range used in Example 6.1 [to be resumed below] for the stan-
dardized difference of the means in the Gaussian shift model.

Table 6.4 *Equivalence ranges for the location parameter ϑ corresponding to*
.30 $< \pi_+ <$ .70 and .3618 $< \pi_+ <$ .7602, respectively, in seven different
models for the two-sample problem with $X_i \sim F_\circ(\cdot - \vartheta)$, $Y_j \sim G_\circ(\cdot)$

Family of Distributions	Equivalence Range $(-\varepsilon_1, \varepsilon_2)$ for ϑ corresponding to $1/2 - \varepsilon_1' < \pi_+ < 1/2 + \varepsilon_2'$, for $(1/2 - \varepsilon_1', 1/2 + \varepsilon_2') =$	
	(0.3000, 0.7000)	(0.3618, 0.7602)
Gaussian	(−0.7416, 0.7416)	(−0.5000, 1.0000)
Cauchy	(−1.4531, 1.4531)	(−0.9274, 2.1324)
Uniform	(−0.2254, 0.2254)	(−0.1494, 0.3075)
Exponential	(−0.5108, 0.5108)	(−0.3235, 0.7348)
Laplace	(−0.8731, 0.8731)	(−0.5770, 1.2070)
Logistic	(−1.2636, 1.2636)	(−0.8491, 1.7127)
$\mathcal{N}(\vartheta, 9)/\mathcal{N}(0, 1)$	(−1.6583, 1.6583)	(−1.1180, 2.2356)

   In the simulation study of the Mann-Whitney test for equivalence, a balanced design was assumed throughout, and the common sample size n was
chosen from the set $\{12, 24, 36\}$. For each of these sample sizes and all
7×2 constellations covered by Table 6.4, the rejection probability of the
test at the usual nominal significance level of 5% under $\vartheta = -\varepsilon_1, \vartheta = \varepsilon_2$ and
$\vartheta = 0 (\Leftrightarrow \pi_+ = 1/2)$ was determined on the basis of 100,000 replications of
the respective Monte Carlo experiment. As can be seen from the results of
this study summarized in Table 6.5, the nominal level is strictly maintained
in all settings with a symmetric choice of the equivalence limits, even for
sample sizes as small as 12. The only cases where the test shows some anticonservative tendency are those where very small samples are used for
establishing an equivalence hypothesis exhibiting marked asymmetry, and
even then the extent of anticonservatism seems not really serious from a
practical point of view. Under the ordinary shift model with a standard
Gaussian cdf as baseline, the loss in power as compared to the optimal
parametric procedure (i.e., the two-sample t-test for equivalence derived in

the preceding section) is roughly of the same order of magnitude as in the analogous paired-sample setting [cf. pp. 88-9].

Table 6.5 *Simulated rejection probabilities of the Mann-Whitney test for equivalence at both boundaries of the hypotheses (columns 5, 6) and $\pi_+ = 1/2$ (rightmost column) with samples of common size n = 12, 24, 36 from distributions belonging to the families listed in Table 6.4 and equivalence range $(1/2 - \varepsilon'_1, 1/2 + \varepsilon'_2) = (.3000, .7000), (.3618, .7602)$ [the italicized values give the power of the two-sample t-test for equivalence at level $\alpha = .05$ against $\pi_+ = 1/2$]*

Family of Distributions	$(1/2 - \varepsilon'_1, 1/2 + \varepsilon'_2)$	m	n	Rejection Probability at $\pi_+ =$		
				$1/2 - \varepsilon'_1$	$1/2 + \varepsilon'_2$	$1/2$
Gaussian	(.3000, .7000)	12	12	.05015	.04941	.22020
						.24605
	"	24	24	.04510	.04565	.57929
						.63971
	"	36	36	.04427	.04476	.82186
						.86027
	(.3618, .7602)	12	12	.05514	.04327	.19727
						.21013
	"	24	24	.05273	.04026	.46811
						.49669
	"	36	36	.04828	.03900	.65010
						.67635
Cauchy	(.3000, .7000)	12	12	.04925	.04780	.20180
	"	24	24	.04644	.04536	.56918
	"	36	36	.04466	.04442	.81617
	(.3618, .7602)	12	12	.05107	.04336	.17994
	"	24	24	.05143	.03939	.45973
	"	36	36	.04967	.03962	.64708
Uniform	(.3000, .7000)	12	12	.04503	.04397	.19944
	"	24	24	.04312	.04282	.56956
	"	36	36	.04267	.04291	.81578
	(.3618, .7602)	12	12	.04872	.03800	.17954
	"	24	24	.04892	.03709	.45624
	"	36	36	.04928	.03824	.64447

Table 6.5 *(continued)*

Family of Distribution	$(1/2 - \varepsilon_1', 1/2 + \varepsilon_2')$	m	n	Rejection Probability at $\pi_+ =$		
				$1/2 - \varepsilon_1'$	$1/2 + \varepsilon_2'$	$1/2$
Exponential	(.3000, .7000)	12	12	.04631	.04557	.20216
"	"	24	24	.04471	.04404	.56989
"	"	36	36	.04285	.04322	.81782
	(.3618, .7602)	12	12	.04949	.04054	.18135
"	"	24	24	.05028	.03879	.45580
"	"	36	36	.04782	.03860	.64542
Laplace	(.3000, .7000)	12	12	.04743	.04745	.20001
"	"	24	24	.04582	.04425	.56931
"	"	36	36	.04255	.04363	.81818
	(.3618, .7602)	12	12	.05138	.04177	.17918
"	"	24	24	.05031	.03961	.46001
"	"	36	36	.04833	.03904	.64797
Logistic	(.3000, .7000)	12	12	.04518	.04577	.20179
"	"	24	24	.04371	.04507	.57006
"	"	36	36	.04324	.04445	.81664
	(.3618, .7602)	12	12	.05102	.03979	.17807
"	"	24	24	.05045	.03922	.45537
"	"	36	36	.04650	.03973	.64290
$\mathcal{N}(\vartheta, 9)/\mathcal{N}(0, 1)$	(.3000, .7000)	12	12	.04862	.05058	.17883
"	"	24	24	.04506	.04605	.47684
"	"	36	36	.04403	.04431	.73950
	(.3618, .7602)	12	12	.05429	.04447	.16224
"	"	24	24	.05090	.04088	.39080
"	"	36	36	.04914	.03921	.58209

All in all the simulation results shown in Table 6.5 allow the following conclusions:

(i) As long as the equivalence range is chosen as an interval symmetric about $1/2$ (which will be the case in the majority of practical applications), sample sizes of one dozen per group are sufficient to ensure that the Mann-Whitney test for equivalence is strictly valid with respect to the significance level. This is even true for pairs of underlying distribution function which satisfy the null hypotheses but exhibit gross departure from homoskedasticity. The anticonservative tendency to be observed in very small samples under some parametric submodels for markedly asymmetric choices of the equivalence limits is only slight and can be ignored for most practical purposes.

(ii) The power attained by the Mann-Whitney test for equivalence under various shift models shows little sensitivity even to gross changes in form of the baseline distribution. Substantial differences in power can only be seen if any of the traditional location shift models is contrasted with the model involving heteroskedasticity in addition to shift in location. In fact, heteroskedasticity (as well as other differences in form of the two distributions to be compared) has a marked negative impact on the efficiency of the test.

(iii) Conclusion (iii) stated on p. 90 with regard to the efficiency of the signed rank test for equivalence under the Gaussian submodel relative to the (paired) t-test applies mutatis mutandis to the Mann-Whitney test for equivalence as well.

By direct analytical arguments, some interesting and intuitively plausible properties of the (exact) power function of the Mann-Whitney test for equivalence can be established which hold under any model obtained by replacing the standard Gaussian cdf with an arbitrary continuous $F_\circ$ in the setting of the ordinary two-sample t-test. To be more specific, let us denote by $\beta_{F_\circ}^{m,n}(\vartheta, \sigma)$ the rejection probability of the test when applied with data such that $X_i = \sigma X_i^\circ + \vartheta$, $X_i^\circ \sim F_\circ \ \forall i = 1, \ldots, m,$ $Y_j = \sigma Y_j^\circ$, $Y_j^\circ \sim F_\circ \ \forall j = 1, \ldots, n$. Then, the following statements hold true:

(a) $F_\circ$ symmetric about 0 or $m = n$

$$\Rightarrow \beta_{F_\circ}^{m,n}(-\vartheta, \sigma) = \beta_{F_\circ}^{m,n}(\vartheta, \sigma) \ \ \forall (\vartheta, \sigma) \in \mathbb{R} \times \mathbb{R}_+ \ ;$$

(b) $\beta_{F_\circ}^{m,n}(\vartheta, \sigma) = \beta_{F_\circ}^{m,n}(\vartheta/\sigma, 1) \ \ \forall (\vartheta, \sigma) \in \mathbb{R} \times \mathbb{R}_+ \ .$

The second of these results implies that in any (not only the Gaussian!) location-scale model for the two-sample setting which assumes homogeneity of the underlying distributions with respect to the scale parameter σ, the equivalence hypothesis which the test presented in this section is tailored for, is a statement about ϑ/σ rather than ϑ per se. This is one of several basic properties distinguishing the testing procedure under consideration from the interval inclusion procedure with Mann-Whitney based confidence limits to ϑ as proposed by Hauschke, Steinijans and Diletti (1990). In fact, the interval estimation method forming the basis of the latter presupposes a simple location shift model as becomes obvious from its construction (cf. Lehmann, 1963). Hence, it cannot be taken for granted that the corresponding interval inclusion test keeps being valid if the underlying nonparametric model covers also pairs of distributions differing in dispersion or other shape parameters in addition to location. Thus, apart from the fact that both approaches relate to totally different formulations of hypotheses, it is clear that the test obtained on the preceding pages is (asymptotically) distribution-free in a much stronger sense than the interval inclusion procedure based on Moses*-Lehmann confidence limits.

6.3 A distribution-free two-sample equivalence test allowing for arbitrary patterns of ties

The assumptions underlying the construction of a nonparametric two-sample test for equivalence described in § 6.2 imply that the occurrence of ties between observations from different samples can be excluded with probability one. Accordingly, the procedure is unsuitable for analyzing data sets made up of independent observations from two different discrete distributions. In this section we show how to generalize the Mann-Whitney test in such a way that arbitrary patterns of ties can be admitted without affecting the (asymptotic) validity of the procedure. In elaborating this idea, basic analogies with the derivation of a generalized signed rank test for equivalence dealt with in § 5.5 will become apparent. Obviously, the definition of the functional π_+ [$\rightarrow$ (6.9)] makes sense for any type of distributions which the X's and Y's are taken from. However, in the noncontinuous case, identity of both distributions no longer implies that π_+ takes on value $1/2$. Instead, in the general case, the relationship $F = G \Rightarrow \pi_+ = 1/2$ has to be replaced with

$$F = G \;\Rightarrow\; \pi_+ = (1/2) \cdot (1 - \pi_0) \tag{6.19}$$

provided we define π_0 as the functional

$$\pi_0 = P[X_i = Y_j] = \int (G - G_-)dF \tag{6.20}$$

assigning each pair of cdf's as its value the probability of a tie between an observation from F and an observation from G independent of the former. (On the right-hand side of the second of the equalities (6.20), G_- stands for the left-continuous version of the cdf G as defined by $G_-(y) = P[Y_j < y]$ $\forall\, y \in \mathbb{R}$.) In view of (6.19), it seems natural to use the distance of $\pi_+/(1 - \pi_0)$ from the point $1/2$ as a measure for the degree of disparity of any two cdf's F and G from which our two samples $(X_1, \ldots X_m)$ and $(Y_1, \ldots Y_n)$ are taken. Adopting this as our basic measure of distance, we are led to formulate our testing problem as

$$H : \pi_+/(1 - \pi_0) \leq 1/2 - \varepsilon_1' \quad \text{or} \quad \pi_+/(1 - \pi_0) \geq 1/2 + \varepsilon_2'$$

$$\text{versus} \quad H_1 : 1/2 - \varepsilon_1' < \pi_+/(1 - \pi_0) < 1/2 + \varepsilon_2'. \tag{6.21}$$

For both of the basic functionals appearing in (6.21), there exists an U-statistic estimator with a kernel which is just the indicator function of

---

* The technique of computing nonparametric confidence limits for the shift in location between two continuous distributions of the same shape and dispersion by means of the Mann-Whitney null distribution has been originally introduced in a textbook chapter authored by Moses (1953, pp. 443-5).

the respective event. Of course, the first of these estimators (for π_+) is the same as that introduced in the previous section [recall (6.11)]. Analogously, a U-statistic estimating π_0 is given by

$$W_0 = \frac{1}{mn} \sum_{i=1}^{m} \sum_{j=1}^{n} I_{\{0\}}(X_i - Y_j), \tag{6.22}$$

with $I_{\{0\}}(u) = 1$ for $u = 0$ and $I_{\{0\}}(u) = 0$ for $u \in (-\infty, 0) \cup (0, \infty)$. Furthermore, it is natural to estimate the target functional in terms of which the hypotheses under assessment now have been formulated, by just plugging in (6.11) and (6.22) into the expression $\pi_+/(1 - \pi_0)$. Denoting this latter estimator by Q, we have by definition

$$Q = W_+/(1 - W_0). \tag{6.23}$$

Now, we proceed by studying the large-sample distribution of (6.23) which is readily obtained as soon as we know the joint asymptotic distribution of the two individual U-statistics involved. Assuming in the sequel that the sequence $(m/N)_{N \in \mathbb{N}}$ of relative sizes of the first sample converges to some nondegenerate limit $\lambda \in (0, 1)$, say, it follows from the asymptotic distribution theory for two-sample U-statistics (see, e.g., Randles and Wolfe, 1979, §3.6) that $\sqrt{N}(W_+ - \pi_+, W_0 - \pi_0)$ converges in law to a centred bivariate normal distribution. The covariance matrix $\Sigma_N = \begin{pmatrix} \sigma_{N;+}^2 & \sigma_{N;+0} \\ \sigma_{N;+0} & \sigma_{N;0}^2 \end{pmatrix}$, say, of this distribution can be computed exactly. The exact formulae contain also terms of order $O(1/N)$:

(i) Variance of $\sqrt{N}(W_+ - \pi_+)$:

$$\sigma_{N;+}^2 = \frac{N}{mn}[\pi_+ - (N-1)\pi_+^2 + (m-1)\Pi_{XXY} + (n-1)\Pi_{XYY}] \tag{6.24a}$$

where
$$\Pi_{XXY} = P[X_{i_1} > Y_j, X_{i_2} > Y_j], \tag{6.24b}$$
$$\Pi_{XYY} = P[X_i > Y_{j_1}, X_i > Y_{j_2}]. \tag{6.24c}$$

(ii) Variance of $\sqrt{N}(W_0 - \pi_0)$:

$$\sigma_{N;0}^2 = \frac{N}{mn}[\pi_0 - (N-1)\pi_0^2 + (m-1)\Psi_{XXY} + (n-1)\Psi_{XYY}] \tag{6.25a}$$

where
$$\Psi_{XXY} = P[X_{i_1} = Y_j, X_{i_2} = Y_j], \tag{6.25b}$$
$$\Psi_{XYY} = P[X_i = Y_{j_1}, X_i = Y_{j_2}]. \tag{6.25c}$$

(iii) Covariance of $\sqrt{N}(W_+ - \pi_+)$ and $\sqrt{N}(W_0 - \pi_0)$:

$$\sigma_{N;+0} = \frac{N}{mn}[(m-1)\Lambda_{XXY} + (n-1)\Lambda_{XYY} - (N-1)\pi_+\pi_0] \tag{6.26a}$$

where

$$\Lambda_{XXY} = P[X_{i_1} > Y_j, X_{i_2} = Y_j], \qquad (6.26b)$$
$$\Lambda_{XYY} = P[X_i > Y_{j_1}, X_i = Y_{j_2}]. \qquad (6.26c)$$

Now let us define the function $q(\cdot, \cdot)$ by $q(\pi_+, \pi_0) = \pi_+/(1 - \pi_0)$ and denote the result of evaluating the quadratic form $\nabla q(\pi_+, \pi_0) \Sigma_N (\nabla q(\pi_+, \pi_0))'$ (with $\nabla q(\pi_+, \pi_0)$ as the gradient (row) vector of $q(\cdot, \cdot)$) by ν_N^2. Then, after straightforward calculations and rearrangements of terms we obtain the expression:

$$\nu_N^2 = \frac{\sigma_{+N}^2}{(1 - \pi_0)^2} + \frac{\pi_+^2 \sigma_{0N}^2}{(1 - \pi_0)^4} + \frac{2\pi_+ \sigma_{+0;N}}{(1 - \pi_0)^3} \, . \qquad (6.27)$$

Resorting to the so-called δ-method (cf. Bishop, Fienberg and Holland, 1975, § 14.6) once more, we can conclude that $\sqrt{N}(Q - \pi_+/(1 - \pi_0)) = \sqrt{N}(q(W_+, W_0) - q(\pi_+, \pi_0))$ converges weakly to a random variable following a centred normal distribution with variance $\nu^2 = \lim_{N \to \infty} \nu_N^2$.

The first step of a natural approach to deriving an estimator for ν_N^2 consists in plugging in U-statistic estimators of all functionals of the underlying cdf's F and G appearing on the right-hand side of equations (6.24) – (6.26). The U-statistic estimators for the functionals indexed by subscript XXY are given by

$$\hat{\Pi}_{XXY} = \frac{2}{m(m-1)n} \sum_{i_1=1}^{m-1} \sum_{i_2=i_1+1}^{m} \sum_{j=1}^{n} \Big[I_{(0,\infty)} \, (X_{i_1} - Y_j) \cdot$$

$$I_{(0,\infty)} \, (X_{i_2} - Y_j) \Big] \qquad (6.28a)$$

$$\hat{\Psi}_{XXY} = \frac{2}{m(m-1)n} \sum_{i_1=1}^{m-1} \sum_{i_2=i_1+1}^{m} \sum_{j=1}^{n} \Big[I_{\{0\}} \, (X_{i_1} - Y_j) \cdot$$

$$I_{\{0\}} \, (X_{i_2} - Y_j) \Big] \qquad (6.28b)$$

$$\hat{\Lambda}_{XXY} = \frac{1}{m(m-1)n} \sum_{i_1=1}^{m} \sum_{i_2 \in \{1,\ldots,m\} \backslash \{i_1\}} \sum_{j=1}^{n} \Big[I_{(0,\infty)} \, (X_{i_1} - Y_j) \cdot$$

$$I_{\{0\}} \, (X_{i_2} - Y_j) \Big]. \qquad (6.28c)$$

The analogous estimators of Π_{XYY}, Ψ_{XYY} and Λ_{XYY} admit the representation:

$$\hat{\Pi}_{XYY} = \frac{2}{m(n-1)n} \sum_{i=1}^{m} \sum_{j_1=1}^{n-1} \sum_{j_2=j_1+1}^{n} \Big[I_{(0,\infty)} \, (X_i - Y_{j_1}) \cdot$$

$$I_{(0,\infty)} \, (X_i - Y_{j_2}) \Big] \qquad (6.29a)$$

$$\widehat{\Psi}_{XYY} = \frac{2}{m(n-1)n} \sum_{i=1}^{m} \sum_{j_1=1}^{n-1} \sum_{j_2=j_1+1}^{n} \left[I_{\{0\}}(X_i - Y_{j_1}) \cdot \right.$$

$$\left. I_{\{0\}}(X_i - Y_{j_2}) \right] \quad (6.29b)$$

$$\widehat{\Lambda}_{XYY} = \frac{1}{m(n-1)n} \sum_{i=1}^{m} \sum_{j_1=1}^{n} \sum_{j_2 \in \{1,\ldots,n\}\setminus\{j_1\}} \left[I_{(0,\infty)}(X_i - Y_{j_1}) \cdot \right.$$

$$\left. I_{\{0\}}(X_i - Y_{j_2}) \right]. \quad (6.29c)$$

Since each of the estimators defined in (6.11), (6.22), (6.28) and (6.29) is (strongly) consistent for its expectation (cf. Lee, 1990, § 3.4.2) , it follows that the plug-in estimator $\hat{\sigma}_{+N}^2$ obtained from (6.24a) by replacing π_+, Π_{XXY} and Π_{XYY} with $W_+, \widehat{\Pi}_{XXY}$ and $\widehat{\Pi}_{XYY}$, respectively, is consistent for σ_{+N}^2, and so on for $\hat{\sigma}_{0N}^2$ and $\hat{\sigma}_{+0;N}$. Finally, consistency of $W_+, W_0, \hat{\sigma}_{+N}^2, \hat{\sigma}_{0N}^2$ and $\hat{\sigma}_{+0;N}$ ensures that the asymptotic variance ν_N^2 of the statistic $\sqrt{N}W_+/(1-W_0)$ (and hence a fortiori its limiting variance ν^2) can be consistently estimated by

$$\hat{\nu}_N^2 = \frac{\hat{\sigma}_{+N}^2}{(1-W_0)^2} + \frac{W_+^2 \hat{\sigma}_{0N}^2}{(1-W_0)^4} + \frac{2W_+ \hat{\sigma}_{+0;N}}{(1-W_0)^3}. \quad (6.30)$$

What is left to do then in order to complete the construction of a Mann-Whitney test for equivalence allowing for arbitrary patterns of ties in the data, is to apply the general approach of § 3.4 to the specific case that $k = 2$, $T_N = W_+/(1-W_0)$, $\theta = \pi_+/(1-\pi_0)$, $\sigma = \nu$ and $\hat{\tau}_N = \hat{\nu}_N/\sqrt{N}$. Accordingly, we end up with the decision rule

Reject $H : \dfrac{\pi_+}{1-\pi_0} \leq \dfrac{1}{2} - \varepsilon_1'$ or $\dfrac{\pi_+}{1-\pi_0} \geq \dfrac{1}{2} + \varepsilon_2'$ if and only if

$$\sqrt{N} \left| W_+/(1-W_0) - (1 - \varepsilon_1' + \varepsilon_2')/2 \right| / \hat{\nu}_N < C_{MW}^*(\alpha; \varepsilon_1', \varepsilon_2'), \quad (6.31)$$

with

$$C_{MW}^*(\alpha; \varepsilon_1', \varepsilon_2') = \left\{ 100\alpha - \text{percentage point of the } \chi^2 - \text{distri-} \right.$$

$$\left. \text{bution with } df = 1 \text{ and } \lambda_{nc}^2 = N(\varepsilon_1' + \varepsilon_2')^2/4\hat{\nu}_N^2 \right\}^{1/2} \quad (6.32)$$

By Theorem A.3.4, it is a fact that the corresponding test is asymptotically valid over the whole class of all pairs (F, G) of distribution functions on the real line such that the limiting variance ν^2 of $\sqrt{N}W_+/(1-W_0)$ does not vanish. Inspecting specific families of discrete distributions corroborates the impression that this regularity condition is actually very mild. Even in the extreme case that both the X_i and the Y_j are Bernoulli variables, the requirement that ν^2 has to be positive rules out merely those constellations in which at least one of the two underlying distributions is degenerate on its own.

In order to reduce the practical effort entailed by carrying out the generalized Mann-Whitney test for equivalence to a minimum, another special *SAS* macro is provided at http://www.zi-mannheim.de/wktsheq. The program for which the name `mwtie_xy` has been chosen, performs all necessary computational steps from scratch, i.e., upon just providing the $m + n$ raw data values as input.

Computational methods for grouped data

Suppose that the set of values taken on by any of the observations in the pooled sample is given by $\{w_1, ..., w_K\}$ such that $w_1 < w_2 < ... < w_K$ and the number K of different groups of values is small compared to both sample sizes. Then, computations can be made considerably faster by reducing the raw data to group frequencies before calculating the various counting statistics involved. For elaborating on this idea, we need some additional notation.

Let M_k and N_k be the number of X's and Y's, respectively, taking on value w_k ($k = 1, ..., K$). Furthermore, define corresponding cumulative frequencies M_k^c and N_k^c by $M_0^c = N_0^c = 0$, $M_k^c = \sum_{l=1}^{k} M_k$, $N_k^c = \sum_{l=1}^{k} N_l$, $k = 1, ..., K$. Then, it is easy to verify that the individual U-statistic estimators required for computing the test statistic of (6.31) admit the following representations:

$$W_+ = \frac{1}{mn} \sum_{k=1}^{K} M_k N_{k-1}^c \;\; , W_0 = \frac{1}{mn} \sum_{k=1}^{K} M_k N_k \;\; ; \tag{6.33}$$

$$\widehat{\Pi}_{XXY} = \frac{1}{m(m-1)n} \sum_{k=1}^{K} (m - M_k^c)(m - M_k^c - 1) N_k \;\; , \tag{6.34a}$$

$$\widehat{\Psi}_{XXY} = \frac{1}{m(m-1)n} \sum_{k=1}^{K} M_k (M_k - 1) N_k \;\; , \tag{6.34b}$$

$$\widehat{\Lambda}_{XXY} = \frac{1}{m(m-1)n} \sum_{k=1}^{K} M_k (m - M_k^c) N_k \;\; ; \tag{6.34c}$$

$$\widehat{\Pi}_{XYY} = \frac{1}{mn(n-1)} \sum_{k=1}^{K} M_k N_{k-1}^c (N_{k-1}^c - 1) \;\; , \tag{6.35a}$$

$$\widehat{\Psi}_{XYY} = \frac{1}{mn(n-1)} \sum_{k=1}^{K} M_k N_k (N_k - 1) \;\; , \tag{6.35b}$$

$$\widehat{\Lambda}_{XYY} = \frac{1}{mn(n-1)} \sum_{k=1}^{K} M_k \, N_k N_{k-1}^c \; . \tag{6.35c}$$

The above identities give rise to a simplified version of the SAS code for the procedure to be found at http://www.zi-mannheim.de/wktsheq under the program name mwtie_fr. The program likewise processes the primary set of raw data. The (cumulative) frequencies appearing in expressions for the U-statistics involved are determined automatically and need not be available as entries in a user-supplied $2 \times K$ contingency table.

Example 6.2

In a recent study (Schumann et al., 2002) of a N-methyl-D-aspartate receptor 2B (NR2B) gene variant as a possible risk factor for alcohol dependence, a single nucleotide polymorphism (SNP) located at position 2873 of the gene was used in genotyping $m = 204$ patients and $n = 258$ unrelated healthy controls. The polymorphism leads to a C (cytosine) to T (thymine) exchange. Table 6.6 shows the frequencies of the 3 possible genotypes found in both samples.

Table 6.6 *Observed distribution of SNP C2873T NR2B genotypes in patients with alcohol dependence and healthy controls*

| | Genotype | | | |
Group	CC	CT	TT	Σ
Patients	103	84	17	$204 = m$
	(50.5)	(41.2)	(8.3)	(100.0)
Controls	135	105	18	$258 = n$
	(52.3)	(40.7)	(7.0)	(100.0)

Since the location of the mutation was suspected to be outside the gene region encoding the domain of an antagonist of the NMDA receptor assumed to play a major role in mediating the reinforcing effects of alcohol abuse, the authors of the study aimed at excluding the existence of a substantial association between SNP C2873T NR2B genotype and alcohol dependence.

In a traditional study of this type being launched with the intention to establish the association, the standard inferential procedure is Armitage's (1955) test for an up- or downward trend in a $2 \times K$ contingency table with ordered column categories and fixed row margins (for more recent reviews of this method focussing on applications to genetic epidemiology see Sasieni, 1997; Devlin and Roeder, 1999). Experience shows that the decision to which this procedure leads rarely differs from that to be taken in a Mann-Whitney test corrected for the large number of ties occurring in a set of data taking on only three different values, namely 0, 1 and 2 (giving simply the number of mutated alleles in an individual's genotype). This fact suggests analyzing the data set underlying Table 6.6 by means of the equivalence counterpart of the tie-corrected Mann-Whitney test derived above.

Let the significance level be chosen as usual, i.e., $\alpha = .05$, and fix the equivalence limits to $\pi_+/(1 - \pi_0) - 1/2$ at $\mp.10$. Running the grouped-data version `mwtie_fr` of the respective SAS macro, we obtain for the genotype frequencies shown above the following estimates:

$$W_+ = .29298, \quad W_0 = .43759, \quad \hat{\nu}_N = .918898.$$

With these values and tolerances $\varepsilon_1' = \varepsilon_2' = .10$, the test statistic to be used according to (6.31) is computed to be

$$\frac{\sqrt{N}\,|W_+/(1 - W_0) - (1 - \varepsilon_1' + \varepsilon_2')/2|}{\hat{\nu}_N} = \frac{\sqrt{462}\,|.52093 - .5|}{.918898} = .489579.$$

As the critical upper bound which $\sqrt{N}\,|W_+/(1 - W_0) - (1 - \varepsilon_1' + \varepsilon_2')/2|/\hat{\nu}_N$ has to be compared to at the 5%-level, the program yields the value 0.70545 which clearly exceeds the observed value of the test statistic. Thus, the results of the study warrant rejection of the null hypothesis that there is a nonnegligible association between the polymorphism under study and alcohol dependence.

Simulation Study

Samples from rounded normal distributions. In numerous applications, occurrence of ties between quantitative observations can suitably be accounted for by numerical rounding processes which the associated "latent" values on some underlying continuous measurement scale are subject to. If the underlying continuous variables have Gaussian distributions with unit variance and rounding is done to the nearest multiple of some fixed rational number r, say, then the distribution of the observable discrete variables is given by a probability mass function of the form

$$p_{\mu;r}(z) = \int_{z-r/2}^{z+r/2} \frac{1}{\sqrt{2\pi}} \exp\{-(u - \mu)^2/2\}\, du\,, \quad z = j\,r, \; j \in \mathbb{Z}. \quad (6.36)$$

In the sequel, we will call any distribution of this form a rounded normal distribution and write $Z \sim \mathcal{N}_r(\mu, 1)$ for a discrete random variable Z having mass function (6.36).

In a first set of simulation experiments on the generalized Mann-Whitney test for equivalence with discretized normally distributed data, rounding was done to nearest multiples of $r = 1/4$. Whereas the Y_j were generated by rounding standard normal random numbers, three different specifications of μ were used for generating the X_i:

$$\text{(a)} \quad \mu = -.695; \quad \text{(b)} \quad \mu = +.695; \quad \text{(c)} \quad \mu = 0.$$

The number $-.695$ was determined by means of a numerical search algorithm as that value of μ which ensures that $X_i \sim \mathcal{N}_{1/4}(\mu, 1)$, $Y_j \sim \mathcal{N}_{1/4}(0, 1) \Rightarrow \pi_+/(1 - \pi_0) = .30$. By symmetry, it follows that $\left(\mathcal{N}_{1/4}(.695, 1), \mathcal{N}_{1/4}(0, 1)\right)$ is a specific pair of distributions belonging to the right-hand boundary of the hypotheses (6.21) for the choice $\varepsilon_1' = \varepsilon_2' = .20$. Of course, generating both the X_i and the Y_j as samples from $\mathcal{N}_{1/4}(0, 1)$ provides a basis for studying the power of the test against the specific alternative that $\pi_+/(1 - \pi_0) = 1/2$.

As another setting involving samples from rounded normal distributions we investigated the case $r = 1$, i.e., rounding to the nearest integer which of course produces a much higher rate π_0 of ties between X's and Y's. For $r = 1$, the nonnull μ's corresponding to $\pi_+/(1-\pi_0) = .30$ and $\pi_+/(1-\pi_0) = .70$ are computed to be $\mp.591$. The mass functions of the three elements of the family $\{\mathcal{N}_1(\mu, 1) \,|\, \mu \in \mathbb{R}\}$ corresponding to $\mu = -.591$, $\mu = 0$ and $\mu = +.591$ are depicted in Figure 6.1.

Tables 6.7a, b show the rejection probabilities of the generalized Wilcoxon test for equivalence at nominal level $\alpha = .05$ at both boundaries of the hypotheses ($\rightarrow$ size) and the centre of the equivalence range ($\rightarrow$ power) found in $100{,}000$ replications of the simulation experiments performed with data from rounded normal distributions. The results suggest that the test keeps the nominal significance level even when both sample sizes are fairly small. Furthermore, for given sample sizes the power of the test decreases markedly with the proportion of ties between observations from different populations.

Table 6.7a *Simulated rejection probabilities with data from normal distributions rounded to the nearest multiple of .25 (from Wellek and Hampel, 1999, with kind permission by Wiley-VCH)*

m	n	Rejection Prob. at $\pi_+/(1 - \pi_0)$ = .30	Rejection Prob. at $\pi_+/(1 - \pi_0)$ = .70	Power at $\pi_+/(1 - \pi_0)$ = .50
20	20	.04429	.04374	.36408
40	40	.04337	.04279	.79949
60	60	.04245	.04253	.95070
10	90	.04830	.04959	.23361

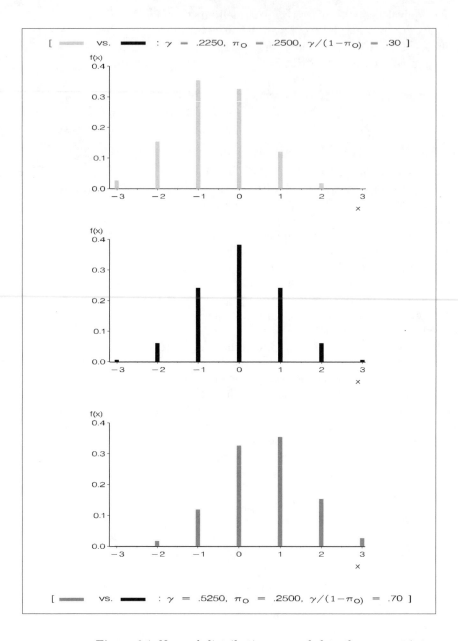

Figure 6.1 *Normal distributions rounded to the nearest integer*
with $\mu = -.695$ (   ), $\mu = 0$ (   ),   and $\mu = .695$ (   ).
(From Wellek and Hampel, 1999, with kind permission by
Wiley-VCH.)

Table 6.7b *Simulated rejection probabilities with data from normal distributions rounded to the nearest integer (from Wellek and Hampel, 1999, with kind permission by Wiley-VCH)*

m	n	Rejection Prob. at $\pi_+/(1-\pi_0)$ = .30	Rejection Prob. at $\pi_+/(1-\pi_0)$ = .70	Power at $\pi_+/(1-\pi_0)$ = .50
20	20	.04277	.04378	.20246
40	40	.04212	.04216	.54873
60	60	.04247	.04248	.80174
10	90	.04664	.04681	.18361

Lehmann alternatives to discrete uniform distributions. Another parametric submodel of considerable interest for purposes of investigating the small sample properties of the test under consideration is given by the class of Lehmann alternatives to the uniform distribution on the set $\{1,\dots,k\}$ of the first k natural numbers ($k \in \mathbb{N}$, fixed). By definition, each distribution belonging to this class has a probability mass function of the form

$$p_{\theta;k}(j) = (j/k)^\theta - ((j-1)/k)^\theta, \quad j = 1,\dots,k, \quad \theta > 0. \quad (6.37)$$

The symbol $\mathcal{U}_k(\theta)$ is to denote any specific distribution of that form.

In the first part of the simulations referring to the model (6.37), the number of mass points was fixed at $k = 6$, and the parameter θ varied over the set $\{\theta_1, \theta_2, \theta_0\}$ with

$$\text{(a)} \quad \theta_1 = .467; \quad \text{(b)} \quad \theta_2 = 2.043; \quad \text{(c)} \quad \theta_0 = 1.$$

These values were determined in such a way that for $\varepsilon_1' = \varepsilon_2' = .20$, the pair $(\mathcal{U}_6(\theta_1), \mathcal{U}_6(\theta_0))$ and $(\mathcal{U}_6(\theta_2), \mathcal{U}_6(\theta_0))$ belongs to the left- and the right-hand boundary of the hypotheses (6.21), respectively. Bar charts of the corresponding probability mass functions are displayed in Figure 6.2.

The second half of the results shown in Table 6.8 for data generated from probability mass functions of the form (6.37) relates to Lehmann alternatives to the uniform distribution on the set $\{1, 2, 3\}$. In the case of these much coarser distributions, the values ensuring that $X_i \sim \mathcal{U}_3(\theta_1), Y_j \sim \mathcal{U}_3(1) \Rightarrow \pi_+/(1-\pi_0) = .30$ and $X_i \sim \mathcal{U}_3(\theta_2), Y_j \sim \mathcal{U}_3(1) \Rightarrow \pi_+/(1-\pi_0) = .70$ were computed to be $\theta_1 = .494$ and $\theta_2 = 1.860$, respectively. Again, the nominal significance level was set to $\alpha = .05$ throughout, and all rejection probabilities listed in the tables are based on 100,000 replications. Essentially, we are led to the same conclusions as suggested by the results for the rounding error model with underlying Gaussian distributions: For balanced designs, the generalized Mann-Whitney test for equivalence guarantees

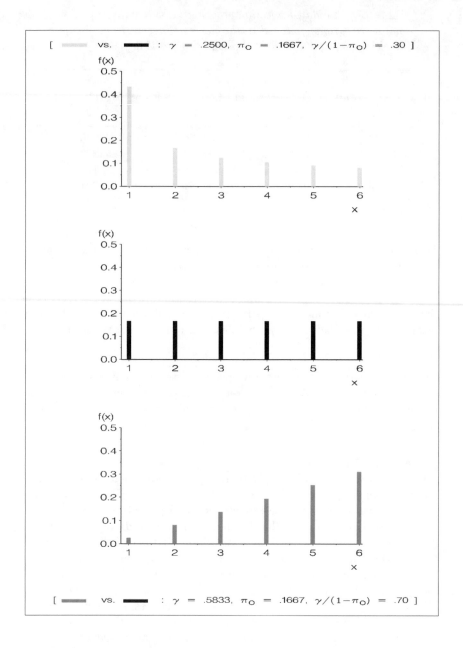

Figure 6.2 *Lehmann alternatives to the uniform distribution on* $\{1,\ldots,6\}$
with $\theta = .467$ (━━), $\theta = 1$ (━━), *and* $\theta = 2.043$ (━━).
(From Wellek and Hampel, 1999, with kind permission by Wiley-VCH.)

Table 6.8a *Simulated rejection probabilities under Lehmann alternatives to the uniform distribution on $\{1, 2, \ldots, 6\}$ (from Wellek and Hampel, 1999, with kind permission by Wiley-VCH)*

m	n	Rejection Prob. at $\pi_+/(1-\pi_0)$ $= .30$	Rejection Prob. at $\pi_+/(1-\pi_0)$ $= .70$	Power at $\pi_+/(1-\pi_0)$ $= .50$
20	20	.04500	.04312	.26757
40	40	.04266	.04202	.68698
60	60	.04184	.04201	.89465
10	90	.04838	.05230	.25194
90	10	.04370	.04544	.24936

Table 6.8b *Simulated rejection probabilities under Lehmann alternatives to the uniform distribution on $\{1, 2, 3\}$ (from Wellek and Hampel, 1999, with kind permission by Wiley-VCH)*

m	n	Rejection Prob. at $\pi_+/(1-\pi_0)$ $= .30$	Rejection Prob. at $\pi_+/(1-\pi_0)$ $= .70$	Power at $\pi_+/(1-\pi_0)$ $= .50$
20	20	.04531	.04566	.17858
40	40	.04270	.04321	.45012
60	60	.04149	.03984	.72160
10	90	.04690	.04772	.15050
90	10	.04203	.04212	.15188

the nominal significance level even when both sample sizes are as small as 20. However, the rejection probability found in the case $k = 6$, $(m, n) = (10, 90)$ at the right-hand boundary of the hypotheses shows that the test is not in general strictly conservative.

Remark. It is worth noticing that ranking the four tables 6.7a – 6.8b with respect to the power of the test at the centre of the equivalence interval yields for every combination of sample sizes the same ordering, namely $(6.8b) \ll (6.7b) \ll (6.8a) \ll (6.7a)$. This is exactly the ordering obtained by arranging the associated values of the tie probability π_0 into a decreasing sequence: Straightforward computations show that π_0 takes on value .333, .250, .167 and .062 for $\mathcal{U}_3, \mathcal{N}_1, \mathcal{U}_6$ and $\mathcal{N}_{1/4}$, respectively.

6.4 Testing for dispersion equivalence of two Gaussian distributions

In routine applications of the most frequently used inferential procedures, the preliminary check on the homogeneity of variances of two Gaussian distributions as a prerequisite for the validity of the classical two-sample t-test consists of an "inverted" conventional test of the null hypothesis of equality of both variances. In other words, the usual F-test is carried out and homogeneity of variances taken for granted whenever the result turns out insignificant. In this section we derive an optimal testing procedure tailored for establishing the alternative hypothesis that the variances, say σ^2 and τ^2, of two normal distributions from which independent samples $X_1, \ldots, X_m$ and $Y_1, \ldots, Y_n$ have been taken, coincide up to irrelevant discrepancies. The region of still tolerable heterogeneity between σ^2 and τ^2 is defined as a sufficiently short interval around 1 which has to cover the true value of the ratio σ^2/τ^2. Accordingly, the present section deals with the problem of testing

$$H : 0 < \sigma^2/\tau^2 \leq \omega_1^2 \quad \text{or} \quad \omega_2^2 \leq \sigma^2/\tau^2 < \infty$$

$$\text{versus} \qquad K : \omega_1^2 < \sigma^2/\tau^2 < \omega_2^2 \tag{6.38}$$

by means of two independent samples $(X_1, \ldots, X_m), (Y_1, \ldots, Y_n)$ such that

$$X_i \sim \mathcal{N}(\xi, \sigma^2), \quad i = 1, \ldots, m, \quad Y_j \sim \mathcal{N}(\eta, \tau^2), \quad j = 1, \ldots, n. \tag{6.39}$$

Of course, the tolerances ω_1^2, ω_2^2 making up the common boundary of the two hypotheses of (6.38) are assumed to be fixed positive numbers satisfying $\omega_1^2 < 1 < \omega_2^2$.

Obviously, (6.38) remains invariant under the same group of transformations as the corresponding one-sided testing problem treated in Lehmann (1986, p. 290, Example 6). By the results established there we know that a test for (6.38) which is uniformly most powerful among all level-α tests invariant under transformations of the form $(X_1, \ldots, X_m, Y_1, \ldots, Y_n) \mapsto (a + bx_1, \ldots, a + bx_m, c + dy_1, \ldots, c + dy_n)$ with $-\infty < a, c < \infty, b, d \neq 0, |b| = |d|$, can be obtained in the following way: In a first step, the raw data $X_1, \ldots, X_m, Y_1, \ldots, Y_n$ are reduced to the statistic

$$Q = S_X^2/S_Y^2 := \frac{n-1}{m-1} \sum_{i=1}^{m} (X_i - \bar{X})^2 / \sum_{j=1}^{n} (Y_j - \bar{Y})^2 \tag{6.40}$$

which the ordinary F-test of the null hypothesis $\sigma^2/\tau^2 = 1$ is based upon. Under The Gaussian model (6.39), the distribution of Q is an element of the scale family associated with the central F-distribution with $\nu_1 = m-1$, $\nu_2 = n-1$ degrees of freedom, and the scale parameter ϱ, say, is related to the variances we want to compare simply by $\varrho = \sigma^2/\tau^2$. Hence, the testing problem (6.38) can be rewritten as

$$\tilde{H} : 0 < \varrho \leq \varrho_1 \vee \varrho_2 \leq \varrho < \infty \text{ versus } \tilde{K} : \varrho_1 < \varrho < \varrho_2 \qquad \widetilde{(6.38)}$$

with $\varrho_k = \omega_k^2$, $k = 1, 2$. If an UMP level-α test exists for $\widetilde{(6.38)}$ and is carried out through Q in terms of the original observations $X_1, \ldots, X_m, Y_1, \ldots, Y_n$, then the result is the desired UMPI test at the same level α for (6.38).

Let $R_\circ$ denote a generic random variable following a central F-distribution with (ν_1, ν_2) degrees of freedom, and $f_{\nu_1,\nu_2}(\,\cdot\,; \varrho)$ the density function of $\varrho R_\circ$ for arbitrary $\varrho > 0$. As is rigorously shown in the Appendix [see p. 250], the family $(f_{\nu_1,\nu_2}(\,\cdot\,; \varrho))_{\varrho>0}$ (sometimes called family of "stretched" F-densities in the literature – cf. Witting, 1985, p. 217) is strictly totally positive of any order and hence in particular STP$_3$. Furthermore, continuity of the standard F-density $f_{\nu_1,\nu_2}(\,\cdot\,; 1)$ with the respective numbers of degrees of freedom obviously implies that the function $(q, \varrho) \mapsto f_{\nu_1,\nu_2}(q; \varrho)$ is continuous in both of its arguments. Thus, the family $(f_{\nu_1,\nu_2}(\,\cdot\,; \varrho))_{\varrho>0}$ of densities satisfies all conditions of Theorem A.1.5 [$\to$ p. 251]. Consequently, the desired UMP level-α test for $\widetilde{(6.38)}$ exists indeed and is given by the rejection region

$$\left\{ \tilde{C}^{(1)}_{\alpha;\nu_1,\nu_2}(\varrho_1, \varrho_2) < Q < \tilde{C}^{(2)}_{\alpha;\nu_1,\nu_2}(\varrho_1, \varrho_2) \right\} . \qquad (6.41)$$

The critical constants $\tilde{C}^{(1)}_{\alpha;\nu_1,\nu_2}(\varrho_1, \varrho_2), k = 1, 2$, have to be determined by solving the equations

$$F_{\nu_1,\nu_2}(\tilde{C}_2/\varrho_1) - F_{\nu_1,\nu_2}(\tilde{C}_1/\varrho_1) = \alpha =$$
$$F_{\nu_1,\nu_2}(\tilde{C}_2/\varrho_2) - F_{\nu_1,\nu_2}(\tilde{C}_1/\varrho_2), \ 0 < \tilde{C}_1 < \tilde{C}_2 < \infty, \qquad (6.42)$$

with $F_{\nu_1,\nu_2}(\cdot)$ denoting the cdf of the standard central F-distribution with (ν_1, ν_2) degrees of freedom.

The algorithm for computing the optimal critical constants admits considerable simplification along the lines described on p. 41 provided the equivalence range for ϱ has been chosen as symmetric on the log-scale, and the underlying parallel-group design is balanced with respect to the sample sizes so that the distribution of Q has the same number of degrees of freedom for numerator and denominator, respectively. In fact, for $\nu_1 = \nu_2 = \nu$, we obviously have $Q^{-1} \overset{d}{=} Q$ under $\varrho = 1$, and this implies that the distribution of Q under any $\varrho > 0$ coincides with that of Q^{-1} under ϱ^{-1}. Hence, for $\nu_1 = \nu_2 = \nu$, $\varrho_1 = \varrho_\circ^{-1}$, $\varrho_2 = \varrho_\circ > 1$, specifying $T(\mathbf{X}) = Q$, $\theta = \log \varrho$, $\varepsilon = \log \varrho_\circ$ yields a setting which satisfies both of the conditions (3.10a), (3.10b) for symmetrizing the critical region of the corresponding uniformly most powerful test. Thus, by (3.11), we may reduce (6.41) and (6.42) in the case of a balanced design and symmetric equivalence limits to

$$\left\{ 1/\tilde{C}^{(\mathrm{o})}_{\alpha;\nu}(\varrho_\mathrm{o}) < Q < \tilde{C}^{(\mathrm{o})}_{\alpha;\nu}(\varrho_\mathrm{o}) \right\} , \qquad (6.43)$$

and

$$F_{\nu,\nu}(\tilde{C}/\varrho_\mathrm{o}) - F_{\nu,\nu}(\tilde{C}^{-1}/\varrho_\mathrm{o}) = \alpha , \quad \tilde{C} > 1 , \qquad (6.44)$$

respectively.

Of course, in (6.43), $\tilde{C}^{(\mathrm{o})}_{\alpha;\nu}(\varrho_\mathrm{o})$ stands for the (unique) solution to equation (6.44).

Reducibility of (6.41) to (6.43) in the special case $\nu_1 = \nu_2 = \nu$, $\varrho_1 = \varrho_\mathrm{o}^{-1}$, $\varrho_2 = \varrho_\mathrm{o}$ means that we may write both for $k = 1$ and $k = 2$: $\tilde{C}^{(k)}_{\alpha;\nu,\nu}(\varrho_\mathrm{o}^{-1},\varrho_\mathrm{o}) = 1/\tilde{C}^{(3-k)}_{\alpha;\nu,\nu}(\varrho_\mathrm{o}^{-1},\varrho_\mathrm{o})$. In view of the obvious fact that for any random variable Z_{ν_1,ν_2} following a central F-distribution with (ν_1,ν_2) degrees of freedom, we have $Z_{\nu_1,\nu_2} \overset{d}{=} 1/Z_{\nu_2,\nu_1}$, this reciprocity relation generalizes to

$$\tilde{C}^{(k)}_{\alpha;\nu_1,\nu_2}(\varrho_1,\varrho_2) = 1/\tilde{C}^{(3-k)}_{\alpha;\nu_2,\nu_1}(\varrho_2^{-1},\varrho_1^{-1}), \quad k = 1,2 . \qquad (6.45)$$

Table 6.9 shows the value of the critical constant $\tilde{C}^{(\mathrm{o})}_{.05;\nu}(\varrho_\mathrm{o})$ to be used in the F-test for equivalence at level $\alpha = .05$ in symmetric settings with $\nu_1 = \nu_2 = \nu$ and $\varrho_2 = 1/\varrho_1 = \varrho_\mathrm{o}$, for $\nu = 10(5)75$ and $\varrho_\mathrm{o} = 1.50(.25)2.50$. The corresponding values of the power attained against the alternative that the population variances under comparison are equal ($\leftrightarrow \varrho = 1$), are given in Table 6.10.

In contrast to (6.44) which, in view of monotonic increasingness in $\tilde{C}$ of the expression on the left-hand side, can be solved more or less by trial and error, solving the system (6.42) to be treated in the general case requires appropriate software tools. The SAS program `fstretch` to be found at http://www.zi-mannheim.de/wktsheq, provides for arbitrary choices of α, ν_k and $\varrho_k \, (k = 1,2)$ both the critical constants $\tilde{C}^{(k)}_{\alpha;\nu_1,\nu_2}(\varrho_1,\varrho_2)$ determining the UMPI critical region (6.41), and the power against $\varrho = 1 \, (\leftrightarrow \sigma^2 = \tau^2)$. Basically, the algorithm used by the program is an adaptation of the iteration scheme described in general terms on pp. 39-40, to the specific case that the STP$_3$ family which the distribution of the test statistic belongs to is generated by rescaling a standard central F-distribution with the appropriate numbers of degrees of freedom, in all possible ways.

Table 6.9 *Critical constant* $\tilde{C}^{(\mathrm{o})}_{.05;\,\nu}(\varrho_{\mathrm{o}})$ *of the F-test for dispersion equivalence of two Gaussian distributions at level* $\alpha = 5\%$ *with common sample size* $m = n = \nu + 1$ *and symmetric equivalence range* $(\varrho_{\mathrm{o}}^{-1}, \varrho_{\mathrm{o}})$ *for* $\varrho = \sigma^2/\tau^2$, *for* $\nu = 10(5)75$ *and* $\varrho_{\mathrm{o}} = 1.50(.25)2.50$

			$\varrho_{\mathrm{o}} =$		
ν	1.50	1.75	2.00	2.25	2.50
10	1.05113	1.06165	1.07593	1.09448	1.11796
15	1.04572	1.06048	1.08259	1.11432	1.15830
20	1.04362	1.06328	1.09561	1.14600	1.21867
25	1.04307	1.06849	1.11396	1.18805	1.29055
30	1.04346	1.07566	1.13724	1.23644	1.36110
35	1.04450	1.08461	1.16457	1.28538	1.42349
40	1.04605	1.09529	1.19424	1.33075	1.47701
45	1.04803	1.10756	1.22424	1.37118	1.52302
50	1.05040	1.12122	1.25297	1.40685	1.56300
55	1.05314	1.13590	1.27963	1.43839	1.59816
60	1.05623	1.15116	1.30399	1.46647	1.62939
65	1.05967	1.16654	1.32612	1.49167	1.65740
70	1.06344	1.18165	1.34626	1.51445	1.68272
75	1.06754	1.19620	1.36464	1.53518	1.70576

Example 6.3

In a laboratory specialized in testing basic physical and chemical properties of innovative materials for potential use in dental medicine, the existing device for taking measurements of breaking strengths of solid plastic elements had to be replaced with technically modernized equipment of the same kind. Two systems A and B, say, were taken into final consideration with A being priced markedly lower than B. In view of this, the head of the laboratory decided to take his own data in order to assess the equivalence of both devices with respect to precision of the measurements they provide. For that purpose, a total of 100 sample elements made of the same material were prepared. For one half of the elements, breaking strength was to be measured by means of A, for the other by means of B, respectively. Since all sample elements could be considered identical in physical properties, it was reasonable to regard pure measurement error as the only source of

Table 6.10 *Power attained at $\varrho = 1$ when using the critical constants shown in Table 6.9 for the F-statistic*

ν	$\varrho_o =$ 1.50	1.75	2.00	2.25	2.50
10	.06129	.07350	.08986	.11071	.13650
15	.06786	.08905	.12011	.16328	.22032
20	.07511	.10778	.15978	.23646	.33743
25	.08313	.13024	.21057	.33006	.47162
30	.09198	.15699	.27303	.43531	.59665
35	.10174	.18852	.34530	.53850	.69906
40	.11250	.22510	.42279	.62999	.77824
45	.12433	.26666	.49986	.70663	.83793
50	.13732	.31260	.57194	.76907	.88235
55	.15156	.36179	.63666	.81917	.91509
60	.16710	.41267	.69332	.85903	.93904
65	.18402	.46361	.74219	.89053	.95644
70	.20234	.51317	.78396	.91529	.96902
75	.22207	.56028	.81944	.93466	.97805

variability found in both sequences of values. Out of the 50 measurements to be taken by means of A, only $m = 41$ came to a regular end since the remaining 9 elements broke already during insertion into the device's clamp. By the same reason, the number of values eventually obtained by means of device B was $n = 46$ rather than 50. All measurement values were assumed to be realizations of normally distributed random variables with parameters (ξ, σ^2) [$\leftrightarrow$ device A] and (η, τ^2) [$\leftrightarrow$ device B], respectively. Precision equivalence of both devices was defined through the condition $.75 < \sigma/\tau < 1.33$ on the standard deviations of the underlying distributions. From the raw data [given in kiloponds], the following values of the sample means and variances were computed:

Device A: $\bar{X} = 5.0298$, $S_X^2 = .0766$;
Device B: $\bar{Y} = 4.8901$, $S_Y^2 = .0851$.

Running the *SAS*-macro `fstretch`, one reads from the output list that in the UMPI test at level $\alpha = .05$ for $\sigma^2/\tau^2 \leq .75^2$ or $\sigma^2/\tau^2 \geq 1.33^2$ versus $.75^2 < \sigma^2/\tau^2 < 1.33^2$, the statistic $Q = S_X^2/S_Y^2$ has to be checked for inclusion between the critical bounds $\tilde{C}_{.05;40,45}^{(1)} (.5625, 1.7689) = .8971$, $\tilde{C}_{.05;40,45}^{(2)} (.5625, 1.7689) = 1.1024$. Since the observed value was $Q = .0766/$

.0851 = .9001, the data satisfy the condition for rejecting nonequivalence. However, the power to detect even strict equality of variances was only 26.10 % under the specifications made in this example.

Exploiting the results of Section 6.4 for testing for equivalence of hazard rates in the two-sample setting with exponentially distributed data

There is a close formal relationship between the testing problem put forward at the beginning of this section, and that of testing for equivalence of the hazard rates of two exponential distributions from which independent samples are obtained. In order to make this relationship precise, let us assume that instead of following normal distributions, the observations making up the two samples under analysis satisfy

$$X_i \sim \mathcal{E}(\sigma), \ i = 1, \ldots, m, \quad Y_j \sim \mathcal{E}(\tau), \ j = 1, \ldots, n, \qquad (6.46)$$

where, as before [recall p. 51], $\mathcal{E}(\theta)$ symbolizes a standard exponential distribution with hazard rate $\theta^{-1} > 0$. Let us assume further that the hypotheses on (σ, τ) between which we want to decide by means of these samples, read

$$H : 0 < \sigma/\tau < \varrho_1 \text{ or } \varrho_2 \leq \sigma/\tau < \infty \text{ versus } K : \varrho_1 < \sigma/\tau < \varrho_2. \quad (6.47)$$

Another application of the general results proved in § 6.5 of the book of Lehmann (1986) shows that carrying out the UMP level α-test for (6.38) in terms of $m^{-1} \sum_{i=1}^{m} X_i/n^{-1} \sum_{j=1}^{n} Y_j$ yields a UMPI test for (6.47) at the same level, provided the numbers of degrees of freedom are specified as $\nu_1 = 2m$, $\nu_2 = 2n$ in (6.41) and (6.42). The group of transformations with respect to which the invariance property holds, consists this time of all homogeneous dilations of any point in $(m+n)$-dimensional real space $\mathbb{R}^{m+n}$. In other words, the practical implementation of the UMPI level-α test for equivalence of two exponential distributions with respect to the hazard rates differs from that of the modified F-test for dispersion equivalence of two Gaussian distributions only with respect to the rule for computing the test statistic from the raw observations and for counting the numbers of degrees of freedom. Thus, it is in particular clear that the program `fstretch` also enables us to carry out an optimal two-sample equivalence test for exponentially distributed data.

6.5 Equivalence tests for two binomial samples

6.5.1 Exact tests for equivalence with respect to the odds ratio

As to the assumed basic structure of the data to be analyzed, the present section resumes the exposition given in § 2.3. Thus, we suppose that we are given a 2×2 contingency table of the form shown in Table 2.2 [$\rightarrow$ p. 21]. But now we are interested in establishing two-sided equivalence of the underlying binomial distributions rather than noninferiority of $\mathcal{B}(m, p_1)$ to $\mathcal{B}(n, p_2)$. Measuring, as in § 2.3.1, the distance between both distributions in terms of $|\varrho - 1|$ with $\varrho = p_1(1 - p_2)/(1 - p_1)p_2$, and p_1 and p_2 as the probability of a favourable response to treatment A and B, respectively, the problem of testing for equivalence in the strict sense reads

$$H : 0 < \varrho \leq \varrho_1 \text{ or } \varrho_2 \leq \varrho < \infty \quad \text{versus} \quad K : \varrho_1 < \varrho < \varrho_2 . \qquad (6.48)$$

Of course, the limits ϱ_1, ϱ_2 of the equivalence range for the odds ratio ϱ have to be specified as positive real numbers satisfying $\varrho_1 < 1 < \varrho_2$. If we keep denoting the number of experimental units responding to treatment A and B by X and Y, respectively, then independence of X and Y implies that the joint probability mass function of both variables can be written

$$P[X = x, Y = y] = \binom{m}{x} \binom{n}{y} (1 - p_1)^m (1 - p_2)^n$$

$$\exp \left\{ x \log \left[\frac{p_1(1 - p_2)}{(1 - p_1)p_2} \right] + (x + y) \log[p_2/(1 - p_2)] \right\},$$

$$(x, y) \in \{0, \ldots, m\} \times \{0, \ldots, n\} . \quad (6.49)$$

Letting $\theta = \log \varrho = \log[p_1(1 - p_2)/(1 - p_1)p_2]$, $\vartheta = \log[p_2/(1 - p_2)]$, it is easily verified that we have $1 - p_1 = (1 + e^{\theta + \vartheta})^{-1}$, $1 - p_2 = (1 + e^{\vartheta})^{-1}$ and hence $(1 - p_1)^m (1 - p_2)^n = (1 + e^{\theta + \vartheta})^{-m} (1 + e^{\vartheta})^{-n}$. If the joint density of (X, Y) is defined with respect to the measure $B^{(2)} \mapsto \sum_{(x,y) \in B^{(2)} \cap \{0,\ldots,m\} \times \{0,\ldots,n\}} \binom{m}{x} \binom{n}{y}$ on the σ-algebra of Borel sets in $\mathbb{R}^2$ rather than the counting measure of the set $\{0, 1, \ldots, m\} \times \{0, 1, \ldots, n\}$, we thus obtain the expression

$$p_{\theta, \vartheta}(x, y) = (1 + e^{\theta + \vartheta})^{-m} (1 + e^{\vartheta})^{-n} \exp\{x\theta + (x + y)\vartheta\} . \qquad (6.50)$$

Obviously, (6.50) defines the generic element of a family of densities of the form considered in § A.2 [see in particular equation (A.16)] with $k = 1$, $T = X$, $S = X + Y$. In other words, the densities (6.50) make up a two-parameter exponential family in $\theta = \log \varrho$, $\vartheta = \log[p_2/(1 - p_2)]$ with X and $S = X + Y$ as a statistic sufficient for θ and ϑ, respectively.

Hence, Theorem A.2.2 [$\rightarrow$ p. 255] does apply implying that a uniformly most powerful unbiased (UMPU) level-α test for (6.48) is obtained by proceeding for each of the possible values $s \in \{0, 1, \ldots, m + n\}$ of the first column total S according to the following decision rule:

$$
\begin{cases}
\text{Rejection of } H & \text{if } C_{1;\alpha}^{m,n}(s;\, \varrho_1, \varrho_2) < \\
& \qquad X < C_{2;\alpha}^{m,n}(s;\, \varrho_1, \varrho_2) \\
\text{Reject with prob. } \gamma_{1;\alpha}^{m,n}(s;\, \varrho_1, \varrho_2) & \text{if } X = C_{1;\alpha}^{m,n}(s;\, \varrho_1, \varrho_2) \\
\text{Reject with prob. } \gamma_{2;\alpha}^{m,n}(s;\, \varrho_1, \varrho_2) & \text{if } X = C_{2;\alpha}^{m,n}(s;\, \varrho_1, \varrho_2) \\
\text{Acceptance of } H & \text{if } X < C_{1;\alpha}^{m,n}(s;\, \varrho_1, \varrho_2) \\
& \qquad \text{or } X > C_{2;\alpha}^{m,n}(s;\, \varrho_1, \varrho_2)
\end{cases}
\qquad (6.51)
$$

The critical constants $C_{\nu;\alpha}^{m,n}(s;\, \varrho_1, \varrho_2)$, $\gamma_{\nu;\alpha}^{m,n}(s;\, \varrho_1, \varrho_2)$, $\nu = 1, 2$, have to be determined for each s by solving the equations

$$
\sum_{x=C_1+1}^{C_2-1} h_s^{m,n}(x;\, \varrho_1) + \sum_{\nu=1}^{2} \gamma_\nu h_s^{m,n}(C_\nu;\, \varrho_1) = \alpha = \sum_{x=C_1+1}^{C_2-1} h_s^{m,n}(x;\, \varrho_2)
$$

$$
+ \sum_{\nu=1}^{2} \gamma_\nu h_s^{m,n}(C_\nu;\, \varrho_2), \quad 0 \le C_1 \le C_2 \le m, \ 0 \le \gamma_1, \gamma_2 < 1. \quad (6.52)
$$

For any value $\varrho \in \mathbb{R}_+$ taken on by the true population odds ratio $p_1(1 - p_2)/(1 - p_1)p_2$, $h_s^{m,n}(\,\cdot\,;\varrho)$ stands for the probability mass function of the distribution of X conditional on the event $\{S = s\}$. As was already stated in § 2.3, this conditional distribution is a so-called extended hypergeometric distribution given by

$$
h_s^{m,n}(x;\, \varrho) = \binom{m}{x}\binom{n}{s-x}\varrho^x \Big/ \sum_{j=\max\{0,s-n\}}^{\min\{s,m\}} \binom{m}{j}\binom{n}{s-j}\varrho^j,
$$

$$
\max\{0, s - n\} \le x \le \min\{s, m\}. \quad (6.53)
$$

In the balanced case of equal sample sizes $m = n$, it is easy to verify that the conditional distributions of X satisfy the symmetry relation

$$
h_s^{n,n}(s - x;\, \varrho^{-1}) = h_s^{n,n}(x;\, \varrho),
$$

$$
\max\{0, s - n\} \le x \le \min\{s, n\}, \ s = 0, 1, \dots, 2n. \quad (6.54)
$$

In view of (6.54) and Corollary A.1.7 [$\to$ p. 252–3], in the case of a balanced design with common size n of both samples and a symmetric equivalence range, say $(\varrho_\circ^{-1}, \varrho_\circ)$ for the population odds ratio ϱ, the decision rule (6.51) defining a UMPU level-α test for (6.48) can be simplified to

$$
\begin{cases}
\text{Rejection of } H & \text{if } |X - s/2| < C(n, s;\, \varrho_\circ, \alpha) \\
\text{Reject with prob. } \gamma(n, s;\, \varrho_\circ, \alpha) & \text{if } |X - s/2| = C(n, s;\, \varrho_\circ, \alpha) \\
\text{Acceptance of } H & \text{if } |X - s/2| > C(n, s;\, \varrho_\circ, \alpha)
\end{cases}
\quad (6.55)
$$

Of the two critical constants appearing in (6.54), the first one has to be determined as

$$C(n, s; \varrho_\mathrm{o}, \alpha) = C^* = \max \left\{ C \,\middle|\, s/2 - C, s/2 + C \in \mathbb{N}_\mathrm{o}, \, s/2 - C \geq \right.$$

$$\left. \max\{0, s - n\}, s/2 + C \leq \min\{s, n\}, \sum_{x=s/2-C+1}^{s/2+C-1} h_s^{n,n}(x; \varrho_\mathrm{o}) \leq \alpha \right\}. \quad (6.56)$$

As soon as the correct value of the critical upper bound $C^* \equiv C(n, s; \varrho_\mathrm{o}, \alpha)$ to $|X - s/2|$ has been found, the randomization probability $\gamma(n, s; \varrho_\mathrm{o}, \alpha)$ can be computed by means of the explicit formula

$$\gamma(n, s; \varrho_\mathrm{o}, \alpha) = \left(\alpha - \sum_{x=s/2-C^*+1}^{s/2+C^*-1} h_s^{n,n}(x; \varrho_\mathrm{o}) \right) \Big/$$

$$\left(h_s^{n,n}(s/2 - C^*; \varrho_\mathrm{o}) + h_s^{n,n}(s/2 + C^*; \varrho_\mathrm{o}) \right). \quad (6.57)$$

Furthermore, the condition for sure rejection of the null hypothesis given in (6.55) can alternatively be expressed in terms of a conditional p-value to be computed as

$$p_{n;\varrho_\mathrm{o}}(x|s) = \sum_{j=s-\tilde{x}_s}^{\tilde{x}_s} h_s^{n,n}(j; \varrho_\mathrm{o}) \quad (6.58)$$

where $h_s^{n,n}(x; \varrho_\mathrm{o})$ is obtained by specializing (6.53) in the obvious way, and the upper summation limit is given by

$$\tilde{x}_s = \max\{x, s - x\} \, . \quad (6.59)$$

In fact, it is readily verified that the observed value x of X satisfies $|x - s/2| < C(n, s; \varrho_\mathrm{o}, \alpha)$ if and only if the conditional p-value (6.58) does not exceed α.

The system (6.51) of equations which determines the critical constants of the exact Fisher type equivalence test in the general case, is of the same form as that which had to be treated in a previous chapter [see p. 56, (4.19)] in the context of the one-sample binomial test for equivalence. Correspondingly, the algorithm proposed for solving the latter can be adopted for handling (6.51) with comparatively few modifications. Of course, the most conspicuous change is that the functions $x \mapsto h_s^{m,n}(x; \varrho_\nu)$ have to replace the binomial probability mass functions $x \mapsto b(x; n, p_\nu)$ ($\nu = 1, 2$). Since the equivalence range for ϱ was assumed to be an interval covering unity, we can expect that an interval (C_1, C_2) satisfying (6.51) when combined with a suitable $(\gamma_1, \gamma_2) \in [0, 1)^2$, contains that point $x_\mathrm{o} \in [\max\{0, s - n\}, \min\{s, m\}]$ which, as an entry into a contingency table with first column total s, yields an observed odds ratio exactly equal to 1. Elementary algebra shows that this number is $x_\mathrm{o} = ms/(m + n)$. For the purpose of searching iteratively for the solution of (6.51), $C_1^\circ = [\![x_\mathrm{o}]\!] + 5$ proved to be a suitable choice of an initial value of the left-hand critical bound to X in numerous trials of the algorithm. Once more, *SAS* provides a particularly well suited programming environment for the implementation of such a numerical procedure. The reason is that the *SAS* system has built in an intrinsic function for the cdf of any extended hypergeometric distribution with probability mass function given by (6.53). A complete *SAS* macro allowing to compute for any $s \in \{0, 1, \ldots, m+n\}$ the critical constants of the optimal conditional test for equivalence of $\mathcal{B}(m, p_1)$ and $\mathcal{B}(n, p_2)$ with respect to the odds ratio, can be found at http://www.zi-mannheim.de/wktsheq under the program name `bi2st`.

The computational issues to be tackled in connection with power analysis and sample size determination for the exact Fisher type test for equivalence are basically the same as those we had to consider in §2.3 with regard to the noninferiority version of the procedure. The major modification to be effected in the two-sided case is that in the numerator of the expression for the conditional power $[\to$ p. 23, (2.4)$]$, $\{j \geq k_\alpha(s) + 1\}$ has to be replaced with the summation region $\{C_{1;\alpha}^{m,n}(s; \varrho_1, \varrho_2) + 1 \leq j \leq C_{2;\alpha}^{m,n}(s; \varrho_1, \varrho_2) - 1\}$ bounded on both sides, and the properly weighted probability of the single point $k_\alpha(s)$ with a weighted sum of the probabilities of the two boundary points of the s-section of the critical region. As before the nonconditional power is obtained by integrating the function $s \mapsto \beta(p_1^*, p_2^* | s)$ assigning to each $s \in \{0, 1, \ldots, m + n\}$ the conditional power given $\{S = s\}$, with respect to the distribution of $S = X + Y$ under the specific alternative $(p_1^*, p_2^*) \in (0, 1)^2$ of interest. In view of the large number of steps involving computation of extended hypergeometric and binomial probabilities, respectively, the results obtained by means of this algorithm will be numerically reliable only if the precision of each intermediate result is kept as high as possible. This is again a reason for not relying on predefined procedures for the respective cdf's as provided by *SAS* but to use self-written routines exploiting extended-precision floating-point arithmetic from the beginning. Accordingly, the programs provided at http://www.zi-mannheim.de/wktsheq for computing power and minimally required sample sizes for the Fisher type test for equivalence of two binomial distributions were coded in Fortran. The procedure named `bi2aeq1` performs the task of computing the power against any specific alternative $(p_1^*, p_2^*) \in \{(p_1, p_2) \in (0, 1)^2 | (p_1(1 - p_2)/(1 - p_1)p_2) \in (\varrho_1, \varrho_2)\}$. It accommodates total sample sizes $N = m + n$ of up to 2000. The other program, `bi2aeq2`, determines for a given specific alternative (p_1^*, p_2^*) and prespecified power β^* to be attained against it, the smallest sample sizes (m^*, n^*) required to guarantee that the rejection probability of the test does not fall short of β^*, subject to the side condition that the ratio of both sample sizes equals some arbitrarily fixed positive value λ. Except for the iterative determination of the critical constants to be used at each possible value of the conditioning statistic S and the above-mentioned modifications referring to the computation of the conditional power, the Fortran program `bi2aeq1` and `bi2aeq2` is a direct analogue of the corresponding program `bi2ste1` and `bi2ste2` for the exact Fisher type test for noninferiority, respectively.

Example 6.4

In a test preliminary to the final confirmatory assessment of the data obtained from a controlled comparative multicenter trial of the calcium blocking agent verapamil and a classical diuretic drug with respect to antihypertensive efficacy, it was the aim to rule out the possibility that patients with and without some previous antihypertensive treatment differ to a relevant extent in the probability of a favourable response to the actual medication. Table 6.11 shows the frequencies of responders and nonresponders observed in both strata of the study population during an 8 weeks' titration period. The equivalence range for the odds ratio ϱ characterizing the underlying (sub–)populations was set to $(\varrho_1, \varrho_2) = (.6667, 1.5000)$, following the

Table 6.11 *Responder rates observed in the VERDI trial (Holzgreve et al., 1989) during an 8 weeks' titration period in patients with and without previous antihypertensive treatment*

Previous treatment with antihypertensive drugs	Response to trial medication +	–	Σ
yes	108 (48.00%)	117 (52.00%)	225 (100.0%)
no	63 (52.94%)	56 (47.06%)	119 (100.0%)
Σ	171	173	344

tentative guidelines of § 1.5 for specifying the tolerances in formulating equivalence hypotheses about target parameters and functionals frequently studied in practice. The significance level was chosen as usual specifying $\alpha = .05$. With $m = 225$, $n = 119$, $s = 179$ and the specified values of the ϱ_ν, the *SAS* macro `bi2st` outputs the critical interval (110, 113) and the probabilities .0021, .6322 of a randomized decision in favour of equivalence to be taken if it happens that $X = 110$ and $X = 113$, respectively. Since the observed value of X remained below the left-hand limit of the critical interval, the data shown in Table 6.11 do not allow to reject the null hypothesis that there are relevant differences between patients with and without previous antihypertensive treatment with respect to the probability of a positive response to the study medication. Running the Fortran program bi2aeq1, the power of the UMPU test against the specific alternative that the true responder rates p_1 and p_2 coincide with the observed proportions .4800 and .5294, is computed to be as small as 16.19%. If the nonrandomized conservative version of the test is used this value drops even to 10.70%.

A selection of results on sample sizes required in the exact Fisher type test for equivalence to maintain some prespecified power against fixed alternatives on the diagonal of the unit square are shown in Table 6.12. All entries into the rightmost columns have been computed by means of the Fortran program bi2aeq2. One interesting fact becoming obvious from these results is that the efficiency of the test decreases with the distance of the common value of p_1 and p_2 from the centre of the unit interval. Furthermore, the order of magnitude of the sample sizes appearing in the lower half of the table corroborates the view that the requirement $2/3 < \varrho < 3/2$ corresponds to a rather strict criterion of equivalence of two

Table 6.12 *Sample sizes required in the exact Fisher type test for equivalence at level $\alpha = .05$ to maintain a prespecified power against selected alternatives $p_1 = p_2 = p_*$ on the diagonal of the unit square, for the balanced $[\leftrightarrow \lambda = m/n = 1]$ and various unbalanced designs $[\leftrightarrow \lambda > 1]$*

(ϱ_1, ϱ_2)	p_*	POW	λ	m	n	$N = m + n$
$(.4286, 2.3333)^\dagger$	.50	.80	1.00	98	98	196
"	.40	"	1.00	102	102	204
"	.30	"	1.00	117	117	234
"	.20	"	1.00	156	156	312
"	.10	"	1.00	281	281	562
$(.6667, 1.5000)$	.50	.60	1.00	302	302	604
"	.50	"	1.25	340	272	612
"	.50	"	1.50	377	251	628
"	.50	"	2.00	454	227	681
"	.50	"	3.00	606	202	808

$^\dagger \approx (3/7, 7/3)$ – cf. p. 12

binomial distributions, as suggested in § 1.5 [recall Table 1.1 (iii)]. Finally, it is worth noticing that keeping both the equivalence range (ϱ_1, ϱ_2) and the specific alternative of interest fixed, the total sample size $N = m + n$ increases with the ratio λ of the larger over the smaller of both group sizes.

6.5.2 An improved nonrandomized version of the UMPU test

Nonrandomized versions of UMPU tests for discrete families of distributions obtained by incorporating the whole boundary of the rejection into the acceptance region, are notoriously conservative except for unusually large sample sizes. This is in particular true for the exact Fisher type test for equivalence in the strict, i.e., two-sided sense of two binomial distributions as presented in the previous subsection. Fortunately, it will turn out that the conceptually most simple trick of raising the nominal conditional significance level by the maximum allowable amount, which leads to considerable improvements to the nonrandomized Fisher type test for the noninferiority setting [recall § 2.3.2], works in the present context as well. Apart from showing also the power of both the conventional and the improved nonrandomized version of the UMPU test, Table 6.13 is the direct two-sided analogue to Table 2.4 of § 2.3.2. It refers likewise to balanced designs with common sample sizes ranging over the whole spectrum of what is realistic for practical applications. The upper and the lower half of the table refers to what has been proposed in § 1.5 as a strict and liberal choice of a symmetric equivalence range for the odds ratio, respectively.

All values appearing in the third column of Table 6.13 as a maximally raised nominal significance level α^* have been computed by means of another Fortran program named bi2aeq3 which is the analogue to bi2ste3 for equivalence testing in the strict sense. The program enables its user to find maximally increased nominal levels for arbitrary combinations of values of $\alpha, \varrho_{\circ}, m$ and n, provided the total sample size $N = m + n$ does not exceed 2000. As to the numerical accuracy attained in computing a maximally raised nominal level for any given configuration $(\alpha, \varrho_{\circ}, m, n)$, the situation is once more strictly analogous to that described in connection with the noninferiority case: there is always a whole interval of nominal levels over which the exact size of the nonrandomized conditional test remains constant so that it suffices to ensure that the resulting value is contained in that interval. Furthermore, a tolerance of 0.1% was specified throughout for a practically negligible anticonservatism of the improved nonrandomized test.

Going through the fourth and fifth column of Table 6.13, one finds that even with sample sizes as large as 250 there remains a substantial margin for adjusting the size of the nonrandomized conditional test. In many cases, the gain in power achieved by raising the nominal over the target significance

Table 6.13 *Nominal significance level, size and power against $p_1 = p_2 = 1/2$ of an improved nonrandomized Fisher type test for the problem (6.48) maintaining significance level $\alpha = 5\%$, for $\varrho_1 = \varrho_\circ^{-1}$, $\varrho_2 = \varrho_\circ = 1.5000, 2.3333$, and $m = n = 25(25)100(50)250$ [Numbers in parentheses refer to the ordinary nonrandomized version of the exact Fisher type test using nominal level .05]*

$\varrho_\circ$	n	α^*	Size		Power against $p_1 = p_2 = 1/2$	
1.5000	25	.17300	.03717	(.00000)	.04804	(.00000)
"	50	.12000	.05017	(.00000)	.07959	(.00000)
"	75	.12000	.04582	(.00000)	.06504	(.00000)
"	100	.08188	.05052	(.03915)	.13916	(.05635)
"	150	.06500	.05079	(.04059)	.22695	(.13747)
"	200	.05875	.05041	(.04153)	.34462	(.27361)
"	250	.05891	.05005	(.04199)	.47284	(.43801)
2.3333	25	.14989	.04893	(.00000)	.13629	(.00000)
"	50	.07500	.05054	(.02910)	.38233	(.23560)
"	75	.06875	.05060	(.03576)	.63079	(.53742)
"	100	.06250	.05020	(.03834)	.81869	(.77034)
"	150	.05875	.04941	(.04064)	.95357	(.94298)
"	200	.06000	.04972	(.04104)	.98929	(.98580)
"	250	.05812	.04968	(.04352)	.99771	(.99721)

level exhibits an order of magnitude in view of which one has clearly to discourage from using the nonrandomized test in its conventional form for real applications.

6.5.3 Tests for equivalence with respect to the difference of success probabilities

On the one hand, we argued in § 1.4 [recall in particular Figure 1.1 of p. 9] that the odds ratio is much better suited for measuring the dissimilarity of any two binomial distributions $\mathcal{B}(m, p_1)$ and $\mathcal{B}(n, p_2)$ than the raw difference $p_1 - p_2$ of both success probabilities. On the other hand, experience of consulting statisticians shows that there is still a large number of applied researchers considering the odds ratio as a mysterious mathematical construct whose introduction into real data analysis should better be avoided. Although the reservation about relying on the parametrization through $p_1 - p_2$ does not lose its justification by this fact, one can hardly ignore that there is considerable practical need for establishing a satisfactory solution also for the problem of testing

$$H : -1 < \delta \leq -\delta_1 \text{ or } \delta_2 \leq \delta < 1 \text{ versus } K : -\delta_1 < \delta < \delta_2 , \qquad (6.60)$$

where

$$\delta = p_1 - p_2 , \qquad (6.61)$$

and δ_1, δ_2 denote fixed numbers to be chosen from the open unit interval.

In contrast to the odds ratio $\varrho = p_1(1 - p_2)/(1 - p_1)p_2$, the simple difference δ of both success probabilities is not a mathematically natural parameter for the underlying class of products of two binomial distributions. Accordingly, we will not be able to exploit one of the major theoretical results presented in the Appendix for deriving an optimal solution to (6.60). Instead, we will adopt the basic idea behind the approach taken in § 5.2 to constructing a valid test for equivalence with respect to δ of two binomial distributions from which a sample of paired observations is available. In the case of two independent samples we have now to deal with, a test statistic for (6.60) which satisfies the conditions of Theorem A.3.4 is given by

$$\frac{|T_N - (\delta_2 - \delta_1)/2|}{\hat{\tau}_N} =$$

$$\frac{|(X/m - Y/n) - (\delta_2 - \delta_1)/2|}{[(1/m)(X/m)(1 - X/m) + (1/n)(Y/n)(1 - Y/n)]^{1/2}} , \qquad (6.62)$$

where the subscript N to which all limiting operations apply, denotes this time the total sample size $m + n$. Accordingly, the two-sample analogue of the decision rule (5.9) obtained in the McNemar setting, reads as follows:

Reject nonequivalence if and only if

$$\frac{|(X/m - Y/n) - (\delta_2 - \delta_1)/2|}{[(1/m)(X/m)(1 - X/m) + (1/n)(Y/n)(1 - Y/n)]^{1/2}} <$$

$$C_\alpha\left(\frac{(\delta_1 + \delta_2)/2}{[(1/m)(X/m)(1 - X/m) + (1/n)(Y/n)(1 - Y/n)]^{1/2}}\right) . \qquad (6.63)$$

The function $C_\alpha(\cdot)$ to be evaluated for determining the critical upper bound to the test statistic is defined as before so that the expression on the right-hand side of (6.63) stands for the square root of the α-quantile of a χ^2-distribution with 1 degree of freedom and (random) noncentrality parameter $(\delta_1 + \delta_2)^2/\left(4\left[(1/m)(X/m)(1 - X/m) + (1/n)(Y/n)(1 - Y/n)\right]\right)$. By Theorem A.3.4, we know that the testing procedure corresponding to (6.63) has asymptotic significance level α whenever it can be taken for granted that the variance of the statistic $\sqrt{N}T_N = \sqrt{N}(X/m - Y/n)$ converges to a positive limit as $N \to \infty$. Since we obviously have that $Var[\sqrt{N}(X/m - Y/n)] = (N/m)p_1(1 - p_1) + (N/n)p_2(1 - p_2)$, this simply requires that the relative size m/N of sample 1 converges to some nondegenerate limit and at least one of the two binomial distributions under comparison be nondegenerate. In other words, (6.63) defines a test of asymptotic level α provided there exists some $\lambda \in (0,1)$ such that $m/N \to \lambda$ as $N \to \infty$, and at least one of the primary parameters p_1 and p_2 is an interior point of the unit interval.

A straightforward approach to *transforming the asymptotic testing procedure (6.63) into an exactly valid test* for the problem (6.60) starts from establishing an algorithm for the exact computation of its rejection probability under any fixed parameter constellation (p_1, p_2). For brevity, let us write

$$Q_{\alpha;m,n}^{\delta_1,\delta_2}(p_1,p_2) =$$
$$P_{(p_1,p_2)}\left[\frac{|X/m - Y/n - (\delta_2 - \delta_1)/2|}{[(1/m)(X/m)(1-X/m) + (1/n)(Y/n)(1-Y/n)]^{1/2}} \right.$$
$$\left. < C_\alpha\left(\frac{(\delta_1 + \delta_2)/2}{[(1/m)(X/m)(1-X/m) + (1/n)(Y/n)(1-Y/n)]^{1/2}} \right) \right] . \quad (6.64)$$

A representation of $Q_{\alpha;m,n}^{\delta_1,\delta_2}(p_1,p_2)$ which proves particularly convenient for computational purposes reads

$$Q_{\alpha;m,n}^{\delta_1,\delta_2}(p_1,p_2) = \sum_{x=0}^{m} \left\{ \sum_{y \in \mathcal{U}_{\alpha,n}^{\delta_1,\delta_2}(x)} b(y; n, p_2) \right\} \cdot b(x; m, p_1) , \quad (6.65)$$

where

$$\mathcal{U}_{\alpha;m,n}^{\delta_1,\delta_2}(x) = \left\{ y \in \mathbb{N}_\circ \;\middle|\; y \leq n, \right.$$
$$\frac{|x/m - y/n - (\delta_2 - \delta_1)/2|}{[(1/m)(x/m)(1-x/m) + (1/n)(y/n)(1-y/n)]^{1/2}}$$
$$\left. < C_\alpha\left(\frac{(\delta_1 + \delta_2)/2}{[(1/m)(x/m)(1-x/m) + (1/n)(y/n)(1-y/n)]^{1/2}} \right) \right\}. \quad (6.66)$$

With regard to the form of the sets $\mathcal{U}_{\alpha;m,n}^{\delta_1,\delta_2}(x)$ over which the inner sum has to be extended in computing exact rejection probabilities of the asymptotic test, things are quite the same as found in the analogous setting with paired observations: By explicit construction, the $\mathcal{U}_{\alpha;m,n}^{\delta_1,\delta_2}(x)$ turn out to be intervals in the sample space of the second of the binomial variables involved. Since there is no argument in sight which allows one to assert that this observation reflects a general mathematical fact, both computer programs bi2diffac, bi2dipow involving evaluations of exact rejection probabilities $Q_{\alpha;m,n}^{\delta_1,\delta_2}(p_1,p_2)$ by means of (6.65) are organized as their paired-observations counterparts [cf. the footnote on p. 74].

Now, we are ready to determine once more the largest nominal significance level α^* which has to be substituted for α in order to ensure that the exact size of the asymptotic testing procedure does not exceed the target significance level. For the sake of avoiding excessively long execution times of the *SAS* program `bi2diffac` provided for accomplishing that task,

$$SIZE_\alpha^B(\delta_1, \delta_2; m, n) = \max\left\{ \sup_{0 < p_1 < 1 - \delta_1} Q_{\alpha; m, n}^{\delta_1, \delta_2}(p_1, p_1 + \delta_1) \right. ,$$

$$\left. \sup_{\delta_2 < p_1 < 1} Q_{\alpha; m, n}^{\delta_1, \delta_2}(p_1, p_1 - \delta_2) \right\} \qquad (6.67)$$

rather than

$$SIZE_\alpha(\delta_1, \delta_2; m, n) = \sup\left\{ Q_{\alpha; m, n}^{\delta_1, \delta_2}(p_1, p_2) \;\middle|\; 0 < p_1, p_2 < 1 , \right.$$

$$\left. p_1 - p_2 \le -\delta_1 \text{ or } p_1 - p_2 \ge \delta_2 \right\} \qquad (6.68)$$

is used in the iteration process as primary objective function of α. Obviously, the corrected nominal significance level α^* obtained in this way has the desired property only if it satisfies $SIZE_{\alpha^*}^B(\delta_1, \delta_2; m, n) = SIZE_{\alpha^*}(\delta_1, \delta_2; m, n)$. Although up to now no mathematical proof has been made available for the proposition that the trivial relationship $SIZE_{\alpha^*}^B(\delta_1, \delta_2; m, n) \le SIZE_{\alpha^*}(\delta_1, \delta_2; m, n)$ can always be replaced with the corresponding straight equality under the present circumstances, in extensive numerical investigations not a single counter-example came to light. Nevertheless, `bi2diffac` checks on this condition and provides for putting out an error code rather than a numerical value for α^* in case of finding that the maximum of the probability of a wrong decision in favour of $-\delta_1 < p_1 - p_2 < \delta_2$ is attained at an interior point of the subspace $\{(p_1, p_2) \in (0, 1)^2 \,|\, p_1 - p_2 \le -\delta_1 \text{ or } p_1 - p_2 \ge \delta_2\}$.

For a selection of balanced two-sample designs with binomially distributed data and two specifications of a symmetric equivalence range for $\delta = p_1 - p_2$, Table 6.14 shows the result of reducing the nominal significance level as far as necessary for making an exactly valid test of the asymptotic procedure (6.63). The exact size of the corrected test is also shown and compared to that of the uncorrected procedure using the target significance level of 5% as the nominal level. All entries into columns 3 − 5 have been computed running the *SAS* macro `bi2diffac` with grid span .001 in all steps of searching through the respective parameter subspace for the maximum rejection probability. Qualitatively speaking, the conclusions to be drawn from studying the exact size of the asymptotic test for equivalence with respect to the difference of success rates are quite similar in the two-sample

Table 6.14 *Nominal significance level and exact size of a corrected version of the testing procedure (6.63) maintaining the 5% level in finite samples of common size $m = n = 25(25)200$ for equivalence ranges $(-\delta_1, \delta_2) = (-\delta_\circ, \delta_\circ)$ with $\delta_\circ = .2, .4$ [Number in ( ): size of the critical region of the noncorrected asymptotic testing procedure]*

$\delta_\circ$	n	α^*	$SIZE_{\alpha^*}(\delta_\circ, \delta_\circ; n, n)$	
.20	25	.0134	.0405	(.0944)
"	50	.0228	.0480	(.1034)
"	75	.0164	.0303	(.0928)
"	100	.0340	.0482	(.0804)
"	125	.0359	.0500	(.0700)
"	150	.0322	.0433	(.0625)
"	175	.0278	.0373	(.0750)
"	200	.0389	.0476	(.0657)
.40	25	.0305	.0382	(.0736)
"	50	.0293	.0318	(.0587)
"	75	.0397	.0448	(.0617)
"	100	.0432	.0459	(.0619)
"	125	.0432	.0468	(.0594)
"	150	.0416	.0443	(.0568)
"	175	.0393	.0427	(.0551)
"	200	.0448	.0493	(.0531)

as compared to the McNemar setting: Even with sample sizes located in the extreme upper tail of the distribution of sample sizes available for well-planned clinical trials, the nominal level has to be curtailed substantially in order to obtain a test for equivalence with respect to δ which really maintains the target significance level of 5%. We can only speculate about the reasons why convergence of the exact size to the nominal significance level turns out to be so slow in these two specific applications of the asymptotic theory developed in § 3.4. It seems as if the mathematically unnatural parametrization of the underlying family of distributions through a raw difference of probabilities would be of greater impact than the binary structure of the individual observations.

Provided one is certain about the reduced nominal level α^* to be substituted for α in (6.63), it is of course of considerable practical interest to know with what power the corresponding level-corrected asymptotic test for the equivalence problem (6.60) is able to detect an arbitrarily specified alternative $(p_1, p_2) \in (0,1)^2$ such that $\delta = p_1 - p_2 \in (-\delta_1, \delta_2)$. The *SAS* macro `bi2dipow` enables its user to readily find the correct answer to any question of that type. It returns the exact value of the rejection probability of the test (6.63) at any nominal level $\alpha \in (0,1)$ under any specified parameter constellation $(p_1, p_2) \in (0,1)^2$. Since each such computation amounts to just a single evaluation of the double sum appearing on the right-hand side of equation (6.65), execution times are very short even if both sample sizes run far beyond the upper limit of the range covered by Table 6.14. Given the sample sizes, the equivalence range and the nominal level, the power of the test not only depends on the true value of the target parameter δ, but at the same time on the "baseline" success probability (i.e., p_1 or p_2) as a nuisance parameter. For $m = n = 50$ and $\delta_1 = \delta_2 = .20$, Figure 6.3 represents the changes in power of the level-corrected asymptotic test for equivalence with respect to δ occurring when the true parameter point (p_1, p_2) moves along the main diagonal of the unit square. Apart from being symmetric about $1/2$, the curve is sharply peaked in the neighbourhood

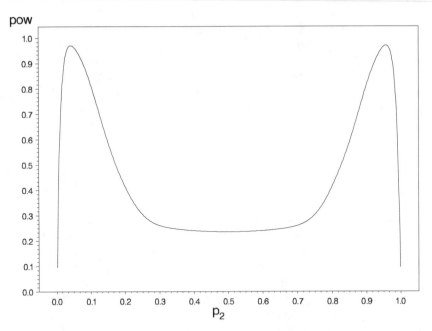

Figure 6.3 *Exact power of the level-corrected version of (6.63) against the alternative $\delta = 0$ $[\Leftrightarrow p_1 = p_2]$ as a function of p_2 as the remaining nuisance parameter, for $m = n = 50$, $\delta_1 = \delta_2 = \delta_\circ = .20$ and $\alpha^* = .0228$.*

of both boundaries of the parameter space flattening out to a minimum of less than $1/3$ of the height of these peaks when approaching the centre from either side.

Discussion

On the one hand, there can be little doubt that it is reasonable to base a test for equivalence of the two binomial distributions $\mathcal{B}(m, p_1)$ and $\mathcal{B}(n, p_2)$ with respect to the raw difference δ of both success probabilities, on the natural estimator of the distance between the true value of δ and the centre of the interval specified under the hypothesis to be established. On the other, inspecting the graph shown in the above figure one can hardly help to concede that the power function of the (level-corrected) testing procedure (6.63) looks fairly strange. Actually, it would be desirable to have an option of replacing the asymptotic procedure with an alternative test giving rise to power curves of much more equalized form, provided the price to pay for this advantage had not been a uniform loss in efficiency.

The only serious competitor to the asymptotic procedure (6.63) and its level-corrected modification we know of is obtained through adopting an idea explained in full detail in the German precursor edition to this book (see Wellek, 1994, § 6.4.2). The key fact one has to exploit in approaching the problem from this alternative point of view is as follows: Given the equivalence limits $-\delta_1$ and δ_2 to δ, one can find equivalence limits $\varrho_1^*(\delta_1, \delta_2)$, $\varrho_2^*(\delta_1, \delta_2)$, say, to the odds ratio such that the associated null hypothesis of nonequivalence with respect to ϱ is the smallest null hypothesis of the kind treated in § 6.5.1 containing the null hypothesis to be tested now. More precisely speaking, by rather elementary analytical arguments it can be shown that defining

$$\varrho_1^*(\delta_1, \delta_2) = \left(\frac{1-\delta_1}{1+\delta_1}\right)^2, \quad \varrho_2^*(\delta_1, \delta_2) = \left(\frac{1+\delta_2}{1-\delta_2}\right)^2 \qquad (6.69)$$

and

$$H^* = \{(p_1, p_2) \in (0,1)^2 \,|\, p_1(1-p_2)/(1-p_1)p_2 \leq \varrho_1^*(\delta_1, \delta_2) \,\vee$$
$$p_1(1-p_2)/(1-p_1)p_2 \geq \varrho_2^*(\delta_1, \delta_2)\} \qquad (6.70)$$

ensures the validity of the following two statements:

(i) $H^* \supseteq H = \{(p_1, p_2) \in (0,1)^2 \,|\, p_1 - p_2 \leq -\delta_1 \,\vee\, p_1 - p_2 \geq \delta_2\}$;

(ii) the common boundary of H and K in the sense of (6.60) contains points which lie also on the common boundary of H^* and the associated alternative hypothesis K^*.

Clearly, part (i) of the result implies that the exact Fisher type level-α test of H^* versus K^* is a fortiori a test for equivalence of $\mathcal{B}(m, p_1)$ and $\mathcal{B}(n, p_2)$ with respect to $\delta = p_1 - p_2$ which will never exceed the prespecified significance level α. Since this test is in particular unbiased for H^* versus K^*, we can conclude from (ii) that even when reinterpreted as a test for equivalence in the sense of $-\delta_1 < p_1 - p_2 < \delta_2$, it exhausts the nominal significance level exhibiting a critical region of a size not falling short of α.

Figure 6.4 contrasts the power function (again restricted to the diagonal of the unit square) of the UMPU test for H^* versus K^* with that of the α-corrected asymptotic test for H versus K in sense of (6.60), for the same specification of the sample sizes and the equivalence range for δ which underlies Figure 6.3. At first glance, the conclusion to be drawn from the graph seems undisputable: The UMPU test of the enlarged null hypothesis H^* looks much too conservative since there are specific alternatives detected by means of the corrected asymptotic test with a power of more than 95% under which its rejection probability fails to substantially exceed the nominal significance level. However, a bit of further reflection reveals reasons for relativizing this unequivocal preference for the modified asymptotic testing procedure: The alternatives under which

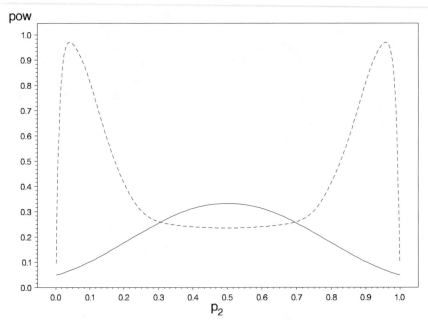

Figure 6.4 *Power of the conservative exact Fisher type test for equivalence with respect to δ against alternatives of the form $p_1 = p_2$, for $\alpha = .05$, $m = n = 50$ and $\delta_1 = \delta_2 = \delta_o = .20$. [Dashed line: Power function of the level-corrected asymptotic test for the same problem, reproduced from Figure 6.3.]*

the corrected asymptotic test so impressively dominates the conservative UMPU test are restricted to rather extreme constellations being of relevance only for the planning of trials such that the baseline responder rate has to be assumed either exceptionally low or near to 100%. In the majority of real clinical trials, prior information suggests to locate the baseline level at a point of the unit interval being nearer to its centre than one of its boundaries, and against alternatives specifying a common response rate in a range of about (.25, .75), the UMPU test of the minimally enlarged null hypothesis in terms of ϱ is at least as powerful as the corrected asymptotic test. Thus, relying on the experience that extreme alternatives are rarely realistic, the conservative approach to testing for equivalence with respect to δ through enclosing the null hypothesis of primary interest by a hypothesis which states inequivalence with respect to the odds ratio, can be regarded as a true alternative to the modified large-sample solution of the testing problem (6.60).

For the sake of completeness, it should be mentioned that the power curve shown in Figure 6.4 for the conservative conditional test, refers to the exact randomized version of the Fisher type test. However, by the means provided in § 6.5.2, the loss in power entailed by dispensing with randomized decisions between the hypotheses can be largely avoided. Hence, the comparative evaluation of the merits of the conservative relative to the direct approach through correcting the large-sample procedure will be little affected by replacing the UMPU test of H^* versus K^* with its improved nonrandomized counterpart.

6.6 Log-rank test for equivalence of two survivor functions

Following Wellek (1993b), we show in this section that the methodology of equivalence testing also extends to situations in which the data are subject to random right-censoring. For this purpose, we adopt the standard framework of statistical survival analysis assuming that the complete information on an arbitrary observational unit is contained in a pair, say (T, C), of random variables such that T denotes the waiting time to some event of interest (usually labelled "death", irrespective of its concrete meaning), and C stands for the time until some censoring event occurs. Of these two variables, only one becomes exactly known to the observer whereas the exact value of the time until the other, later occurring event remains latent. In addition to recording the value of the smaller of both time variables, the observer is also enabled to identify the type of the event (death versus censorship) which occurred at the respective time. As usual, information on the event type is represented by an indicator variable, say $\tilde{D}$, taking on value 1 and 0 if $T \leq C$ and $T > C$, respectively.

For convenience, let us arrange the pooled set of all pairs of time variables underlying a two-sample setting with survival data subject to random right-censoring, into a single sequence $((T_k, C_k))_{1 \leq k \leq N}$. Then, the data effectively available from the first sample are given by the m random pairs $(X_1, \tilde{D}_1^{(1)}), \ldots, (X_m, \tilde{D}_m^{(1)})$ with

$$X_i = \min(T_i, C_i), \quad \tilde{D}_i^{(1)} = \begin{cases} 1 \\ 0 \end{cases} \text{ for } \begin{array}{l} T_i \leq C_i \\ T_i > C_i \end{array}, \quad 1 \leq i \leq m. \qquad (6.71a)$$

Likewise, the censoring process reduces the second sample from $(T_{m+1}, C_{m+1}), \ldots, (T_{m+n}, C_{m+n})$ to $(Y_1, \tilde{D}_1^{(2)}), \ldots, (Y_n, \tilde{D}_n^{(2)})$ where

$$Y_j = \min(T_{m+j}, C_{m+j}),$$

$$\tilde{D}_j^{(2)} = \begin{cases} 1 \\ 0 \end{cases} \text{ for } \begin{array}{l} T_{m+j} \leq C_{m+j} \\ T_{m+j} > C_{m+j} \end{array}, \quad 1 \leq j \leq n. \qquad (6.71b)$$

Of course, the distributions whose equivalence we want to establish are those of the true survival times $T_1, \ldots, T_m$ ($\leftrightarrow$ Sample 1) and $T_{m+1}, \ldots, T_{m+n}$ ($\leftrightarrow$ Sample 2). The survivor functions characterizing these distributions will be denoted by $S_1(\cdot)$ and $S_2(\cdot)$ so that we have by definition:

$$S_1(t) = P[T_i \geq t], \quad t \geq 0, \quad i \in \{1, \ldots, m\}; \qquad (6.72a)$$

$$S_2(t) = P[T_{m+j} \geq t], \quad t \geq 0, \quad j \in \{1, \ldots, n\}. \qquad (6.72b)$$

Both $S_1(\cdot)$ and $S_2(\cdot)$ is assumed to be absolutely continuous and to satisfy an ordinary proportional hazards model (see, e.g., Kalbfleisch and Prentice, 1980, § 2.3.2). With no loss of generality, we treat $S_2(\cdot)$ as the baseline survivor function underlying the model. With this convention, the proportional hazards assumption is equivalent to the condition

$$S_1(t) = [S_2(t)]^\theta \text{ for all } t \geq 0 \text{ and some } \theta > 0. \qquad (6.73)$$

Generally, it seems intuitively plausible to define equivalent survivor functions by requiring the uniform distance between $S_1(\cdot)$ and $S_2(\cdot)$ to be sufficiently small. In other words, we can take equivalence of $S_1(\cdot)$ and $S_2(\cdot)$ for granted if we have

$$\|S_1 - S_2\| \equiv \sup_{t > 0} |S_1(t) - S_2(t)| < \delta \text{ for some } \delta > 0. \qquad (6.74)$$

In view of the continuity of $S_2(\cdot)$, (6.73) implies that

$$\|S_1 - S_2\| = \sup_{0 < u < 1} |u - u^\theta|, \qquad (6.75)$$

and from (6.75) it follows by means of some elementary calculus that

$$\|S_1 - S_2\| = |\theta^{1/(1-\theta)} - \theta^{\theta/(1-\theta)}|. \qquad (6.76)$$

Since, as a function of θ, the right-hand side of equation (6.76) is strictly decreasing (increasing) on $(0, 1)$ (on $(1, \infty)$), and remains invariant under the reparametrization $\theta \mapsto \theta^{-1}$, we can conclude that condition (6.74) is (logically) equivalent to

$$(1 + \varepsilon)^{-1} < \theta < 1 + \varepsilon \text{ for some suitable } \varepsilon > 0. \quad (6.77)$$

Here the constant ε has to be determined from δ by solving the equation

$$(1 + \varepsilon)^{-1/\varepsilon} - (1 + \varepsilon)^{-(1+\varepsilon)/\varepsilon} = \delta. \quad (6.78)$$

Consequently, under the proportional hazards assumption, equivalent survivor functions in the sense of (6.74) are characterized by the fact that the relative risk belongs to a sufficiently small interval around 1 being symmetric on the log scale. Table 6.15 shows the correspondence between δ and ε by (6.78) for a selection of numerical examples, together with the right-hand limit of the equivalence range for $\log \theta$ which in the proportional hazards model corresponds to (6.74) for the specified value of δ. Figure 6.5 visualizes a section through the equivalence region (6.74) obtained by fixing the baseline survivor function $S_2(\cdot)$ and letting $S_1(\cdot)$ vary over the set $\left\{ S_2^\theta(\cdot) \,\middle|\, \theta > 0, \, \| S_2^\theta - S_2 \| < \delta \right\}$.

Table 6.15 *Numerical correspondence between equivalence limits referring to $\|S_1 - S_2\|$ and the parameter θ relating both survivor functions under the proportional hazards model*

δ	.05	.075	.10	.15	.20	.25
ε	.1457	.2266	.3135	.5077	.7341	1.0000
$\log(1 + \varepsilon)$	.1360	.2042	.2727	.4106	.5505	.6931

Since both survivor functions under comparison have been assumed absolutely continuous, each of the true survival times T_k $(k = 1, \ldots, N)$ has a well-defined hazard function, say $\lambda_1(\cdot)$ (for $k = 1, \ldots, m$) and $\lambda_2(\cdot)$ (for $k = m + 1, \ldots, m + n$), where

$$\lambda_\nu(t) = \frac{d}{dt}\left[-\log S_\nu(t) \right], \quad t \geq 0, \quad \nu \in \{1, 2\}. \quad (6.79)$$

By the basic model assumption (6.73), these functions admit the representation

$$\lambda_\nu(t) = \lambda_2(t) e^{z_k \beta}, \quad t \geq 0, \quad \nu \in \{1, 2\}, \quad k \in \{1, \ldots, N\} \quad (6.80)$$

where

$$\beta = \log \theta \text{ and } z_k = \begin{cases} 1 \\ 0 \end{cases} \text{ for } \begin{array}{l} 1 \leq k \leq m \\ m + 1 \leq k \leq N \end{array}. \quad (6.81)$$

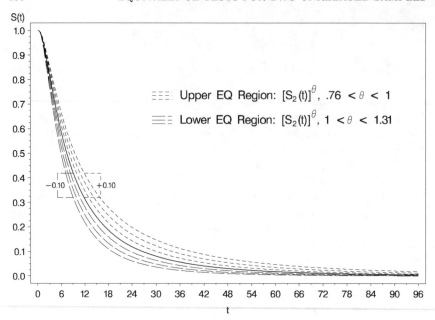

Figure 6.5 *Region of survival curves being equivalent to a given baseline survivor function (solid line) with respect to uniform vertical distance in the proportional hazards model.*

After these preparations, we are ready to construct an asymptotic testing procedure for

$$H : ||S_1 - S_2|| \geq \delta \quad \text{versus} \quad K : ||S_1 - S_2|| < \delta. \tag{6.82}$$

As explained above, under the proportional hazards assumption (6.73), the problem of testing (6.82) is the same as that of testing

$$\tilde{H} : |\beta| \geq \log(1 + \varepsilon) \quad \text{versus} \quad \tilde{K} : |\beta| < \log(1 + \varepsilon) \tag{6.82}$$

provided β is the real-valued regression coefficient appearing in (6.80) and ε is determined as the unique solution to equation (6.78).

It is easy to verify that in the special case of a proportional hazards model given by (6.80) and (6.81), the partial log-likelihood for β simplifies to

$$\log L(\beta) = \tilde{d}^{(1)}\beta - \sum_{q=1}^{\tilde{q}} \log(r_{q1}e^{\beta} + r_{q2}) \tag{6.83}$$

where

$r_{q\nu}$ = number of items at risk in the νth sample at the qth smallest failure time $t_{(q)}$ $(\nu = 1, 2;\ q = 1, \ldots, \tilde{q})$,

$$\tilde{d}^{(1)}_{\cdot} = \sum_{i=1}^{m} \tilde{d}^{(1)}_{i} = \text{total number of failures in Sample 1.} \qquad (6.84)$$

Correspondingly, the maximum partial likelihood estimator $\hat{\beta}$ is found by solving the equation

$$\sum_{q=1}^{\tilde{q}} \frac{r_{q1}\, e^{\beta}}{r_{q1}\, e^{\beta} + r_{q2}} = \tilde{d}^{(1)}_{\cdot}, \quad -\infty < \beta < \infty, \qquad (6.85)$$

and the observed information at $\beta = \hat{\beta}$ is obtained as

$$I_N(\hat{\beta}) = \sum_{q=1}^{\tilde{q}} \frac{r_{q1} r_{q2} e^{\hat{\beta}}}{(r_{q1} e^{\hat{\beta}} + r_{q2})^2}\,. \qquad (6.86)$$

Fairly mild conditions which can be made mathematically precise by specializing the regularity assumptions formulated by Andersen and Gill (1982, § 3) (for additional details see Andersen et al., 1993, § VII.2.2) ensure that there exists a finite positive constant, $\sigma^2_*(\hat{\beta})$ say, such that

$$N^{-1} I_N(\hat{\beta}) \xrightarrow{P} 1/\sigma^2_*(\hat{\beta}) \text{ as } N \to \infty, \qquad (6.87)$$

and

$$\sqrt{N}(\hat{\beta} - \beta)/\sigma_*(\hat{\beta}) \xrightarrow{\mathcal{L}} \mathcal{N}(0,1) \text{ as } N \to \infty, \text{ for all } \beta. \qquad (6.88)$$

In view of these properties of $\hat{\beta}$ and $I_N(\hat{\beta})$, another application of Theorem A.3.4 shows that the rejection region of an asymptotically valid test for $(\widetilde{6.82})$ and hence for (6.82) itself, is given by

$$\left\{ I_N^{1/2}(\hat{\beta})\, |\hat{\beta}| < C_\alpha \big(I_N^{1/2}(\hat{\beta}) \log(1+\varepsilon)\big) \right\}\,. \qquad (6.89)$$

The function $\psi \mapsto C_\alpha(\psi)$ to be evaluated at $\psi = I_N^{1/2}(\hat{\beta}) \log(1 + \varepsilon)$ in order to determine the critical upper bound to the absolute value of the standardized estimate of the regression coefficient is the same as defined in the general description given in § 3.4 of the asymptotic approach to constructing tests for equivalence. In other words, for any $\psi > 0$, $C_\alpha(\psi)$ stands for the square root of the lower 100α percentage point of a χ^2-distribution with $df = 1$ and noncentrality parameter ψ^2. Thus, given the value of $\hat{\beta}$ and its estimated standard error, the practical effort entailed in computing the (random) critical bound to be used in the log-rank test for equivalence with rejection region (6.89) reduces to writing a single line of SAS code invoking the intrinsic function `cinv` with arguments $\alpha, 1$ and $I(\hat{\beta}) \log^2(1+\varepsilon)$, respectively. A standard software package like SAS provides its user also

with an easy to handle tool for finding the solution to the partial likelihood equation (6.85): It suffices to run a procedure tailored for analyzing
standard proportional hazards models with time-independent covariates.
In the output list one will find both the value of $\hat{\beta}$ (usually under the label
"Parameter Estimate") and $I_N^{-1/2}(\hat{\beta})$ (as an entry into the column "Standard Error"). Altogether, these hints should make it sufficiently clear that
the practical implementation of the log-rank test for equivalence as given
by the rejection region (6.89) reduces to steps very easy to carry out by
anybody having access to professional statistics software.

Example 6.5

For the Medulloblastoma II Trial of the SIOP (for details see Bailey et al.,
1995), $N = 357$ children suffering from such malignoma of the cerebellum
were enrolled. At some stage of the statistical analysis of the data obtained
from this long-term trial, it was of interest to establish equivalence with
respect to relapse-free survival between the subgroups of patients treated in
big (8 or more cases accrued into the trial) and small centres, respectively.
Sample 1 ($\leftrightarrow$ patients from big centres) was of size $m = 176$, exhibiting a total of $\tilde{d}^{(1)} = 75$ failure events. In the $n = 181$ patients of Sample 2 ($\leftrightarrow$ small
centres), $\tilde{d}^{(2)} = 70$ relapses were recorded. The complete relapse-free survival curves obtained for both groups by means of standard product-limit
estimation are shown in Figure 6.6. As the maximum distance δ considered
compatible with equivalence of the underlying true survivor functions [re-
call (6.74)] let us choose $\delta = .15$, i.e., the value in the middle between the
two alternative specifications recommended in § 1.5 for defining equivalence
ranges for parameters taking values in (0, 1). By (6.78) and (6.82), this
is the same as specifying the alternative hypothesis $|\beta| < .4106$ [→ Ta-
ble 6.15] about the regression coefficient introduced in (6.81). With the
data underlying Figure 6.6, solving equation (6.85) gives the ML estimate
$\hat{\beta} = .0944$. Using this value in (6.86) yields $I_N(\hat{\beta}) = 36.1981$ as the informa-
tion observed at $\hat{\beta}$ so that we get $I_N^{1/2}(\hat{\beta})|\hat{\beta}| = .5680$. On the other hand,
with $\hat{\psi}_N = \sqrt{36.1981} \cdot .4106 = 2.4704$ and $\alpha = .05$, for the critical bound
which the test statistic $I_N^{1/2}(\hat{\beta})|\hat{\beta}|$ has to be compared with according to
(6.89), we obtain $C_\alpha(\hat{\psi}_N) = \sqrt{.689235} = .8302$ where, in SAS, .689235 is
the value assigned to the variable csq, say, as the result of getting executed
the statement csq=cinv(.05,1,2.4704**2). Since the observed value of
$I_N^{1/2}(\hat{\beta})|\hat{\beta}|$ thus falls short of its critical upper bound, the test decides in
favour of equivalence of the survivor functions under comparison.

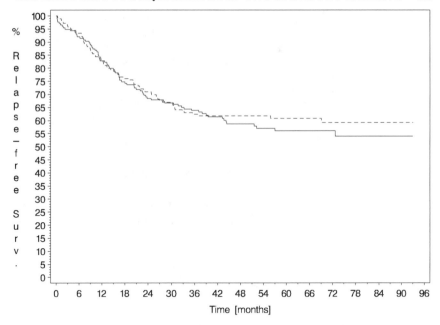

Figure 6.6 *Medulloblastoma Trial SIOP II: Observed relapse-free survival curves by size of treatment centre. Solid line: Big centres having enrolled $\geq$ 8 patients. Dashed line: Small centres with total accrual < 8. (From Wellek, 1993, with kind permission by the International Biometric Society.)*

Simulation results on the size of the log-rank test for equivalence

In order to study the size of the critical region (6.89), two sets of simulation experiments were performed. In the first set, the baseline survivor function was log-normal with parameters $\mu = 2$ and $\sigma^2 = 1$ as given by $S_2(t) = \Phi(2 - \log t)$, whereas the censoring distribution function was specified $C(t) = 1 - e^{-t/50}$ irrespective of the true value of the hazard ratio θ. In the second set of experiments, the log-normal distribution $\mathcal{LN}(2,1)$ was replaced by the Weibull distribution with form parameter $c = 2$ and unit scale parameter. The associated censoring times were generated from two different rectangular distributions inducing baseline ($\leftrightarrow$ Group 2) censoring rates of 20 and 80%, respectively. The results of studying the size of the critical region (6.89) under both types of models are summarized in Tables 6.16 a,b. Each entry is based on $40,000$ replications of the respective simulation experiments and gives the fraction of samples for which the test decides in favour of equivalence. None of the entries into the rightmost columns of the tables indicates relevant anticonservatism so that the level properties of the test are fully satisfactory even when performed with very small samples.

Table 6.16a *Estimated rejection probabilities of the log-rank test for equivalence at nominal level $\alpha = .05$ under the null hypothesis $\|S_1 - S_2\| \geq .15$ ($\leftrightarrow \varepsilon = .5077$) in a model with lognormal baseline survivor function and exponentially distributed censoring times*[†]

m	n	$\theta = 1/(1+\varepsilon)$	$\theta = 1+\varepsilon$
25	25	.04945	.05103
50	25	.05078	.05158
50	50	.05108	.05003
75	50	.04778	.05238
75	75	.05085	.04913
100	75	.04800	.04963
100	100	.04943	.05025

[†] censoring rates: .188 for Group 2; .268 and .133 for Group 1 under $\theta = 1/1.5077$ and $\theta = 1.5077$, respectively

Table 6.16b *Analogue to Table 6.16a for a Weibull baseline survivor function and uniform censoring distributions $\mathcal{U}(0, \tau)$ inducing various group-specific censoring rates ζ_1 and ζ_2.*

m	n	τ	$\theta = 1/(1+\varepsilon)$	$\theta = 1+\varepsilon$
25	25	4.431133*	.04913	.05068
50	25	"	.04703	.05125
50	50	"	.05000	.04843
75	50	"	.04548	.05063
75	75	"	.04940	.05030
100	75	"	.04978	.05110
100	100	"	.04848	.05165
25	25	1.748709**	.04838	.04820
50	25	"	.04875	.05375
50	50	"	.04995	.04850
75	50	"	.04918	.04995
75	75	"	.05050	.05045
100	75	"	.04723	.05028
100	100	"	.05090	.04705

*$(\zeta_1, \zeta_2) = (.2450, .2000)$ and $(.1633, .2000)$ under $\theta = 1/(1+\varepsilon)$ and $\theta = 1+\varepsilon$, respectively

**$(\zeta_1, \zeta_2) = (.5938, .5000)$ and $(.4127, .5000)$ under $\theta = 1/(1+\varepsilon)$ and $\theta = 1+\varepsilon$, respectively

Power approximation and sample size calculation

As usual, for purposes of approximating the power and computing sample sizes required for attaining some prespecified power, we need an expression for the "theoretical" variance of the nonstandardized test statistic under any alternative of potential interest. In view of practical applications to the planning of equivalence trials with survival endpoints, it seems sufficient to restrict the class of alternatives of interest by the following assumptions:

(I) Both groups are subject to the same independent censoring mechanism induced by a recruitment process running uniformly over some fixed accrual period $[0, \tau]$.

(II) The study protocol specifies a minimum follow-up period of length $t^\circ \geq 0$ for each patient. Since t° might also be equal to zero, studies allowing the admission of new patients during the whole duration of the trial are covered as a special case.

(III) The trial under consideration is to be a balanced one, in the sense that we have $m = n$, $N = 2n$.

Applying Theorem VII.2.2 of Andersen et al. (1993) it can be shown that under assumptions (I) – (III), the asymptotic variance of the normalized partial likelihood estimator $\sqrt{N}\,\hat{\beta}$ is given by

$$\sigma_*^2(\hat{\beta}) = \frac{1}{v^2(\beta\,;\,\tau, t^\circ)} \tag{6.90}$$

where

$$v^2(\beta\,;\,\tau, t^\circ) = \frac{e^\beta}{2} \left\{ \int_0^{t^\circ} \left[e^\beta + (S_2(t))^{1-e^\beta} \right]^{-1} f_2(t)\, dt + \right.$$
$$\left. \int_{t^\circ}^{t^\circ+\tau} \left[e^\beta + (S_2(t))^{1-e^\beta} \right]^{-1} \frac{t^\circ + \tau - t}{\tau} f_2(t)\, dt \right\} \tag{6.91}$$

and $f_2(\cdot)$ denotes the density of the baseline survival distribution as assumed for Group 2.

In general, the integral appearing on the right-hand side of (6.91) admits no representation in closed form. However, it is easy to evaluate numerically (e.g., using *Mathematica* or *Maple*). In the specific case $\beta = 0$ [$\leftrightarrow$ alternative of exact coincidence of both survival distributions], (6.91) reduces to

$$v^2(0\,;\,\tau, t^\circ) = \frac{1}{4} P[T < Z] \tag{6.92}$$

where T denotes a random variable with density $f_2(\cdot)$, and Z a censoring variable independent of T and following the uniform distribution over the interval $[t^\circ, t^\circ + \tau]$.

Now, (6.87) and (6.88) suggest that for purposes of power approximation, we replace $I_N^{1/2}(\hat{\beta})$ with $\sqrt{N}/\sigma_*(\hat{\beta})$ everywhere in (6.89) and treat $\sqrt{N}\hat{\beta}/\sigma_*(\hat{\beta})$ as normally distributed with unit variance and mean $\sqrt{N}\beta_\circ/\sigma_*(\hat{\beta})$ where $\beta_\circ \in \mathbb{R}$ denotes the value of the log-hazard ratio β [recall (6.80), (6.81)] specified as the alternative of interest. Denoting the power of the test given by (6.89) against $\beta = \beta_\circ$ by $\Pi_\circ$, this leads to the relationship

$$\Pi_\circ \approx \Phi\Big(C_\alpha\big(\sqrt{N}\log(1+\varepsilon)/\sigma_*(\hat{\beta})\big) - \sqrt{N}\beta_\circ/\sigma_*(\hat{\beta})\Big) - $$
$$\Phi\Big(-C_\alpha\big(\sqrt{N}\log(1+\varepsilon)/\sigma_*(\hat{\beta})\big) - \sqrt{N}\beta_\circ/\sigma_*(\hat{\beta})\Big) \ . \qquad (6.93)$$

A natural way of establishing a method for estimating minimally required sample sizes is now to treat (6.93) as an equation in N with all other quantities as given numbers. The task of formulating an algorithm for finding the solution to this equation can considerably be simplified by making use of another approximation, namely $C_\alpha(\sqrt{N}\log(1+\varepsilon)/\sigma_*(\hat{\beta})) \approx \sqrt{N}\log(1+\varepsilon)/\sigma_*(\hat{\beta}) - u_{1-\alpha}$ [$\to$ p. 61, (4.26) with $\sqrt{N}\log(1+\varepsilon)/\sigma_*(\hat{\beta})$ being substituted for $\sqrt{n}\varepsilon$]. Combining the latter with (6.93) and dropping the distinction between approximate and exact identities yields after a few rearrangements of terms the equation

$$\Phi\left(\frac{\sqrt{N}(\log(1+\varepsilon) - \beta_\circ)}{\sigma_*(\hat{\beta})} - u_{1-\alpha}\right)$$
$$+ \ \Phi\left(\frac{\sqrt{N}(\log(1+\varepsilon) + \beta_\circ)}{\sigma_*(\hat{\beta})} - u_{1-\alpha}\right) \ = 1 + \Pi_\circ \ . \qquad (6.94)$$

In order to determine N from (6.94), it is convenient to proceed as follows: We first treat $\sigma_*(\hat{\beta})/\sqrt{N}$ as an unknown positive number, say $\tilde{\sigma}$, and solve the equation

$$\Phi\left(\frac{\log(1+\varepsilon) - \beta_\circ}{\tilde{\sigma}} - u_{1-\alpha}\right) + \Phi\left(\frac{\log(1+\varepsilon) + \beta_\circ}{\tilde{\sigma}} - u_{1-\alpha}\right) = 1 + \Pi_\circ \quad \widetilde{(6.94)}$$

for $\tilde{\sigma}$ which can be done by elementary numerical techniques since the expression on the left-hand side is obviously decreasing in $\tilde{\sigma}$. Denoting the solution to $\widetilde{(6.94)}$ by $\tilde{\sigma}(\beta_\circ; \alpha, \varepsilon, \Pi_\circ)$, we have to choose N such that it satisfies $\sigma_*(\hat{\beta})/\sqrt{N} = \tilde{\sigma}(\beta_\circ; \alpha, \varepsilon, \Pi_\circ)$. In view of (6.90), this is equivalent to determining the approximate total sample size required for attaining power $\Pi_\circ$ against the specific alternative $\beta_\circ \in (-\log(1+\varepsilon), \log(1+\varepsilon))$ by means of

$$N = \left[\tilde{\sigma}^2(\beta_\circ; \alpha, \varepsilon, \Pi_\circ) \ v^2(\beta_\circ; \tau, t^\circ)\right]^{-1} \ . \qquad (6.95)$$

Through $v^2(\beta_o; \tau, t^\circ)$ [recall (6.91)], the resulting minimum sample size depends both on the selected baseline survival distribution and the censoring mechanism, as has necessarily to be the case.

In the special case of the "null alternative" $\beta_o = 0$ under which both survivor functions actually coincide, $\widetilde{(6.94)}$ reduces to $\Phi\left(\dfrac{\log(1+\varepsilon)}{\tilde{\sigma}} - u_{1-\alpha}\right) = (1+\Pi_o)/2$ so that $\tilde{\sigma}(0; \alpha, \varepsilon, \Pi_o)$ is explicitly given by $\dfrac{1}{\tilde{\sigma}(0;\, \alpha,\, \varepsilon,\, \Pi_o)} = \dfrac{\Phi^{-1}\big((1+\Pi_o)/2\big) + u_{1-\alpha}}{\log(1+\varepsilon)}$. Plugging this expression into (6.95) gives

$$N = \frac{[\Phi^{-1}((1+\Pi_o)/2) + u_{1-\alpha}]^2}{v^2(0; \tau, t^\circ)\log^2(1+\varepsilon)} \qquad (6.95^\circ)$$

as the null alternative version of (6.95). Interestingly it can be shown (for details see Wellek, 2002) that the same formula provides a remarkably accurate approximation to the total sample size required for achieving power $(1 + \Pi_o)/2$ against $\beta = 0$ in the noninferiority version of the test discussed in this section. Furthermore, it follows from (6.92) that (6.95°) exhibits a strict formal analogy with the well-known sample size formula derived by Schoenfeld (1981) for the log-rank test for conventional one-sided hypotheses. In fact, according to Schoenfeld's result, (6.95°) approximates the total sample size required to detect the alternative that the true hazard ratio equals $1 + \varepsilon$, with power $1 - \alpha$ in a test at nominal significance level $1 - (1 + \Pi_o)/2$.

Simulation results on power and sample size approximation

In the majority of real applications of the log-rank test for equivalence, sample size calculation will be done under the assumption that the trial aims at detecting perfect coincidence of the survival distributions under comparison. Accordingly, the bulk of the simulation results presented below as a basis for assessing the accuracy of the sample size approximation (6.95) refers to the special case (6.95°). Table 6.17 contrasts the total sample size computed by means of our approximate formula with the simulated exact N required to attain prespecified power Π_o against $\beta = \beta_o = 0$ for various values of Π_o and common censoring rates ζ. In the Monte Carlo experiments performed to generate the entries in the last two columns of this table, we again assumed both true survival distributions to be Weibull with shape parameter $c = 2.0$ and unit scale parameter. Furthermore,

Table 6.17 *Simulated exact total sample sizes versus sample sizes approximated by means of formula (6.95°), for nominal power $\Pi_\circ = .5, .8, .9$ and common censoring rate $\zeta = .1, .2, .5, .8$ (Survival distributions: Weibull with form parameter $c = 2.0$; censoring distributions: uniform)*

ζ	$\Pi_\circ$	Approx. N	Simulated Exact Power	Simulated Exact N
.10	.50	140	.4779	144
"	.80	226	.7826	230
"	.90	286	.9008	= Approx. N
.20	.50	160	.4834	164
"	.80	254	.7871	258
"	.90	320	.8902	328
.50	.50	256	.5022	= Approx. N
"	.80	406	.7931	408
"	.90	514	.8966	= Approx. N
.80	.50	638	.4994	= Approx. N
"	.80	1016	.7923	1020

the associated values of the censoring variables were generated to satisfy conditions (I) – (III) of p. 155 with $t^\circ = 0$ [↔ no minimum follow-up period, i.e., admission of new patients over the whole duration of the trial] and length τ of accrual period being adjusted to match with the prespecified event rate $1-\zeta$ common to both arms of the trial. The equivalence range for the log-hazard rate β was chosen as in Tables 6.16 a,b so that under the hypothesis to be established, a vertical distance of $\delta = .15$ at most was considered compatible with equivalence between two survivor functions. Each individual simulation experiment was run 10,000 times.

Qualitatively speaking, the accuracy of the suggested approximation to the total sample size required to detect null alternatives in the log-rank test with prespecified power, turns out surprisingly good. In fact, the discrepancy between the approximated and the simulated exact value, if existent at all, is found not to exceed 4 per group which seems negligible for all practical purposes.

The subsequent table suggests that this conclusion is warranted all the more if the alternative $\beta_\circ$ of interest is chosen as some point between the centre and the boundaries of the equivalence range specified for the target parameter under the alternative hypothesis as a whole. The simulation study performed to generate the entries in the rightmost column of Table 6.18 was designed as follows: Both survival distributions were assumed to

Table 6.18 *Exact versus nominal power against nonnull alternatives of the log-rank test for equivalence with total sample size estimated from (6.95) [Baseline survival distribution: exponential with hazard rate .80; censoring distribution: uniform, inducing event rates of $1-\zeta_2 = .50$ under baseline hazard]*

ψ	$\beta_\circ$	$v^2(\beta_\circ; \tau, t^\circ)$	$\Pi_\circ$	$\tilde{\sigma}(\beta_\circ; \alpha, \varepsilon, \Pi_\circ)$	Appr. N	Simul. Ex. Pow.
.1	.049526	.126806	.50	.17497	258	.4995
"	"	"	.80	.13640	424	.7951
"	"	"	.90	.11988	548	.8949
.25	.119499	.129242	.50	.16332	290	.5038
"	"	"	.80	.11676	568	.8010
"	"	"	.90	.09945	782	.8975

be exponential with hazard rate $\lambda_2 = .80$ ($\leftrightarrow$ baseline) and $\lambda_1 = \lambda_2(1 + \psi\varepsilon)$ ($\leftrightarrow$ Group 1), respectively, with ε specified as before (i.e., $\varepsilon = .5077$) and $0 < \psi < 1$. The censoring distribution was assumed uniform over $[0, \tau] = [0, 1.992030]$ for both arms of the trial ensuring that the censoring proportion had exact value $\zeta_2 = .50$ under the baseline hazard rate. The entries in column 3 have been obtained by evaluating the second integral (the first one vanishes for $t^\circ = 0$) on the right-hand side of (6.91) with $S_2(t) = e^{-\lambda_2 t}$, $f_2(t) = \lambda_2 e^{-\lambda_2 t}$, $t > 0$. Column 5 shows the values of $\tilde{\sigma}$ which solve equation (6.94) for the respective combination of $\beta_\circ$ and $\Pi_\circ$ when (α, ε) is fixed at (.05, .5077).

The main conclusion to be drawn from the results shown in Table 6.18 is that the exact power attained with samples of total size estimated by means of formula (6.95) approximates the nominal power even slightly better for nonnull alternatives as compared to settings where perfect coincidence of both survivor functions is the specific alternative of interest. Presumably, this just reflects the obvious fact that given the values of all other parameters involved, the total sample size required to detect the specific alternative $\beta = \beta_\circ$ increases with the distance of $\beta_\circ$ from the centre of the equivalence range for β.

CHAPTER 7

Multisample tests for equivalence

7.1 The intersection-union principle as a general solution to multisample equivalence problems

The existing literature on k-sample equivalence testing procedures is comparatively sparse. A reason for this fact might be that, at least for parametric settings, there is a straightforward yet often overconservative solution to problems of establishing equivalence of k distributions as soon as a test for the corresponding two-sample problem is available. The rationale behind this approach is a result which can appropriately be termed intersection-union principle because of its straight duality with Roy's (1953) well-known union-intersection approach to multiple testing and interval estimation. The scope of potential applications of the principle is fairly wide and goes far beyond the specific multisample settings discussed in the subsequent sections of this chapter.

In order to introduce the general idea, let us assume that we are considering an arbitrary but fixed number $q \geq 2$, say, of elementary null hypotheses $H_1, \ldots, H_q$ to be tested against associated alternatives $K_1, \ldots, K_q$. For each $\nu = 1, \ldots, q$, let H_ν and K_ν denote statements about some parametric function (in nonparametric settings: a functional of the distributions from which the data are taken) η_ν such that there is some testing procedure ϕ_ν, say, valid at the selected nominal significance level $\alpha \in (0,1)$. Finally, suppose that the rejection probability of test ϕ_ν does not exceed α, under any possible parameter constellation $(\eta_1, \ldots \eta_q)$ such that $\eta_\nu \in H_\nu$, *irrespective of how many and what other elementary null hypotheses are true*. Then, the intersection-union principle states that the following decision rule defines a valid level-α test for the "combined" problem

$$H \equiv H_1 \cup H_2 \cup \ldots \cup H_q \quad \text{versus} \quad K \equiv K_1 \cap K_2 \ldots \cap K_q : \qquad (7.1)$$

Reject H in favour of K if and only if

each individual test ϕ_ν rejects the null hypothesis H_ν

which it has been constructed for $(\nu = 1, \ldots q)$. $\qquad (7.2)$

The *proof* of the result is almost trivial, at least if one is willing to adopt some piece of the basic formalism customary in expositions of the abstract theory of statistical hypotheses testing methods. In fact, if we denote the combined test defined by (7.2) ϕ and identify each test involved with its critical function, it is clear that ϕ admits the representation $\phi = \phi_1 \cdot \phi_2 \cdot \ldots \cdot \phi_q$. The condition we have to verify, reads then as follows:

$$E_{(\eta_1,..,\eta_q)}(\phi) \leq \alpha \quad \text{for all} \quad (\eta_1,..,\eta_q) \in H \tag{7.3}$$

where $E_{(\eta_1,...,\eta_q)}(\cdot)$ denotes the expected value computed under the parameter constellation $(\eta_1,\ldots,\eta_q)$. Now, if $(\eta_1,\ldots,\eta_q)$ belongs to H, this means by definition that there is some $\nu \in \{1,\ldots,q\}$ with $\eta_\nu \in H_\nu$. Furthermore, every critical function $\phi_1,\ldots,\phi_q$ takes on values in $[0,1]$ only which implies that $\phi \leq \phi_\nu$ and thus $E_{(\eta_1,...,\eta_q)}(\phi) \leq E_{(\eta_1,...,\eta_q)}(\phi_\nu)$. By assumption, we have $E_{(\eta_1,...,\eta_q)}(\phi_\nu) \leq \alpha$ for every $(\eta_1,\ldots,\eta_q)$ with $\eta_\nu \in H_\nu$, and hence the proof of (7.3) is already complete.

It is interesting to note that the principle of confidence interval inclusion introduced in §3.1 as a general approach to the construction of tests for single equivalence hypotheses, can be viewed as a special case of the intersection-union principle. This follows simply from the fact pointed out on p. 30 that every interval inclusion test admits a representation as a double one-sided testing procedure.

In order to apply the result to multisample equivalence testing problems, let θ_j be the parameter of interest (e.g., the expected value) for the ith distribution under comparison, and require of a pair (i,j) of distributions equivalent to each other that the statement

$$K_{(i,j)} : \quad \rho(\theta_i,\theta_j) < \varepsilon, \tag{7.4}$$

holds true with $\rho(\cdot,\cdot)$ denoting a suitable measure of distance between two parameters. Suppose furthermore that for each (i,j) a test $\phi_{(i,j)}$ of $H_{(i,j)} : \rho(\theta_i,\theta_j) \geq \varepsilon$ versus $K_{(i,j)} : \rho(\theta_i,\theta_j) < \varepsilon$ is available whose rejection probability is $\leq \alpha$ at any point $(\theta_1,\ldots,\theta_k)$ in the full parameter space such that $\rho(\theta_i,\theta_j) \geq \varepsilon$. Then, by the intersection-union principle, deciding in favour of "global equivalence" if and only if equivalence can be established for all $\binom{k}{2}$ possible pairs, yields a valid level-α test for

$$H : \max_{i<j}\{\rho(\theta_i,\theta_j)\} \geq \varepsilon \quad \text{versus} \quad K : \max_{i<j}\{\rho(\theta_i,\theta_j)\} < \varepsilon. \tag{7.5}$$

As a specific instance, we get a quick solution to the problem of testing k Gaussian distributions with common unknown variance σ^2 for equivalence with respect to their unscaled means, say $\mu_1 \ldots,\mu_k$, if we proceed in the following way: Apply for each (i,j) the interval inclusion rule with standard t-based $(1-2\alpha)$-confidence intervals for $\mu_i - \mu_j$. This yields a test for equivalence of $\mathcal{N}(\mu_i,\sigma^2)$ and $\mathcal{N}(\mu_j,\sigma^2)$ in the sense of $|\mu_i - \mu_j| < \varepsilon$ whose validity is not affected by changes of any other functions of the whole vector $(\mu_1,\ldots \mu_k)$ of means except for the difference within the given pair. Thus, deciding in favour of "global" equivalence of all k distributions if and only if all $\binom{k}{2}$ confidence intervals are included in $(-\varepsilon, \varepsilon)$ yields a valid level-α test of $H : |\mu_i - \mu_j| \geq \varepsilon$ for at least one (i, j) versus $K : |\mu_i - \mu_j| < \varepsilon$ for all $(i, j) \in \{1, \ldots, k\}^2$.

More often than not, the obvious advantages of this approach (conceptual simplicity of the underlying principle, ease of practical implementation of the resulting "global" decision rule) will be outweighed by the following drawbacks:

1. The test of $H : \max_{i<j}\{\rho(\theta_i, \theta_j)\} \geq \varepsilon$ versus $K : \max_{i<j}\{\rho(\theta_i, \theta_j)\} < \varepsilon$ obtained by applying the intersection-union principle with $q = \binom{k}{2}$ and $H_{ij} : \rho(\theta_i, \theta_j) \geq \varepsilon$ vs. $K_{ij} : \rho(\theta_i, \theta_j) < \varepsilon$ $(1 \leq i < j \leq k)$ as the elementary testing problems can be markedly overconservative.

2. Looking at the maximum distance between pairs of distributions might not adequately translate an investigator's notion of equivalence between all k distributions into a testable statistical hypothesis; for other distance measures, the intersection-union principle is typically no longer applicable.

In the following sections of the present chapter, we show for selected settings frequently encountered in practice, how to replace the intersection-union test with a less conservative specific multisample test for equivalence.

7.2 F-test for equivalence of k normal distributions

The considerations of this (as well as of the subsequent) section refer to the classical univariate ANOVA one-way layout with normally distributed observations of common (yet unknown) variance $\sigma^2 \in \mathbb{R}_+$. Thus we suppose that the pooled data set to be analyzed exhibits the following structure:

$$
\begin{array}{lll}
X_{11}, \ldots, X_{1n_1} & \leftarrow & \text{1st} \quad \text{sample, from } \mathcal{N}(\mu_1, \sigma^2) \\
X_{21}, \ldots, X_{2n_2} & \leftarrow & \text{2nd} \quad \text{sample, from } \mathcal{N}(\mu_2, \sigma^2) \\
\ldots\ldots\ldots\ldots\ldots & \ldots & \ldots \quad \ldots\ldots\ldots, \ldots\ldots\ldots\ldots\ldots \\
X_{k1}, \ldots, X_{kn_k} & \leftarrow & \text{kth} \quad \text{sample, from } \mathcal{N}(\mu_k, \sigma^2)
\end{array}
$$

In the balanced case $n_1 = \ldots = n_k = n$, a natural measure of the degree to which the true underlying distributions deviate from the "ideal" of perfect pairwise coincidence is given by the squared Euclidean distance of the vector $(\mu_1/\sigma, \ldots, \mu_k/\sigma)$ from the point $(\bar{\mu}./\sigma)\, \mathbf{1}_k$, where $\bar{\mu}.$ and $\mathbf{1}_k$ denotes the ordinary arithmetic mean of the μ_i and the k-vector of ones, respectively. A useful way of extending the definition of this measure to arbitrarily unbalanced designs of the same kind consists of replacing $\bar{\mu}.$ with the average $\tilde{\mu}.$, say, of the sample-size–weighted population means $n_i\mu_i$, and the unit weight to the squared distance in the ith component with $(n_i/\bar{n})$. The resulting generalized squared Euclidean distance is then given by

$$\psi^2 = \sum_{i=1}^{k}(n_i/\bar{n})(\mu_i - \tilde{\mu}.)^2/\sigma^2 , \tag{7.6}$$

with

$$\tilde{\mu}. = \sum_{i=1}^{k} n_i\mu_i / \sum_{i=1}^{k} n_i , \quad \bar{n} = \sum_{i=1}^{k} n_i/k . \tag{7.7}$$

Using ψ^2 as our target parameter leads to the problem of testing

$$H : \psi^2 \geq \varepsilon^2 \quad \text{versus} \quad K : \psi^2 < \varepsilon^2 \tag{7.8}$$

with suitably fixed $\varepsilon > 0$.

Clearly, in any balanced design, equivalence in the sense of (7.8) is satisfied if and only if the point with the standardized population means as coordinates lies in a k-dimensional sphere of radius ε around $(\bar{\mu}./\sigma, \ldots, \bar{\mu}./\sigma)$. In the case of $k = 2$ samples with common size $n_1 = n_2 = n$, this condition simplifies still further in that it turns out equivalent to $|\mu_1 - \mu_2|/\sigma < \sqrt{2}\,\varepsilon$. This suggests adopting the guidance given in Table 1.1(v) for specifying the tolerance ε in the two-sample case, also for arbitrary multisample designs choosing $\varepsilon = .36/\sqrt{2} \approx .25$ and $\varepsilon = .74/\sqrt{2} \approx .50$, depending on whether the equivalence criterion is intended to be rather strict or comparatively weak.

The testing problem (7.8) remains invariant under a large group $\mathcal{G}$, say, of affine transformations which contains in particular arbitrary common rescalings and translations of all observations in the pooled sample (an exhaustive characterization of $\mathcal{G}$ involves canonical coordinates and is not required in the present context; for full mathematical details see Lehmann, 1986, § 7.1) . The usual F-statistic for the one-way fixed-effects ANOVA is a maximal invariant with respect to this group of transformations. Dropping the constant factor $\bar{n}/(k-1)$, it can be viewed as an estimator of the target parameter ψ^2 so that we write

$$\hat{\psi}^2 = \frac{\displaystyle\sum_{i=1}^{k}(n_i/\bar{n})(\bar{X}_i - \bar{X}..)^2}{(N-k)^{-1}\displaystyle\sum_{i=1}^{k}\sum_{\nu=1}^{n_i}(X_{i\nu} - \bar{X}_i)^2} \tag{7.9}$$

The distribution of $(\bar{n}/(k-1))\hat{\psi}^2$ depends on the μ_i and σ^2 only through ψ^2 and is noncentral F with $k-1, N-k$ degrees of freedom (where N denotes the total sample size $\sum_{i=1}^{k} n_i$) and noncentrality parameter $\lambda_{nc}^2 = \bar{n}\psi^2$. It is thus an element of a family with strictly monotone likelihood ratios, and it follows that the class of all level-α tests for (7.8) which depend on the raw data only through $\hat{\psi}^2$ contains a uniformly most powerful one. The critical region of this optimal test is given by

$$\left\{ \hat{\psi}^2 < ((k-1)/\bar{n})F_{k-1,N-k;\,\alpha}(\bar{n}\varepsilon^2) \right\} \qquad (7.10)$$

with

$$
\begin{aligned}
F_{k-1,N-k;\,\alpha}(\bar{n}\varepsilon^2) \;\equiv\; &\text{lower } 100\alpha\text{-percentage point of a non-}\\
&\text{central } F\text{-distribution with } k-1, N-k\\
&\text{degrees of freedom and noncentrality}\\
&\text{parameter } \bar{n}\varepsilon^2\,. \qquad\qquad\qquad (7.11)
\end{aligned}
$$

In view of the maximal invariance of the statistic $\hat{\psi}^2$ with respect to the group $\mathcal{G}$ of all transformations of the full sample space leaving the testing problem invariant, the rejection region (7.10) defines an UMPI level-α test for (7.8). Its size is exactly equal to α, and the power against any specific alternative is strictly greater than the significance level ($\rightarrow$ strictly unbiased testing procedure). The exact rejection probability under any parameter constellation depends only on ψ^2 and can easily be computed by means of the formula:

$$\beta(\psi^2) = P\left[\,\mathcal{F}_{k-1,N-k}(\bar{n}\psi^2) < F_{k-1,N-k;\,\alpha}(\bar{n}\varepsilon^2)\,\right] \qquad (7.12)$$

where $\mathcal{F}_{k-1,N-k}(\tilde{\psi}^2)$ stands for a variable which has an F-distribution with $k-1, N-k$ degrees of freedom and noncentrality parameter $\tilde{\psi}^2$. In particular, using *SAS* one will obtain the value of $\beta(\psi^2)$ simply by submitting the statements

```
c=finv(alpha,k-1,N-k,n_*eps**2);

beta=probf(c,k-1,N-k,n_*psi**2);
```

provided, the value specified for α, k, N, $\bar{n}$, ε and ψ has been previously assigned to the variable alpha, k, N, n_, eps and psi, respectively.

Example 7.1

In a comparative clinical trial of 4 different antihypertensive treatments, blood pressure was recorded continuously over 24 hours in each patient enrolled. The AUC (area under the curve) for the diastolic value divided by the length of the measurement interval was defined as the primary endpoint for assessing efficacy of treatment. The raw data [mm Hg] obtained in this way are listed in the following table:

Table 7.1 *Raw data of a 4-arm trial using the average of diastolic blood pressure recorded continuously over 24 hours as primary endpoint*

Sample 1

112.488,	103.738,	86.344,	101.708,	95.108,	105.931,
95.815,	91.864,	102.479,	102.644		

Sample 2

100.421,	101.966,	99.636,	105.983,	88.377,	102.618,
105.486,	98.662,	94.137,	98.626,	89.367,	106.204

Sample 3

84.846,	100.488,	119.763,	103.736,	93.141,	108.254,
99.510,	89.005,	108.200,	82.209,	100.104,	103.706,
107.067					

Sample 4

100.825,	100.255,	103.363,	93.230,	95.325,	100.288,
94.750,	107.129,	98.246,	96.365,	99.740,	106.049,
92.691,	93.111,	98.243			

The sample means and standard deviations computed from these raw data are shown in Table 7.2. Hence, in the present example, we have:

$$N = 50\,, \quad k = 4\,, \quad \bar{n} = 12.5\,; \qquad \bar{X}_{..} = 99.3849\,;$$

$$\sum_{i=1}^{k} (n_i/\bar{n})(\bar{X}_i - \bar{X}_{..})^2 = 1.2157\,;$$

$$(N-k)^{-1} \sum_{i=1}^{k} \sum_{\nu=1}^{n_i} (X_{i\nu} - \bar{X}_i)^2 = 54.6976\,;$$

$$\Rightarrow \qquad \hat{\psi}^2 = 1.2157/54.6976 = .0222\,.$$

Specifying $\alpha = .05$ and $\varepsilon = .50$, the critical upper bound of (7.10) comes out (using *SAS*) as

$$c = (3/12.5) \cdot F_{4-1, 50-4;\,.05}(12.5 \cdot .25) = .24 \cdot \mathtt{finv}(.05, 3, 46, 3.125)$$
$$= .24 \cdot .30833 = .0740\,.$$

Since the observed value of the test statistic $\hat{\psi}^2$ falls below this bound, the UMPI test rejects nonequivalence.

Table 7.2 *Summary statistics for the raw data of Table 7.1*
[with i numbering the individual samples]

i	n_i	$\bar{X}_i$	S_i
1	10	99.8120	7.5639
2	12	99.2903	5.9968
3	13	100.0024	10.4809
4	15	98.6407	4.5309

Finally, evaluating the right-hand side of equation (7.12) yields for the power of the test against the specific alternative of identical distributions:
$\beta(0) = P\left[\mathcal{F}_{3,46}(0) < (12.5/3) \cdot c\right] = \texttt{probf(.30833,3,46,0)} = 18.08\%$.

7.3 Modified studentized range test for equivalence

Under the additional assumption that the one-way ANOVA layout we are dealing with is a *balanced* one satisfying $n_1 = \ldots = n_k = n$, an alternative approach to testing for equivalence of an arbitrary number k of normal distributions with means $\mu_i \in \mathbb{R}$ and common variance $\sigma^2 > 0$ can be based on the studentized range statistic. Of course, such a change in the test statistic would make little if any sense without a corresponding reformulation of hypotheses in terms of a different parametric function viewed as the basic measure of dissimilarity of the distributions under assessment. In the present context, this measure is chosen to be the maximum of all pairwise distances between standardized population means which leads to replacing (7.8) with the testing problem

$$\tilde{H}_\mu : \max_{i<j} |\mu_i - \mu_j|/\sigma \geq \delta \quad \text{versus} \quad \tilde{K}_\mu : \max_{i<j} |\mu_i - \mu_j|/\sigma < \delta, \quad (7.13)$$

with arbitrarily fixed equivalence margin $\delta > 0$. The studentized range statistic which will be denoted R_s in the sequel, is obtained by simply replacing both $\max_{i<j} |\mu_i - \mu_j|$ and σ with its sample analogue yielding

$$R_s = \frac{\bar{X}_{(k)} - \bar{X}_{(1)}}{S} \qquad (7.14)$$

where $\bar{X}_{(i)}$ stands for the ith-smallest $(i = 1, \ldots, k)$ among the k sample means, and S^2 is the usual ANOVA estimator of the error variance as appearing in the denominator to (7.9).

In the equivalence case, determining a suitable critical constant for the statistic R_s is a rather complicated problem which has been solved by Giani and Finner (1991). As shown by these authors, the critical bound $r_{\alpha;\delta}(n,k)$, say, which the studentized range statistic has to be compared with in order to obtain a valid test for (7.13), has to be computed as the αth quantile of the distribution of R_s under the specific parameter constellation $(\mu_1/\sigma, \ldots, \mu_k/\sigma) = (-\delta/2, 0, \ldots, 0, \delta/2)$. Fortunately, a program has been made available by the same group of authors (Giani, Straßburger and Seefeldt, 1997) which computes $r_{\alpha; \delta}(n, k)$ for arbitrary combinations of α, δ, n and k by numerical integration. Table 7.3 shows the critical upper bounds to R_s to be used in equivalence testing at level $\alpha = .05$ for $\delta \in \{1/2, 1\}$ with up to 5 samples of size 10 and 50, respectively.

Table 7.3 *Critical bounds for the studentized range test for equivalence at level $\alpha = .05$, for $\delta = 1/2$, 1, $\quad n = 10$, 50 and $k = 3$, 4, 5 [computed by means of the program SeParATe, Version 2.0B (Giani, Straßburger and Seefeldt, 1997)]*

δ	n	k	$r_{\alpha; \delta}(n, k)$
.50	10	3	.185896
"	10	4	.293307
"	10	5	.376803
"	50	3	.221237
"	50	4	.255186
"	50	5	.281114
1.00	10	3	.407372
"	10	4	.494329
"	10	5	.559521
"	50	3	.669046
"	50	4	.673074
"	50	5	.676400

Example 7.1 (continued)

Suppose 99.8120 ± 7.5639, 99.2903 ± 5.9968, 100.0024 ± 10.4809, 98.6407 ± 4.5309 [cf. Table 7.2] would actually describe (in terms of $\bar{X}_i \pm S_i$) the data obtained in a *balanced* trial involving $k = 4$ groups of size $n = 10$ each. Then, the estimator of the error variance would take on the value $S^2 = (7.5639^2 + 5.9968^2 + 10.4809^2 + 4.5309^2)/4 = 55.8881$, and for the studentized range statistic we would have

$$R_s = (\bar{X}_{(4)} - \bar{X}_{(1)})/S = (100.0024 - 98.6407)/\sqrt{55.8881} = .1821.$$

On the other hand, the critical bound to which R_s must be compared in a test at level $\alpha = .05$ of $\max_{i<j} |\mu_i - \mu_j|/\sigma \geq 1.00$ versus $\max_{i<j} |\mu_i - \mu_j|/\sigma < 1.00$ with four groups of 10 observations each is seen from the above table to be $r_{.05; 1.00}(10, 4) = .494329$. Hence, with the data and the specifications of this (synthetic) example, the modified studentized range test decides in favour of equivalence again.

Before concluding the discussion of approaches to testing for equivalence of several homoskedastic normal distributions with respect to their standardized means, it seems worthwhile to point out the *most important differences and similarities between the modified studentized range and the noncentral F-test* of § 7.2:

- Both tests are exactly valid with respect to the significance level, provided there are no deviations from the basic assumptions of the classical ANOVA model.

- The critical constant of the noncentral F-test can easily be computed without recourse to nonstandard software.

- The applicability of the studentized range statistic is restricted to balanced designs whereas the noncentral F-test allows for arbitrary imbalances between the sample sizes.

- Power comparisons between the procedures are futile since the hypotheses they are tailored for are of grossly different shape (except for $k = 2$).

7.4 Testing for dispersion equivalence of more than two Gaussian distributions

If homoskedasticity of the normal distributions behind the samples $(X_{11}, \ldots, X_{1n_1}), \ldots, (X_{k1}, \ldots, X_{kn_k})$ cannot be taken for granted a priori, then it is natural that one tries to establish it by means of the actual data. In order to keep the description of a large-sample procedure for an equivalence hypothesis specifying homoskedasticity except for negligible heterogeneity of the variances as simple as possible, we restrict consideration first to balanced designs. Furthermore, it will be convenient to use the following additional notation:

$$\zeta_i = \log \sigma_i, \quad \bar{\zeta} = k^{-1} \sum_{i=1}^{k} \log \sigma_i ; \tag{7.15a}$$

$$Z_i = \log S_i, \quad \bar{Z} = k^{-1} \sum_{i=1}^{k} \log S_i . \tag{7.15b}$$

A reasonable way of translating the phrase "homoskedastic except for irrelevant differences in variability" into a formal statement about a suitable parametric function consists in requiring that all logarithmic standard deviations ζ_i lie in a sphere of sufficiently small radius ε_* around their average $\bar{\zeta}$. This leads to proposing the problem of testing

$$H_\sigma : \sum_{i=1}^{k} (\zeta_i - \bar{\zeta})^2 \geq \varepsilon_*^2 \quad \text{versus} \quad K_\sigma : \sum_{i=1}^{k} (\zeta_i - \bar{\zeta})^2 < \varepsilon_*^2 \tag{7.16}$$

with some suitably fixed $\varepsilon_* > 0$. Some guidance for choosing the equivalence margin for $\sum_{i=1}^{k}(\zeta_i - \bar\zeta)^2$ can be provided by noting that in the two-sample case, dispersion equivalence in the sense of the above alternative hypothesis K_σ reduces to the condition $(1 + \varepsilon)^{-1} < \sigma_1/\sigma_2 < 1 + \varepsilon$ with ε being related to ε_* by the equation $\varepsilon_* = (1/\sqrt{2}) \log(1 + \varepsilon)$. In view of this fact, generalizing the suggestions given in Table 1.1 for choosing the equivalence margin for the case of $k = 2$ variances leads to specifying $\varepsilon_* = .2867$ or $\varepsilon_* = .4901$, depending on whether a rather strict or more liberal criterion of equivalence is intended to apply.

In order to construct a large-sample test for (7.16), we exploit the well-known fact (see, e.g., Lehmann, 1986, p. 376) that the observed log-standard deviations $Z_1 = \log S_1, \ldots, Z_k = \log S_k$ are asymptotically normal and mutually independent estimators of the corresponding population parameters $\zeta_1 = \log \sigma_1, \ldots, \zeta_k = \log \sigma_k$. Since all of these estimators have the same asymptotic variance $(2n)^{-1}$, this means that for large n, the $Z_i = \log S_i$ have distributions $\mathcal{N}(\log \sigma_i, 1/2n)$. In view of the mutual independence of all statistics depending on individual variables from different samples, this implies that for arbitrary values of the true σ_i's, we have

$$P\left[2n \sum_{i=1}^{k}(Z_i - \bar Z)^2 \le v^2\right] \approx G_{k-1, \lambda_{nc}^2}(v^2) \ \forall \ v^2 > 0 \qquad (7.17)$$

with $\lambda_{nc}^2 = 2n \sum(\zeta_i - \bar\zeta)^2$ and $G_{k-1, \lambda_{nc}^2}(\cdot)$ as the cdf of a χ^2-distribution with $df = k - 1$ and noncentrality parameter λ_{nc}^2.

In view of (7.17), an approximately valid test at level α for (7.16) is given by the rejection region

$$\left\{Q_{k,n} < q_{k,n;\,\alpha}(\varepsilon_*)\right\} \qquad (7.18)$$

where

$$Q_{k,n} = 2n \sum_{i=1}^{k}\left[\log S_i - (1/k)\sum_{\iota=1}^{k}\log S_\iota\right]^2 \qquad (7.19)$$

and

$$q_{k,n;\,\alpha}(\varepsilon_*) = \chi_{k-1;\,\alpha}^2(2n\varepsilon_*^2) \equiv \text{lower } 100\alpha \text{ percentage point}$$
$$\text{of a } \chi^2\text{-distribution with } k - 1 \text{ degrees of freedom}$$
$$\text{and noncentrality parameter } \lambda_{nc}^2 = 2n\varepsilon_*^2. \qquad (7.20)$$

The power of this test against any alternative $(\sigma_1, \ldots, \sigma_k) \in \mathbb{R}_+^k$ such that $2n \sum_{i=1}^{k}\left[\log \sigma_i - (1/k)\left(\sum_{\iota=1}^{k}\log \sigma_\iota\right)\right]^2 = \tilde\lambda_{nc}^2 < 2n\varepsilon_*^2$ can be approximated as

$$\beta(\tilde\lambda_{nc}^2) \approx G_{k-1;\tilde\lambda_{nc}^2}\left(\chi_{k-1;\,\alpha}^2(2n\varepsilon_*^2)\right). \qquad (7.21)$$

Example 7.2

The data displayed in Table 7.4 are sample variances and corresponding log-standard deviations observed in $k = 4$ groups of common size $n = 50$. The Gaussian distributions behind the samples are to be tested for dispersion equivalence in the sense of (7.16) where the radius ε_* of the equivalence sphere centred at the mean of the logarithmic population standard deviations is specified $\varepsilon_* = .2867$ corresponding to a ratio of 1.5 at most in the two-sample case. The significance level is once more fixed at $\alpha = .05$.

Table 7.4 *Variances and logarithmic standard deviations computed from a raw data set consisting of $k = 4$ independent samples of common size $n = 50$*

i	1	2	3	4
S_i^2	49.4	45.7	43.1	53.6
Z_i	1.9500	1.9110	1.8818	1.9908

For this data set, the value of the test statistic turns out as

$$2 \cdot 50 \cdot \sum_{i=1}^{k} (Z_i - \bar{Z})^2 = 100 \cdot .006735 = .6735 \,.$$

On the other hand, the critical upper bound which $2n \sum_{i=1}^{k} (Z_i - \bar{Z})^2$ has to be compared to, is readily computed (using once more the respective *SAS* function) to be

$$\chi^2_{3;.05}(2 \cdot 50 \cdot .2867^2) = \texttt{cinv(.05,3,8.2197)} = 2.85636 \,.$$

Since the value observed for the test statistic clearly falls short of this bound, the data set shown in the above table falls in the rejection region (7.18) so that we have to decide in favour of dispersion equivalence of the underlying normal distributions. In order to approximate the power of the test against the alternative of exact homoskedasticity, we invoke the *SAS* intrinsic function for the cdf rather the quantile function of the χ^2-distribution with $k - 1 = 3$ degrees of freedom, giving

$$\beta(0) \approx G_{3;0}(2.85636) = \texttt{probchi(2.85636,3,0)} = 58.57\% \,.$$

Although it is not our intention here to enter into a detailed investigation of the accuracy of the approximation (7.17) underlying the testing procedure given by (7.18) – (7.20), it should be mentioned that sufficient simulation results are available to justify the following qualitative statements: Even for large numbers k of distributions to compare, the probability of rejecting the null hypothesis of (7.16) according to (7.18) approaches the nominal significance level α rather quickly with increasing common sample size n, under parameter configurations lying on the common boundary of H_σ and K_σ. Furthermore, if nonnegligible discrepancies between α and exact rejection probabilities under parameter configurations $(\sigma_1, \ldots, \sigma_k)$ satisfying $\sum_{i=1}^{k} \left[\log \sigma_i - (1/k) \sum_{\iota=1}^{k} \log \sigma_\iota \right]^2 = \varepsilon_*^2$ occur at all, the testing procedure is found to be over- rather that anticonservative throughout.

Generalization to the unbalanced case

Unbalancedness of the design requires only minor modifications to the test. It suffices to replace in all sums appearing in the formula for the test statistic and the noncentrality parameter, unit weights by the weighing factors $n_i/\bar{n}$, with $\bar{n} = N/k = \sum_{i=1}^{k} n_i/k$.

By plugging in these weights the alternative hypothesis of dispersion equivalence takes on the form

$$K_\sigma' : \sum_{i=1}^{k} (n_i/\bar{n}) \left(\zeta_i - \sum_{\iota=1}^{k} n_\iota \zeta_\iota/N \right)^2 , \tag{7.16'}$$

and the test statistic has to be computed as

$$Q_{k,n}' \equiv 2 \sum_{i=1}^{k} n_i \left[\log S_i - \sum_{\iota=1}^{k} n_\iota \log S_\iota/N \right]^2 . \tag{7.19'}$$

Finally, the critical upper bound to which the observed value of $Q_{k,n}'$ has to be compared, is given by

$$q_{k,n;\,\alpha}'(\varepsilon_*) = \chi_{k-1;\alpha}^2 (2\bar{n}\varepsilon_*^2) . \tag{7.20'}$$

7.5 A nonparametric k-sample test for equivalence

The approach to multisample equivalence testing to be discussed in this section can be viewed as a natural extension of the Mann-Whitney test for equivalence of two continuous distributions of arbitrary shape as described in § 6.2. Although the basic idea behind this extension is almost self-explanatory, the construction is technically rather intricate involving a lengthy sequence of formulae for the various entries in the covariance matrix of a vector of U-statistics whose dimension grows with the square of the number of distributions under comparison. Instead of writing down all these details which would be rather tedious, we confine the exposition to an outline of major steps to be taken in carrying out the construction.

First of all, we must define a sensible nonparametric measure of distance between all k distributions. This can be obtained by measuring the distance between each individual pair of distributions in the same way as in the two-sample case and combining the resulting $k(k-1)/2$ functionals into a single overall measure by means of a suitable algebraic operation. In order to make this idea precise, let us define for any $1 \leq i < j \leq k$

$$\pi_{ij}^+ = P[X_i > X_j] = \int F_j \, dF_i \qquad (7.22)$$

where X_i and X_j denote "generic" observations, independent of each other, from population i and j with cdf F_i and F_j, respectively. In view of the obvious fact that $F_i = F_j \Rightarrow \pi_{ij}^+ = 1/2$, we proposed in §6.2 $|\pi_{ij}^+ - 1/2|$ as a suitable nonparametric distance measure for the case of two samples. A natural generalization to the k-sample setting is to replace $|\pi_{ij}^+ - 1/2|$ with the Euclidean distance between the vector $(\pi_{12}^+, \ldots, \pi_{1k}^+, \pi_{23}^+, \ldots, \pi_{k-1,k}^+)$ of all pairwise proversion probabilities (7.22), and that point in the $(k(k-1)/2)$-dimensional unit interval whose coordinates all equal $1/2$. Using this distance in its squared form (which turns out technically a bit more convenient), we are lead to formulate the testing problem

$$H : \sum_{i<j}(\pi_{ij}^+ - 1/2)^2 \geq \tilde{\varepsilon}^2 \quad \text{versus} \quad K : \sum_{i<j}(\pi_{ij}^+ - 1/2)^2 < \tilde{\varepsilon}^2 \qquad (7.23)$$

with suitably specified equivalence margin $\tilde{\varepsilon}^2 > 0$.

In order to keep notation sufficiently compact, we introduce an extra symbol for representing the squared Euclidean distance between any two vectors in $(k(k-1)/2)$-dimensional space defining

$$d^2(\boldsymbol{u}, \boldsymbol{v}) = \sum_{i=1}^{k(k-1)/2} (u_i - v_i)^2, \quad \boldsymbol{u}, \boldsymbol{v} \in \mathbb{R}^{k(k-1)/2}. \qquad (7.24)$$

Using this convention, the condition assumed to be satisfied under the alternative hypothesis of (7.23) can be written $d^2(\boldsymbol{\pi}^+, \boldsymbol{1/2}) < \tilde{\varepsilon}^2$, provided the symbols appearing as arguments to $d^2(\,\cdot\,,\,\cdot\,)$ in that inequality are read as

$$\boldsymbol{\pi}^+ = (\pi_{12}^+, \ldots, \pi_{1k}^+, \pi_{23}^+, \ldots, \pi_{k-1,k}^+), \ \ \boldsymbol{1/2} = (1/2) \cdot \boldsymbol{1}_{k(k-1)/2}, \qquad (7.25)$$

with $\boldsymbol{1}_m$ denoting the vector of m 1's for arbitrary $m \in \mathbb{N}$.

Now, a natural choice of a statistic which an asymptotic test for establishing the hypothesis $K : d^2(\boldsymbol{\pi}^+, \boldsymbol{1/2}) < \tilde{\varepsilon}^2$ can be based upon, is this: We estimate the squared distance between $\boldsymbol{\pi}^+$ and $\boldsymbol{1/2}$ by that between the corresponding vector $\boldsymbol{W}^+$, say, of two-sample U-statistics, and the same point of reference in the parameter space $[0, 1]^{k(k-1)/2}$. Of course, for any $1 \leq i < j \leq k$, the (i, j)-component of $\boldsymbol{W}^+$ has to be defined by

$$W_{ij}^+ = \frac{1}{n_i n_j} \sum_{\mu=1}^{n_i} \sum_{\nu=1}^{n_j} I_{(0,\infty)}(X_{i\mu} - X_{j\nu}) \qquad (7.26)$$

[recall (6.11)].

The most tedious part of the construction consists in establishing a procedure for estimating the asymptotic standard error of the estimated distance $d^2(\mathbf{W}^+, 1/2)$. For that purpose, we need to know the full covariance matrix, say $\mathbf{\Sigma}^{(N)} = (\sigma^{(N)}_{(i_1,j_1),(i_2,j_2)})_{1 \leq i_1 < j_1 \leq k,\, 1 \leq i_2 < j_2 \leq k}$, of $\sqrt{N}\mathbf{W}^+$. For each element of $\mathbf{\Sigma}^{(N)}$, an exact expression can be found which is a function of the sizes of the samples involved, the appropriate components of $\boldsymbol{\pi}^+$, and functionals of the form $P[X_{i_1} > X_{j_1}, X_{i_2} > X_{j_2}]$. The resulting formulae for $\sigma^{(N)}_{(i_1,j_1),(i_2,j_2)}$ differ markedly in structure, depending on the number of common elements in the set $\{i_1, j_1, i_2, j_2\}$ of indices involved. For $i_1 \neq i_2$, $j_1 \neq j_2$, $W^+_{i_1 j_1}$ and $W^+_{i_2 j_2}$ refer to four different samples, which trivially implies that we have

$$\sigma^{(N)}_{(i_1,j_1),(i_2,j_2)} = 0 \text{ for all } (i_1, j_1), (i_2, j_2) \text{ with } i_1 \neq i_2 \text{ and } j_1 \neq j_2. \quad (7.27)$$

The other extreme is given by the diagonal elements of $\mathbf{\Sigma}^{(N)}$: In this case, $\{i_1, j_1, i_2, j_2\}$ reduces to a set of cardinality 2, say $\{i, j\}$, and $\sigma^{(N)}_{(i,j),(i,j)}$ is readily obtained by applying formulae (6.12), (6.13) for the computation of the exact variance of a single Mann-Whitney statistic. If the pairs (i_1, j_1) and (i_2, j_2) coincide with respect to the first component but differ in the second, we have

$$\sigma^{(N)}_{(i_1,j_1),(i_2,j_2)} = (N/n_i)\left(P[X_i > X_{j_1}, X_i > X_{j_2}] - \pi^+_{ij_1}\pi^+_{ij_2}\right)$$

$$= (N/n_i)\left(\int F_{j_1} F_{j_2}\, dF_i - \int F_{j_1}\, dF_i \int F_{j_2}\, dF_i\right)$$

$$\text{for} \quad i = i_1 = i_2, \qquad\qquad\qquad (7.28)$$

and so on for the other possible constellations with $\#(\{i_1, j_1\} \cap \{i_2, j_2\}) = 1$.

Obviously, all these expressions converge to well-defined limits, say $\sigma_{(i_1,j_1),(i_2,j_2)}$, as $N \to \infty$, provided the relative size n_i/N of each sample converges to some nondegenerate limit $\lambda_i \in (0,1)$ as the total sample size grows to infinity. Furthermore, it follows from well-known results of the asymptotic theory of generalized U-statistics (cf. Lee, 1990, § 3.7.1) that the existence of nondegenerate limits for all n_i/N ensures weak convergence of the normalized vector $\sqrt{N}(\mathbf{W}^+ - \boldsymbol{\pi}^+)$ of pairwise Mann-Whitney statistics to a centred $(k(k-1))$-variate normal distribution with covariance matrix $\mathbf{\Sigma} = \lim_{N\to\infty} \mathbf{\Sigma}^{(N)}$. Hence, another application of the δ-method yields

$$\sqrt{N}\big(d^2(\mathbf{W}^+, 1/2) - d^2(\boldsymbol{\pi}^+, 1/2)\big)$$

$$\xrightarrow{d} \mathcal{N}\big(0, \sigma^2[d^2(\mathbf{W}^+, 1/2)]\big) \text{ as } N \to \infty \qquad (7.29)$$

with

$$\sigma^2\big[d^2(\mathbf{W}^+, 1/2)\big] = 4(\boldsymbol{\pi}^+ - 1/2)\mathbf{\Sigma}(\boldsymbol{\pi}^+ - 1/2)'. \qquad (7.30)$$

Finally, under mild additional regularity conditions, each entry $\sigma^{(N)}_{(i_1,j_1),(i_2,j_2)}$ in the exact covariance matrix $\mathbf{\Sigma}^{(N)}$ can be consistently estimated by means of a suitable function of two-sample ($\rightarrow$ diagonal elements) or two- and three-sample U-statistics ($\rightarrow$ off-diagonal elements). In view of $\sigma^{(N)}_{(i_1,j_1),(i_2,j_2)} \rightarrow \sigma_{(i_1,j_1),(i_2,j_2)} \forall \big((i_1,j_1),(i_2,j_2) \big)$, these estimators are a fortiori consistent for the respective elements of the limiting covariance matrix Σ. Thus, if we denote by $\widehat{\Sigma}^{(N)}$ the matrix obtained by replacing each $\sigma^{(N)}_{(i_1,j_1),(i_2,j_2)}$ with its consistent estimator, the asymptotic variance (7.30) of $\sqrt{N} d^2(\boldsymbol{W}^+, \boldsymbol{1/2})$ can be consistently estimated by

$$\hat{\sigma}^2_N \big[d^2(\boldsymbol{W}^+, \boldsymbol{1/2}) \big] = 4(\boldsymbol{W}^+ - \boldsymbol{1/2}) \widehat{\Sigma}^{(N)}(\boldsymbol{W}^+ - \boldsymbol{1/2})' . \tag{7.31}$$

Hence, we have

$$\frac{\sqrt{N}\big(d^2(\boldsymbol{W}^+, \boldsymbol{1/2}) - d^2(\boldsymbol{\pi}^+, \boldsymbol{1/2}) \big)}{\hat{\sigma}_N\big[d^2(\boldsymbol{W}^+, \boldsymbol{1/2}) \big]} \xrightarrow{\mathcal{L}} \mathcal{N}(0,1) \text{ as } N \to \infty \tag{7.32}$$

under any k-tuple $(F_1, \ldots, F_k)$ of continuous cdf's such that Σ is positive definite and $\boldsymbol{\pi}^+ \neq \boldsymbol{1/2}$. Accordingly, an approximate level-α test for (7.23) can be based on the decision rule:

Reject nonequivalence in the sense of $d^2(\boldsymbol{\pi}^+, \boldsymbol{1/2}) \geq \tilde{\varepsilon}^2$ iff

$$d^2(\boldsymbol{W}^+, \boldsymbol{1/2}) < \tilde{\varepsilon}^2 - u_{1-\alpha} \cdot \hat{\sigma}_N\big[d^2(\boldsymbol{W}^+, \boldsymbol{1/2}) \big] \big] / \sqrt{N} . \tag{7.33}$$

Example 7.1 (continued)

To illustrate the nonparametric approach to multisample equivalence testing described above, we reanalyze the data set introduced in Example 7.1. With the entries in Table 7.1, the $k(k-1)/2 = 6$ pairwise Mann-Whitney statistics are computed to be:

$$W^+_{12} = .52500, \ W^+_{13} = .49231, \ W^+_{14} = .57333;$$

$$W^+_{23} = .44231, \ W^+_{24} = .56667, \ W^+_{34} = .58974.$$

Thus, the result of estimating the squared distance between $\boldsymbol{\pi}^+$ and $\boldsymbol{1/2}$ is

$$\begin{aligned}
d^2(\boldsymbol{W}^+, \boldsymbol{1/2}) &= (.52500 - .5)^2 + (.49231 - .5)^2 + (.57333 - .5)^2 \\
&\quad + (.44231 - .5)^2 + (.56667 - .5)^2 + (.58974 - .5)^2 \\
&= .021888 .
\end{aligned}$$

For the estimated exact covariance matrix $\widehat{\Sigma}^{(N)}$ of $\sqrt{N}\,\boldsymbol{W}^+$, we obtain

$$N^{-1}\hat{\mathbf{\Sigma}}^{(N)} = \begin{pmatrix} .01392 & .00704 & .01112 & -.00386 & -.00650 & .00000 \\ .00704 & .01271 & .00777 & .01012 & .00000 & -.01026 \\ .01112 & .00777 & .01487 & .00000 & .00371 & .00214 \\ -.00386 & .01012 & .00000 & .01227 & .00440 & -.01142 \\ -.00650 & .00000 & .00371 & .00440 & .01195 & .00276 \\ .00000 & -.01026 & .00214 & -.01142 & .00276 & .01257 \end{pmatrix}$$

Plugging in the observed values of $\boldsymbol{W}^+$ and $N^{-1}\hat{\mathbf{\Sigma}}^{(N)}$ on the right-hand side of (7.31), the empirical standard error of $d^2(\boldsymbol{W}^+, \mathbf{1/2})$ is found to be

$$\hat{\sigma}_N\left[d^2(\boldsymbol{W}^+, \mathbf{1/2})\right]/\sqrt{N} =$$

$$2 \cdot \left[(.02500, -.00769, .07333, -.05769, .06667, .08974)(N^{-1}\hat{\mathbf{\Sigma}}^{(N)})\right.$$

$$\left. (.02500, -.00769, .07333, -.05769, .06667, .08974)'\right]^{1/2} = .045094 \,.$$

Fixing the significance level at the conventional value $\alpha = .05$, there remains to specify the equivalence margin $\tilde{\varepsilon}^2$ for $d^2(\boldsymbol{\pi}^+, \mathbf{1/2})$. For the two-sample case, $|\pi_+ - 1/2| < .20$ has been proposed in § 1.5 as a reasonable criterion of equivalence. This motivates to choose $\tilde{\varepsilon}$ as the radius of the smallest sphere around $\mathbf{1/2}$ in $(k(k-1))$-dimensional space which contains all points with every coordinate equal to $1/2 \pm .20$. This leads to the specification $\tilde{\varepsilon}^2 = (k(k-1))/2 \cdot .20^2$ so that we use $\tilde{\varepsilon}^2 = 6 \cdot .04 = .24$ in the present example.

With $\alpha = .05$, $\tilde{\varepsilon}^2 = .24$ and $\hat{\sigma}_N\left[d^2(\boldsymbol{W}^+, \mathbf{1/2})\right]/\sqrt{N} = .045094$, the critical upper bound which the observed value of $d^2(\boldsymbol{W}^+, \mathbf{1/2})$ has to be compared to according to (7.33), is $.24 - 1.644854 \cdot .045094 = .165827$. Hence, the raw data shown in Table 7.1 fall in the rejection region of our nonparametric test at level $\alpha = .05$ for equivalence of the distributions from which the $k = 4$ samples under analysis are taken.

CHAPTER 8

Tests for establishing goodness of fit

8.1 Testing for equivalence of a single multinomial distribution with a fully specified reference distribution

In their simplest form, problems of testing for goodness rather than lack of fit involve a fully specified multinomial distribution, together with some sufficiently small "neighbourhood" of distributional models of the same kind which according to the alternative hypothesis to be established by means of the data, contains the true distribution from which the sample has been taken. In such a setting the primary data set consists of n mutually independent random vectors $(Y_{11}, \ldots, Y_{1k}), \ldots, (Y_{n1}, \ldots, Y_{nk})$ of dimension $k \geq 2$ where $(Y_{i1}, \ldots, Y_{ik})$ indicates in what out of k mutually exclusive categories the ith sampling unit is observed to be placed. Thus, $(Y_{i1}, \ldots, Y_{ik})$ consists of exactly $k - 1$ zeros and a single one, and the probability that the nonzero component appears at the jth position is assumed to be the same number $\pi_j \in [0, 1]$ for each element of the sample. As usual in the analysis of categorical data, these vectors are aggregated to the corresponding cell counts $(X_1, \ldots, X_k)$ form the beginning defining $X_j \equiv \#\{i \mid i \in \{1, \ldots, n\}, Y_{ij} = 1\}$ for $j = 1, \ldots, k$. Then, we have $\sum_{j=1}^{k} X_j = n$, and the distribution of $(X_1, \ldots, X_k)$ is multinomial with parameters n and $\boldsymbol{\pi} = (\pi_1, \ldots, \pi_k)$ given by the probability mass function

$$P\left[X_1 = x_1, \ldots, X_k = x_k\right] = n! \prod_{j=1}^{k} \pi_j^{x_j} / x_j! \,,$$

$$(x_1, \ldots, x_k) \in \left\{(\tilde{x}_1, \ldots, \tilde{x}_k) \mid \tilde{x}_j \in \mathbb{N}_\circ \, \forall \, j = 1, \ldots, k, \sum_{j=1}^{k} \tilde{x}_j = n\right\}. \quad (8.1)$$

The usual shorthand notation for this distribution is $\mathcal{M}(n; \pi_1, \ldots, \pi_k)$.

The reference distribution of $(X_1, \ldots, X_k)$ to which the true one is asserted to fit sufficiently well under the alternative hypothesis to be established by assessing the observed cell counts, is simply given by some specific choice of the parameter (row-) vector $\boldsymbol{\pi}$, say $\boldsymbol{\pi}^\circ = (\pi_1^\circ, \ldots, \pi_k^\circ) \in \left\{(p_1, \ldots, p_k) \in [0, 1]^k \mid \sum_{j=1}^{k} p_j = 1\right\}$. In order to quantify the degree of dissimilarity between the true and the target distribution of $(X_1, \ldots, X_k)$, it seems reasonable to use the ordinary Euclidean distance between the associated parameter vectors which leads to the following formulation of the problem of testing for goodness of fit of $\mathcal{M}(n; \pi_1, \ldots, \pi_k)$ to $\mathcal{M}(n; \pi_1^\circ, \ldots, \pi_k^\circ)$:

$$H : d^2(\boldsymbol{\pi}, \boldsymbol{\pi}^\circ) \geq \varepsilon^2 \quad \text{versus} \quad K : d^2(\boldsymbol{\pi}, \boldsymbol{\pi}^\circ) < \varepsilon^2. \qquad (8.2)$$

As before [recall (7.24)], $d^2(\cdot, \cdot)$ denotes the square of the metric in the Euclidean space of prespecified dimension. In other words, (8.2) has to be read with

$$d^2(\boldsymbol{\pi}, \boldsymbol{\pi}^\circ) = \sum_{j=1}^{k} (\pi_j - \pi_j^\circ)^2 \quad \forall \ \boldsymbol{\pi} \in \boldsymbol{\Pi} \qquad (8.3)$$

where $\boldsymbol{\Pi}$ denotes the parameter space for the underlying family of distributions, i.e., the hyperplane $\{(p_1, \ldots, p_k) \in [0,1]^k | \sum_{j=1}^{k} p_j = 1\}$ in the k-dimensional unit-cube.

In the special case that there are just 2 different categories, (8.2) reduces to the problem considered in § 4.3, with $(\pi_1^\circ - \varepsilon/\sqrt{2}, \pi_1^\circ + \varepsilon/\sqrt{2})$ as the equivalence range to the binomial parameter $p = \pi_1$. For larger values of k, there is no hope of being able to solve (8.2) in a way yielding an exact optimal testing procedure. Instead, we will rely again on asymptotic methods starting from the well-known fact (see, e.g., Bishop, Fienberg and Holland, 1975, Theorem 14.3–4) that the normalized vector

$$\sqrt{n}(\hat{\pi}_1 - \pi_1, \ldots, \hat{\pi}_k - \pi_k) \equiv \sqrt{n}(X_1/n - \pi_1, \ldots, X_k/n - \pi_k) \qquad (8.4)$$

of relative frequencies converges in law (as $n \to \infty$) to a random variable which follows a k-dimensional Gaussian distribution with mean $\mathbf{0}$ and covariance matrix

$$\boldsymbol{\Sigma}_{\boldsymbol{\pi}} = \boldsymbol{D}_{\boldsymbol{\pi}} - \boldsymbol{\pi}'\boldsymbol{\pi} \equiv \begin{pmatrix} \pi_1 & 0 & \cdots & 0 \\ 0 & \pi_2 & \cdots & 0 \\ \vdots & \vdots & & \vdots \\ 0 & 0 & \cdots & \pi_k \end{pmatrix} - \begin{pmatrix} \pi_1^2 & \cdots & \pi_1\pi_k \\ \pi_2\pi_1 & \cdots & \pi_2\pi_k \\ \vdots & & \vdots \\ \pi_k\pi_1 & \cdots & \pi_k^2 \end{pmatrix}. \qquad (8.5)$$

Furthermore, it is obvious that $\boldsymbol{\pi} \mapsto d^2(\boldsymbol{\pi}, \boldsymbol{\pi}^\circ)$ is totally differentiable on $\boldsymbol{\Pi}$ with gradient vector $\nabla d^2(\boldsymbol{\pi}, \boldsymbol{\pi}^\circ) = 2(\boldsymbol{\pi} - \boldsymbol{\pi}^\circ)$. These facts imply that we can exploit once more the so-called δ-method to derive the asymptotic distribution of the estimated squared distance $d^2(\hat{\boldsymbol{\pi}}, \boldsymbol{\pi}^\circ)$ between true and target parameter vector. Writing

$$\sigma_a^2\big[\sqrt{n}\, d^2(\hat{\boldsymbol{\pi}}, \boldsymbol{\pi}^\circ)\big] = 4\,(\boldsymbol{\pi} - \boldsymbol{\pi}^\circ)(\boldsymbol{D}_{\boldsymbol{\pi}} - \boldsymbol{\pi}'\boldsymbol{\pi})(\boldsymbol{\pi} - \boldsymbol{\pi}_\circ)', \qquad (8.6)$$

we may thus conclude that

$$\sqrt{n}\big(d^2(\hat{\boldsymbol{\pi}}, \boldsymbol{\pi}^\circ) - d^2(\boldsymbol{\pi}, \boldsymbol{\pi}^\circ)\big) \overset{\mathcal{L}}{\to} Z \sim \mathcal{N}\Big(0, \sigma_a^2\big[\sqrt{n}\, d^2(\hat{\boldsymbol{\pi}}, \boldsymbol{\pi}^\circ)\big]\Big)$$

$$\text{as} \quad n \to \infty. \qquad (8.7)$$

Next, the expression on the right-hand side of (8.6) is readily expanded into $4\big[\sum_{j=1}^{k}(\pi_j - \pi_j^\circ)^2\pi_j - \sum_{j_1=1}^{k}\sum_{j_2=1}^{k}(\pi_{j_1} - \pi_{j_1}^\circ)(\pi_{j_2} - \pi_{j_2}^\circ)\pi_{j_1}\pi_{j_2}\big]$ which is obviously a polynomial in $(\pi_1, \ldots, \pi_k)$. Since $\hat{\pi}_j$ is a consistent estimator of π_j for each $j = 1, \ldots, k$, the asymptotic variance (8.6) can be consistently estimated by replacing in this latter expression each cell probability with the homologous relative frequency. Denoting the resulting variance estimator by $v_n^2(\hat{\boldsymbol{\pi}}, \boldsymbol{\pi}^\circ)$, we have

$$v_n^2(\hat{\boldsymbol{\pi}}, \boldsymbol{\pi}^\circ) = 4\left[\sum_{j=1}^{k}(\hat{\pi}_j - \pi_j^\circ)^2\, \hat{\pi}_j - \right.$$

$$\left. \sum_{j_1=1}^{k}\sum_{j_2=1}^{k}(\hat{\pi}_{j_1} - \pi_{j_1}^\circ)(\hat{\pi}_{j_2} - \pi_{j_2}^\circ)\hat{\pi}_{j_1}\hat{\pi}_{j_2} \right]. \qquad (8.8)$$

In view of (8.7) and the consistency of $v_n^2(\hat{\boldsymbol{\pi}}, \boldsymbol{\pi}^\circ)$ for $\sigma_a^2\big[\sqrt{n}\, d^2(\hat{\boldsymbol{\pi}}, \boldsymbol{\pi}^\circ)\big]$, an asymptotically valid test for the goodness-of-fit problem (8.2) is obtained by treating $d^2(\hat{\boldsymbol{\pi}}, \boldsymbol{\pi}^\circ)$ as a normally distributed statistic with known variance $n^{-1}v_n^2(\hat{\boldsymbol{\pi}}, \boldsymbol{\pi}^\circ)$ and unknown expected value θ, say, about which the one-sided null hypothesis $\theta \geq \varepsilon^2$ has been formulated. Accordingly, an asymptotic solution to (8.2) can be based on the following decision procedure:

Reject lack of fit of $\quad \mathcal{M}(n; \pi_1, \ldots, \pi_k) \;\text{ to }\; \mathcal{M}(n; \pi_1^\circ, \ldots, \pi_k^\circ)$

iff it turns out that $\quad d^2(\hat{\boldsymbol{\pi}}, \boldsymbol{\pi}^\circ) < \varepsilon^2 - u_{1-\alpha}\, v_n(\hat{\boldsymbol{\pi}}, \boldsymbol{\pi}^\circ)/\sqrt{n}\ , \qquad (8.9)$

with $u_{1-\alpha} = \Phi^{-1}(1 - \alpha)$.

Example 8.1

For the purpose of illustrating the use of the testing procedure derived in this section, it is tempting to revisit the elementary class-room example of assessing the compatibility of the results of casting the same play dice independently a given number n of times, with the Laplacean "equal likelihood" definition of probability. Suppose, the number of casts performed in such an experiment was $n = 100$, and the following frequencies of the possible elementary outcomes were recorded:

Table 8.1 *Absolute frequencies observed in a sequence of n = 100 casts of a given play dice*

j	1	2	3	4	5	6	Σ
x_j	17	16	25	9	16	17	100

With these data, the traditional χ^2-test for lack of fit yields 7.7600 as the observed value of the test statistic. The associated p-value, i.e., the upper tail-probability of 7.7600 under a central χ^2-distribution with 5 degrees of freedom, is computed to be $p = .16997$, indicating that the observed frequencies do not deviate significantly from those expected for an ideal dice. But is this really sufficient for asserting positively that the dice under assessment is approximately fair?

In order to obtain a conclusive answer to this question, we perform the testing procedure defined by (8.9), at the conventional significance level $\alpha = .05$ and with tolerance $\varepsilon = .15$ which corresponds in the binomial case to a theoretical equivalence interval of length $\approx 2 \cdot .10$. The necessary computational steps are readily carried out by means of the procedure $\tt gofsimpt$, another SAS macro provided at http://www.zi-mannheim.de/wktsheq. The squared distance between the empirical distribution shown in Table 8.1 and the theoretical distribution given by $\pi_j^\circ = 1/6 \; \forall j = 1, \ldots, 6$, turns out to be $d^2(\hat{\boldsymbol{\pi}}, \boldsymbol{\pi}^\circ) = .012933$ with an estimated standard error of $n^{-1/2} v_n(\hat{\boldsymbol{\pi}}, \boldsymbol{\pi}^\circ) = .009200$. Hence, with the suggested specifications of α and ε, the critical upper bound which the observed value of $d^2(\hat{\boldsymbol{\pi}}, \boldsymbol{\pi}^\circ)$ has to be compared to according to (8.9), is $.15^2 - 1.644854 \cdot .009200 = .007367$. Since the observed value of the test statistic clearly exceeds this bound, at the 5% level the data of Table 8.1 do not allow us to decide in favour of the (alternative) hypothesis that the dice under assessment is approximately fair. Thus, the example gives a concrete illustration of the basic general fact (obvious enough from a theoretical viewpoint) that the traditional χ^2-test of goodness of fit to a fully specified multinomial distribution is inappropriate for *establishing* the hypothesis of (approximate) fit of the true to the prespecified distribution.

Some simulation results on the finite-sample behaviour of the test

As is the case for every multiparameter problem with a composite null hypothesis specifying an uncountable subspace of parameter values, performing a high-resolution search for the maximum exact rejection probability on the common boundary of the hypotheses of (8.2) or, still more, on H as a whole in a simulation study would entail a tremendous computational effort. Therefore, for the purpose of throwing some light on the effective size of the critical region of the test (8.9) when applied to finite samples, we confine ourselves to present simulated rejection probabilities only under a small yet sufficiently diversified selection of parameter configurations $\boldsymbol{\pi} \in \boldsymbol{\Pi}$ with $d(\boldsymbol{\pi}, \boldsymbol{\pi}^\circ) = \varepsilon$. Tables 8.2 a and b show such a representative set of rejection probabilities simulated under the null hypothesis for the "equal likelihood" problem with $k = 4$ and $k = 6$ categories, respectively, for the same specification of α and ε as in the above dice-casting example.

Table 8.2a *Simulated exact rejection probability of the test (8.9) at nominal level $\alpha = .05$ with $n = 100$ observations, under selected null configurations for $k = 4$, $\pi_j^\circ = 1/4$ $\forall j = 1, \ldots, 4$, and $\varepsilon = .15$ [40,000 replications of each Monte Carlo experiment]*

π_1	π_2	π_3	π_4	Rejection Probability
.28879	.13000	.25000	.33121	.03025
.29655	.15000	.21000	.34345	.04250
.21029	.20000	.21000	.37971	.06513
.25388	.22000	.16000	.36612	.05098
.14393	.25000	.25000	.35607	.04143
.17500	.32500	.17500	.32500	.04540

Table 8.2b *Analogue to Table 8.2a for $k = 6$*

π_1	π_2	π_3	π_4	π_5	π_6	Rejection Probability
.21057	.05000	.15000	.15000	.20000	.23943	.00835
.12296	.05000	.20000	.20000	.20000	.22704	.00833
.17296	.10000	.10000	.15000	.20000	.27704	.02685
.10283	.15000	.10000	.15000	.25000	.24717	.02575
.10211	.15000	.15000	.15000	.15000	.29789	.03943
.10543	.22790	.10543	.22790	.10543	.22790	.02113

The results displayed in the above pair of tables suggest that, given the sample size, the signed difference between nominal significance level and exact size of the critical region increases quite rapidly with the number of cells of the underlying contingency table. In fact, whereas for $k = 4$ the tabulated rejection probabilities indicate some tendency towards anti-conservatism (whose extent seems to cause little harm for most practical purposes, to be sure), under the conditions of Example 8.1 the test fails to exhaust the target significance level by about 1%. Clearly, both of these undesirable effects can be removed at least in part by adjusting the nominal level to the maximum admissible degree, but working out the details is beyond our scope here.

Tables 8.3 a and b give results from simulation experiments performed in order to study the second basic property of the test (8.9), namely, the relationship between its power against the specific alternative of perfect coincidence between true and model-derived distribution of $(X_1, \ldots, X_k)$, and size n of the available sample. These latter data point to an interesting relationship corroborated by the results of additional simulation experi-

Table 8.3a *Simulated exact power $POW_\circ$ of the test (8.9) at nominal level $\alpha = .05$ against the alternative that $\pi_j = \pi_j^\circ = 1/k \; \forall j = 1, \ldots, k$, for $k = 4$, $\varepsilon = .15$ and $n = 50(25)200$ [40,000 replications of each experiment]*

n	50	75	100	125	150	175	200
$POW_\circ$	.23798	.44120	.63673	.77330	.87213	.92868	.96388

Table 8.3b *Analogue to Table 8.3a for $k = 6$*

n	50	75	100	125	150	175	200
$POW_\circ$	.16030	.42943	.66795	.83120	.92620	.96913	.98710

ments with other values of k: The larger the number of categories, the steeper the increase of the power against $\pi = \pi^\circ$ as a function of n. Both in the tetra- and the hexanomial case, $n = 150$ observations turn out sufficient to guarantee satisfactory power of the test (8.9) against the specific alternative of primary interest.

8.2 Testing for approximate collapsibility of multiway contingency tables

The concept of collapsibility plays an important role within the literature on log-linear models for multiway contingency tables (cf. Bishop, Fienberg and Holland, 1975, § 2.5). The precise meaning of the term in its strict sense is as follows: Let $(X_{1\ldots1}, \ldots, X_{k_1 \ldots k_q})$ be the vector of frequencies counted in the $\prod_{\nu=1}^q k_\nu$ cells of a higher-order contingency table formed by cross-classifying each of n sampling units with respect to q categorical variables $C_1, \ldots, C_q$ with possible values $\{1, \ldots, k_1\}, \ldots, \{1, \ldots, k_q\}$, respectively. Then, the set $\{C_1, \ldots, C_q\}$ is called strictly collapsible across C_ν

(for prespecified $\nu \in \{1, \ldots, q\}$) if the log-linear model for the reduced table $(X_{1\ldots+\ldots1}, \ldots, X_{k_1\ldots k_{\nu-1}+k_{\nu+1}\ldots k_q})$ obtained by taking for each $(i_1, \ldots, i_{\nu-1}, i_{\nu+1}, \ldots, i_q)$ the sum $\sum_{i_\nu=1}^{k_\nu} X_{i_1\ldots i_{\nu-1}i_\nu i_{\nu+1}\ldots i_q}$ contains exactly the same parameters as that for the original table, except for those related to C_ν. It can be shown (see Bishop et al., loc. cit., p. 47) that this holds true if and only if C_ν is independent of $\{C_1, \ldots, C_{\nu-1}, C_{\nu+1}, \ldots, C_q\}$. Accordingly, strict collapsibility of a set of categorical variables defining a given multiway contingency table is a special case of independence of a couple of such variables, so that the general problem raised in the title of this section can be solved by constructing a test for approximate independence of two categorical variables A and B say, with possible values $1, \ldots, r$ and $1, \ldots, s$, respectively.

As usual, we denote by π_{ij} the probability, that a specific sampling unit is observed to belong to cell (i, j) of the corresponding two-way table, and X_{ij} stands for the number of sampling units counted in that cell. Of course, independence of the two characteristics A and B holds if and only if we may write $\pi_{ij} = \pi_{i+}\pi_{+j} \equiv (\sum_{\nu=1}^{s} \pi_{i\nu})(\sum_{\mu=1}^{r} \pi_{\mu j}) \, \forall \, (i,j) \in \{1, \ldots, r\} \times \{1, \ldots, s\}$. Thus, the target distribution to which the true distribution of the primary observations is asserted to be sufficiently similar under any hypothesis formalizing the notion of approximate independence, depends on the unknown parameters π_{ij} rather than being completely specified. Nevertheless, it will turn out comparatively easy to accommodate the approach of the preceding section to this more complicated situation.

In order to give the details of the construction, we have to adapt the notation for the primary parameter vector by defining $\boldsymbol{\pi}$ as the vector of dimension $r \times s$ formed by putting the rows of the matrix $(\pi_{ij})_{(r,s)}$ of cell probabilities one after the other. Furthermore, it will be convenient to use the following extra symbols for additional parametric functions to be referred to repeatedly in defining the hypotheses, as well as in deriving a test statistic which an asymptotically valid test for approximate independence of A and B can be based upon:

$$\varrho_i(\boldsymbol{\pi}) \equiv \sum_{\nu=1}^{s} \pi_{i\nu}, \quad i = 1, \ldots, r; \tag{8.10a}$$

$$\zeta_j(\boldsymbol{\pi}) \equiv \sum_{\mu=1}^{r} \pi_{\mu j}, \quad j = 1, \ldots, s; \tag{8.10b}$$

$$\mathbf{g}(\boldsymbol{\pi}) \equiv \big(\varrho_1(\boldsymbol{\pi})\zeta_1(\boldsymbol{\pi}), \ldots, \varrho_1(\boldsymbol{\pi})\zeta_s(\boldsymbol{\pi}),$$
$$\ldots, \varrho_r(\boldsymbol{\pi})\zeta_1(\boldsymbol{\pi}), \ldots, \varrho_r(\boldsymbol{\pi})\zeta_s(\boldsymbol{\pi})\big) . \tag{8.10c}$$

By analogy with the way of approaching the problem of testing for consistency with a fully specified distribution considered in § 8.1, it seems sensible to base the criterion for approximate independence of the classifications under consideration on the squared Euclidean distance

$$d^2\big(\boldsymbol{\pi}, \mathbf{g}(\boldsymbol{\pi})\big) = \sum_{i=1}^{r}\sum_{j=1}^{s}\big(\pi_{ij} - \varrho_i(\boldsymbol{\pi})\zeta_j(\boldsymbol{\pi})\big)^2 \qquad (8.11)$$

between the vector $\boldsymbol{\pi}$ of true cell probabilities and the associated vector $\mathbf{g}(\boldsymbol{\pi})$ of products of marginal totals. Again, a natural estimator of that distance is obtained by substituting the vector $\hat{\boldsymbol{\pi}}$ of observed relative frequencies for $\boldsymbol{\pi}$ throughout, where the components of $\hat{\boldsymbol{\pi}}$ have this time to be written $\hat{\pi}_{ij} = X_{ij}/n$. Except for obvious changes in notation, the asymptotic distribution of $\sqrt{n}(\hat{\boldsymbol{\pi}} - \boldsymbol{\pi})$ is the same as in the one-dimensional case [recall (8.5)]. This implies that $\sqrt{n}\big(d^2\big(\hat{\boldsymbol{\pi}}, \mathbf{g}(\hat{\boldsymbol{\pi}})\big) - d^2\big(\boldsymbol{\pi}, \mathbf{g}(\boldsymbol{\pi})\big)\big)$ is asymptotically normal with expectation 0 and variance $\sigma_a^2\big[\sqrt{n}\,d^2\big(\hat{\boldsymbol{\pi}}, \mathbf{g}(\hat{\boldsymbol{\pi}})\big)\big]$, say, which can be computed by means of the δ-method as

$$\sigma_a^2\big[\sqrt{n}\,d^2\big(\hat{\boldsymbol{\pi}}, \mathbf{g}(\hat{\boldsymbol{\pi}})\big)\big] = \sum_{i=1}^{r}\sum_{j=1}^{s}\Big[\frac{\partial}{\partial\pi_{ij}}d^2\big(\boldsymbol{\pi}, \mathbf{g}(\boldsymbol{\pi})\big)\Big]^2\pi_{ij}$$

$$-\sum_{i_1=1}^{r}\sum_{j_1=1}^{s}\sum_{i_2=1}^{r}\sum_{j_2=1}^{s}\frac{\partial}{\partial\pi_{i_1j_1}}d^2\big(\boldsymbol{\pi}, \mathbf{g}(\boldsymbol{\pi})\big)\frac{\partial}{\partial\pi_{i_2j_2}}d^2\big(\boldsymbol{\pi}, \mathbf{g}(\boldsymbol{\pi})\big)\pi_{i_1j_1}\pi_{i_2j_2}. \quad (8.12)$$

For the purpose of deriving explicit expressions for the individual components of the gradient of $\boldsymbol{\pi} \mapsto d^2\big(\boldsymbol{\pi}, \mathbf{g}(\boldsymbol{\pi})\big)$, we start with determining the partial derivatives of the (i, j)th term of the double sum appearing on the right-hand side of (8.11) [for arbitrarily fixed $(i, j) \in \{1, \ldots, r\} \times \{1, \ldots, s\}$] with respect to $\pi_{\mu\nu}$ for $\mu = 1, \ldots, r$, $\nu = 1, \ldots, s$. From (8.10a), (8.10b) it is obvious that we have

$$\frac{\partial\big(\varrho_i(\boldsymbol{\pi})\zeta_j(\boldsymbol{\pi})\big)}{\partial\pi_{\mu\nu}} = \begin{cases} 0 & \mu \neq i, \ \nu \neq j \\ \zeta_j(\boldsymbol{\pi}) & \mu = i, \ \nu \neq j \\ \varrho_i(\boldsymbol{\pi}) & \mu \neq i, \ \nu = j \\ \varrho_i(\boldsymbol{\pi}) + \zeta_j(\boldsymbol{\pi}) & \mu = i, \ \nu = j \end{cases} \quad \text{for} \qquad (8.12a)$$

Using (8.12a), it is readily verified that

$$\frac{1}{2}\frac{\partial\big(\pi_{ij} - \varrho_i(\boldsymbol{\pi})\zeta_j(\boldsymbol{\pi})\big)^2}{\partial\pi_{\mu\nu}} =$$

$$\begin{cases} 0 & \mu \neq i, \ \nu \neq j \\ -\big(\pi_{ij} - \varrho_i(\boldsymbol{\pi})\zeta_j(\boldsymbol{\pi})\big)\zeta_j(\boldsymbol{\pi}) & \mu = i, \ \nu \neq j \\ -\big(\pi_{ij} - \varrho_i(\boldsymbol{\pi})\zeta_j(\boldsymbol{\pi})\big)\varrho_i(\boldsymbol{\pi}) & \mu \neq i, \ \nu = j \\ \big(\pi_{ij} - \varrho_i(\boldsymbol{\pi})\zeta_j(\boldsymbol{\pi})\big)\big(1 - \varrho_i(\boldsymbol{\pi}) - \zeta_j(\boldsymbol{\pi})\big) & \mu = i, \ \nu = j \end{cases} \quad \text{for} \qquad (8.12b)$$

Summing (8.12b) over $(i, j) \in \{1, \ldots, r\} \times \{1, \ldots, s\}$ gives:

$$\frac{\partial}{\partial \pi_{\mu\nu}} d^2\big(\boldsymbol{\pi}, \mathbf{g}(\boldsymbol{\pi})\big) = 2\bigg\{ \big(\pi_{\mu\nu} - \varrho_\mu(\boldsymbol{\pi})\zeta_\nu(\boldsymbol{\pi})\big) - \sum_{i=1}^{r} \Big[\big(\pi_{i\nu} - $$

$$\varrho_i(\boldsymbol{\pi})\zeta_\nu(\boldsymbol{\pi})\big)\varrho_i(\boldsymbol{\pi}) \Big] - \sum_{j=1}^{s} \Big[\big(\pi_{\mu j} - \varrho_\mu(\boldsymbol{\pi})\zeta_j(\boldsymbol{\pi})\big)\zeta_j(\boldsymbol{\pi}) \Big] \bigg\} . \quad (8.13)$$

Of course, what we eventually need is a consistent estimator, say $v_n^2(\hat{\boldsymbol{\pi}}, \mathbf{g}(\hat{\boldsymbol{\pi}}))$, of $\sigma_a^2\big[\sqrt{n}\, d^2(\hat{\boldsymbol{\pi}}, \mathbf{g}(\hat{\boldsymbol{\pi}}))\big]$. In view of (8.12) and (8.13), for achieving this goal, it is sufficient to plug in the homologous relative frequency at every place on the right-hand side of both equations where a population parameter, i.e., a component of the vector $\boldsymbol{\pi}$ appears. More precisely speaking, for any $(\mu, \nu) \in \{1, \ldots, r\} \times \{1, \ldots, s\}$, the (μ, ν)-component of the gradient vector of $\boldsymbol{\pi} \mapsto d^2\big(\boldsymbol{\pi}, \mathbf{g}(\boldsymbol{\pi})\big)$ can be consistently estimated by

$$\hat{d}_{\mu\nu} \equiv 2\bigg\{ \big(\hat{\pi}_{\mu\nu} - \varrho_\mu(\hat{\boldsymbol{\pi}})\zeta_\nu(\hat{\boldsymbol{\pi}})\big) - \sum_{i=1}^{r} \Big[\big(\hat{\pi}_{i\nu} - \varrho_i(\hat{\boldsymbol{\pi}})\zeta_\nu(\hat{\boldsymbol{\pi}})\big) \cdot $$

$$\varrho_i(\hat{\boldsymbol{\pi}}) \Big] - \sum_{j=1}^{s} \Big[\big(\hat{\pi}_{\mu j} - \varrho_\mu(\hat{\boldsymbol{\pi}})\zeta_j(\hat{\boldsymbol{\pi}})\big)\zeta_j(\hat{\boldsymbol{\pi}}) \Big] \bigg\} . \quad (8.14)$$

Finally, the desired estimator of the asymptotic variance of $\sqrt{n}\, d^2\big(\hat{\boldsymbol{\pi}}, \mathbf{g}(\hat{\boldsymbol{\pi}})\big)$ is obtained by substituting $\hat{d}_{11}, \ldots, \hat{d}_{rs}$ and $\hat{\pi}_{11}, \ldots, \hat{\pi}_{rs}$ for $\frac{\partial}{\partial \pi_{11}} d^2\big(\boldsymbol{\pi}, \mathbf{g}(\boldsymbol{\pi})\big)$, $\ldots, \frac{\partial}{\partial \pi_{rs}} d^2\big(\boldsymbol{\pi}, \mathbf{g}(\boldsymbol{\pi})\big)$ and $\pi_{11}, \ldots, \pi_{rs}$, respectively, on the right-hand side of (8.12), yielding

$$v_n^2\big(\hat{\boldsymbol{\pi}}, \mathbf{g}(\hat{\boldsymbol{\pi}})\big) = \sum_{i=1}^{r} \sum_{j=1}^{s} \hat{d}_{ij}^2\, \hat{\pi}_{ij} - $$

$$\sum_{i_1=1}^{r} \sum_{j_1=1}^{s} \sum_{i_2=1}^{r} \sum_{j_2=1}^{s} \hat{d}_{i_1 j_1} \hat{d}_{i_2 j_2} \hat{\pi}_{i_1 j_1} \hat{\pi}_{i_2 j_2} . \quad (8.15)$$

Now we are ready to formulate the decision rule of an asymptotically valid test of

$$H : d^2\big(\boldsymbol{\pi}, \mathbf{g}(\boldsymbol{\pi})\big) \geq \varepsilon^2 \quad \text{versus} \quad K : d^2\big(\boldsymbol{\pi}, \mathbf{g}(\boldsymbol{\pi})\big) < \varepsilon^2 \quad (8.16)$$

for fixed $\varepsilon > 0$ to be chosen a priori. The alternative hypothesis we want to establish according to (8.16) specifies that the true distribution is in acceptably close agreement with that hypothesized by the model of independence given both vectors of marginal probabilities, which seems to be an adequate translation of the notion of approximate validity of that model into a statement about the parameter characterizing the distribution from which the data are taken. After the technical preparations made in the preceding paragraphs, we know that asymptotically, the estimated squared distance of π from $\mathbf{g}(\pi)$ can be viewed as a normally distributed variable with $d^2(\pi, \mathbf{g}(\pi))$ as unknown expected value and fixed known variance $n^{-1} v_n^2(\hat{\pi}, \mathbf{g}(\hat{\pi}))$. Hence, we get a test of asymptotic level α for the problem (8.16) by applying the decision rule:

Reject existence of relevant discrepencies between true distribution and independence model iff

$$d^2(\hat{\pi}, \mathbf{g}(\hat{\pi})) < \varepsilon^2 - u_{1-\alpha} v_n(\hat{\pi}, \mathbf{g}(\hat{\pi}))/\sqrt{n} . \qquad (8.17)$$

Example 8.2

In one out of four different arms of a large multicentre trial of drugs used as first-choice medication for mild arterial hypertension, classifying the patients by gender and outcome of short-term treatment gave the 2×4 contingency table shown below as Table 8.4. It covers all patients who were randomized for administration of the calcium-entry blocking agent nitrendipine and treated in compliance with the study protocol. At a certain stage of their work, the statisticians responsible for the analysis of the results of the trial were confronted also with the problem of identifying those treatment arms for which a relevant gender-by-outcome interaction could be excluded. For the nitrendipine group, this question can be suitably addressed by applying decision rule (8.17) to the data of Table 8.4. Once more, we set the significance level to $\alpha = .05$, and specify $\varepsilon = .15$ as the largest tolerable distance between the vector of true cell probabilities and the associated vector of products of marginal probabilities.

Table 8.4 *2×4 contingency table relating gender and treatment outcome on nitrendipine monotherapy in patients suffering from mild arterial hypertension.* (Source: Philipp et al. (1997); Numbers in ( ): relative frequencies with respect to the overall total n)

		Outcome Category				
		1[*)]	2[**)]	3[***)]	4[†)]	Σ
Gender	Female	9	13	13	48	83
		(.042)	(.060)	(.060)	(.221)	(.382)
	Male	24	18	20	72	134
		(.111)	(.083)	(.092)	(.332)	(.618)
	Σ	33	31	33	120	217
		(.152)	(.143)	(.152)	(.553)	(1.000)

[*)]…[***)] Response at lowest, middle and highest dose step, respectively
[†)] Failure to reach target level of diastolic blood pressure at all three dose steps

With $X_{11} = 9, \ldots, X_{24} = 72$, the estimated distance between $\boldsymbol{\pi} = (\pi_{11}, \ldots, \pi_{24})$ and $\mathbf{g}(\boldsymbol{\pi}) = (\pi_{1+}\pi_{+1}, \ldots, \pi_{2+}\pi_{+4})$ is readily computed to be $d(\hat{\boldsymbol{\pi}}, \mathbf{g}(\hat{\boldsymbol{\pi}})) = .028396$. Evaluating formula (8.15) for the squared standard error of the statistic $\sqrt{n}\, d^2(\hat{\boldsymbol{\pi}}, \mathbf{g}(\hat{\boldsymbol{\pi}}))$ by hand or by means of a pocket calculator is a rather tedious process, even if the total number of cells of the contingency table under analysis is comparatively small. So we leave this job to another computer program ready for being downloaded from http://www.zimannheim.de/wktsheq. It is again written in *SAS*, with `gofind_t` as program name. Running this macro, we read from the output $v_n = .017016$. Thus, at the 5%-level and with $\varepsilon = .15$, the critical upper bound which the observed value of $d^2(\hat{\boldsymbol{\pi}}, \mathbf{g}(\hat{\boldsymbol{\pi}}))$ has to be compared to, is computed to be $.15^2 - 1.644854 \cdot .017016/\sqrt{217} = .020600$. Since $.028396^2 = .000806$ is clearly smaller than this critical bound, we have to decide in favour of approximate independence between gender and treatment outcome in hypertensive patients taking nitrendipine according to the prescriptions of the protocol of the trial from which the data of Table 8.4 are taken (for details see Philipp et al., 1997).

Example 8.3

In the light of the introductory remarks at the beginning of this section, we now turn to illustrating the use of decision rule (8.17) for testing for approximate collapsibility in the strict sense of a higher-order contingency table across a prespecified element of the set $\{C_1, \ldots, C_q\}$ of categorical variables involved. For this purpose, we confine ourselves to a brief discussion of a synthetic data set. Suppose the format of the table under analysis is $2 \times 2 \times 2$ with observed cell frequencies as shown below, and the variable with respect to which we aim to establish collapsibility, is the first one. Suppose further that α and ε have been specified as in the previous example.

Table 8.5a *Observed $2 \times 2 \times 2$ table to be tested for approximate collapsibility in the strict sense across the first binary classification*

C_1		C_2	C_3 +	C_3 −
+	+	+	8	13
		−	15	6
−		+	19	21
		−	31	7

In a preliminary step we have to rearrange the original array in a 2×4 table with the combination of C_2 and C_3 defining the columns. Using the entries in the rearranged Table 8.5b as input data to the SAS macro gofind_t we obtain $d\big(\hat{\boldsymbol{\pi}}, \mathbf{g}(\hat{\boldsymbol{\pi}})\big) = .030332$ and $v_n = .019190$. Hence, the condition for rejecting the null hypothesis of relevant deviations from collapsibility is in the present case that $d^2\big(\hat{\boldsymbol{\pi}}, \mathbf{g}(\hat{\boldsymbol{\pi}})\big) < .15^2 - 1.644854 \times .019190/\sqrt{120} = .019619$ which in view of $.030332^2 < .001$ is clearly satisfied.

Table 8.5b *Rearrangement of Table 8.5a in a 2×4 array*

		1	2	3	4	$\sum$
		B ($\leftrightarrow C_2 \times C_3$)				
A ($\leftrightarrow C_1$)	1	8	13	15	6	42
	2	19	21	31	7	78
$\sum$		27	34	46	13	120

Simulation results on size and power

Table 8.6 is an analogue to Tables 8.2 a, b for the testing procedure (8.17) as applied to a 2×4 contingency table containing roughly the same total number of observations as had been available in the real application described in Example 8.2. Of course, for the problem of testing for approximate independence of two categorical variables, a numerically accurate search for the maximum rejection probability on the common boundary of the hypotheses is still farther beyond the scope of computational feasibility than for the problem of establishing goodness of fit to a fully specified multinomial distribution. In fact, in the independence case, the alternative hypothesis is an uncountable union of hyperspheres of radius ε rather than a single set of that form. Accordingly, the simulation results displayed in the rightmost column of the next table allow only a rough qualitative assessment of the finite-sample behaviour of the testing procedure (8.17) under the null hypothesis H of (8.16). Again we find some anticonservative tendency whose extent seems small enough for being ignored in the majority of practical applications, but is clearly outside the range of deviations which can be accounted for by the simulation error. Since the results of additional simulation experiments not reproduced in detail here suggest that the convergence of the exact size of the asymptotic test to the target significance level is quite slow, it is recommended to rely on an adjusted nominal level $\alpha^* < \alpha$ whenever strict maintenance of the prespecified level is felt to be an indispensible requirement. For instance, replacing $\alpha = .05$

with $\alpha^* = .025$ suffices for ensuring that even for the least favourable of the parameter constellations covered by Table 8.6 [$\rightarrow$ row 1], the (simulated) exact rejection probability with a sample of size $n = 200$ no longer exceeds the 5%-bound.

Table 8.6 *Simulated exact rejection probability of the test (8.17) at nominal level $\alpha = .05$, with $r = 2$, $s = 4$, $\varepsilon = .15$ and $n = 200$, under various parameter configurations on the common boundary of the hypotheses (8.16) [40,000 replications per Monte Carlo experiment]*

π_{11}	π_{12}	π_{13}	π_{14}	π_{21}	π_{22}	π_{23}	π_{24}	P [Rejection]
.05	.05	.05	.05	.65923	.05	.05	.04077	.07153
.05	.05	.05	.10	.48723	.05	.15	.06277	.06718
.05	.15	.10	.35	.07878	.05	.15	.07122	.06218
.10	.05	.25	.15	.18082	.10	.05	.11918	.05405
.10	.10	.10	.15	.24850	.10	.20	.00150	.05680
.05	.10	.15	.20	.23229	.05	.10	.11771	.05803
.25	.25	.05	.05	.04030	.20	.15	.00970	.05615
.15	.15	.15	.15	.25308	.05	.05	.04692	.06573
.20	.05	.05	.05	.16601	.30	.15	.03399	.06993
.20	.05	.05	.20	.27247	.05	.15	.02753	.05895

For completeness, we finish our discussion of (asymptotic) testing procedures tailored for establishing the approximate validity of customary models for contingency tables, with presenting some simulation results on the power of the procedure (8.17) to detect that the true parameter configuration π fits the model of independence exactly. Obviously, given the format of the two-way tables to be analyzed, there is an uncountable manifold of specific alternatives of that type. Singling out once more the case $(r, s) = (2, 4)$, we studied the power under three configurations of marginal probabilities $\pi_{1+}, \pi_{2+}; \pi_{+1}, \ldots, \pi_{+4}$ determining extremely different joint distributions of the X_{ij}. Table 8.7 shows the rejection probabilities simulated under these parameter configurations for $n \in \{50, 100, 150\}$, $\varepsilon = .15$ and nominal levels α^* which, according to our results on the size of the test (8.17), are small enough to ensure that the target level of 5% is maintained at least at all points on the common boundary of the hypotheses covered by Table 8.6.

Not surprisingly, the power against alternatives π such that $d\left(\pi, \mathbf{g}\left(\pi\right)\right)$ vanishes turns out to be very sensitive against gross changes to the shape of the marginal distributions. Furthermore, even if the nominal significance level α^* is downgraded as far as necessary for ensuring that the rejection probability keeps below the target level of 5% under all null constellations studied for assessing the level properties of the test, a sample size of 100 seems sufficient for achieving reasonable power against alternatives satisfying the model of independence exactly.

Table 8.7 *Simulated exact power of the test (8.17) against three alternatives satisfying* $\pi_{ij} = \pi_{i+}\pi_{+j} \ \forall \ (i,j)$ *for* 2×4 *arrays, with* $\varepsilon = .15$, $n = 50, 100, 150$ *and corrected nominal significance level* α^* *[40,000 replications per Monte Carlo experiment]*

n	α^*	π_{1+}	π_{2+}	π_{+1}	π_{+2}	π_{+3}	π_{+4}	P [Rejection]
50	.01	.25	.75	.10	.40	.30	.20	.39788
"	"	.50	.50	.25	.25	.25	.25	.25395
"	"	.33	.67	.15	.15	.15	.55	.43115
100	.02	.25	.75	.10	.40	.30	.20	.87578
"	"	.50	.50	.25	.25	.25	.25	.84405
"	"	.33	.67	.15	.15	.15	.55	.90630
150	.025	.25	.75	.10	.40	.30	.20	.97925
"	"	.50	.50	.25	.25	.25	.25	.98458
"	"	.33	.67	.15	.15	.15	.55	.98758

8.3 Establishing goodness of fit of linear models for normally distributed data

8.3.1 An exact optimal test for negligibility of interactions in a two-way ANOVA layout

Presumably, more often than not, existence of interaction effects will be considered as an undesirable lack of fit to the model which an investigator applying standard ANOVA techniques would like to rely upon. The obvious reason is that in presence of interactions, the main effects do not admit a direct interpretation. In fact, only in absence of interactions, a positive main effect associated with some level of a given factor justifies the conclusion that on an average, all experimental units assigned to that level do better than those assigned to another level with a negative effect of the same factor. Adopting this perspective, it is natural to consider that part of the analysis of an ANOVA two-way layout which deals with the interaction effects, as a preliminary check carried out with the intention to establish that the "ideal" additive model fits the data sufficiently well.

For the moment, we restrict the description of a testing procedure, which allows us to exclude relevant deviations from additivity of the main effects, to the case of a strictly balanced design. In other words, we assume that the data set under analysis consists of $r \cdot s$ independent samples of common size n from normal distributions with the same unknown variance $\sigma^2 > 0$. Denoting the kth observation in group (i,j) by X_{ijk}, we suppose that for each $(i,j) \in \{1, \ldots, r\} \times \{1, \ldots, s\}$, the cell mean $\mu_{ij} = E(X_{ij1}) = \ldots = E(X_{ijk})$ can be additively decomposed in the usual way leading to the representation

$$\mu_{ij} = \mu + \alpha_i + \beta_j + \gamma_{ij} \ . \tag{8.18}$$

Of course, the parameters coming into play according to this basic model equation are assumed to satisfy the usual side conditions $\sum_{i=1}^{r} \alpha_i = 0 = \sum_{j=1}^{s} \beta_j$, $\sum_{j=1}^{s} \gamma_{ij} = 0 \ \forall \, i = 1, \ldots, r$, $\sum_{i=1}^{r} \gamma_{ij} = 0 \ \forall \, j = 1, \ldots, s$.

Now, it seems reasonable to consider the interaction effects negligible as soon as it can be taken for granted that the standardized γ_{ij} are the coordinates of a point in rs-dimensional Euclidean space which lies in a spherical neighbourhood of $\mathbf{0}$ of sufficiently small radius $\varepsilon > 0$. Accordingly, our alternative hypothesis of absence of relevant interactions specifies that $\sum_{i=1}^{r} \sum_{j=1}^{s} (\gamma_{ij}/\sigma)^2 < \varepsilon^2$, so that the testing problem as a whole reads

$$H : d^2(\boldsymbol{\gamma}/\sigma, \mathbf{0}) \geq \varepsilon^2 \quad \text{versus} \quad K : d^2(\boldsymbol{\gamma}/\sigma, \mathbf{0}) < \varepsilon^2 \,, \tag{8.19}$$

provided $\boldsymbol{\gamma}$ stands for the vector consisting of the rows of the matrix $(\gamma_{ij})_{(r,s)}$, $\mathbf{0}$ for the null vector in rs-dimensional space, and $d(\mathbf{u}, \mathbf{v})$ denotes the Euclidean distance between arbitrary points $\mathbf{u}, \mathbf{v} \in \mathbb{R}^{rs}$. It is easily verified that this pair of hypotheses remains invariant under the same group of $1 : 1$ transformations of the sample space $\mathbb{R}^{nrs}$ onto itself as the problem of testing the conventional null hypothesis that all interaction parameters vanish. (As is generally the case with problems exhibiting the same invariance structure as a pair of linear hypotheses about the mean of an independent vector of homoskedastic Gaussian variables, a precise characterization of this transformation group requires the introduction of a canonical coordinate system for the observed vector which would lead the exposition away from what our real issue is here.) Hence, any invariant test of (8.19) is necessarily a function of the classical F-ratio for testing $\gamma_{ij} = 0 \ \forall (i,j)$ vs. $\gamma_{ij} \neq 0$ for some $(i,j) \in \{1, \ldots, r\} \times \{1, \ldots, s\}$. Discarding the constant factor $n/(r-s)(s-1)$, this statistic can be viewed as the squared Euclidean distance from the origin of the least squares estimator of $\boldsymbol{\gamma}$ standardized with respect to the length of the residual vector for the nonrestricted model as the standard estimator of σ. Using a notation which is to be suggestive of this interpretation of the rescaled F-ratio, we write

$$d^2(\hat{\gamma}/S, \mathbf{0}) = \frac{\sum_{i=1}^{r} \sum_{j=1}^{s} (\bar{X}_{ij} - \bar{X}_{i.} - \bar{X}_{.j} + \bar{X}_{..})^2}{\sum_{i=1}^{r} \sum_{j=1}^{s} \sum_{k=1}^{n} (X_{ijk} - \bar{X}_{ij})^2/(n-1)\,rs} , \tag{8.20}$$

with $\bar{X}_{ij} \equiv \sum_{k=1}^{n} X_{ijk}/n$, $\bar{X}_{i.} \equiv \sum_{j=1}^{s} \bar{X}_{ij}/s$, $\bar{X}_{.j} \equiv \sum_{i=1}^{r} \bar{X}_{ij}/r$, and $\bar{X}_{..} \equiv \sum_{i=1}^{r} \sum_{j=1}^{s} \bar{X}_{ij}/rs$.

The distribution of $nd^2(\hat{\gamma}/S, \mathbf{0})/((r-1)(s-1))$ is well known (see, e.g., Lehmann, 1986, p. 394) to be noncentral F with $(r-1)(s-1)$, $(n-1)rs$ degrees of freedom and noncentrality parameter $\lambda_{nc}^2 = nd^2(\gamma/\sigma, \mathbf{0})$, under any parameter constellation $(\mu, \alpha_1, \ldots, \alpha_r, \beta_1, \ldots, \beta_s, \gamma_{11}, \ldots, \gamma_{rs}) \in \mathbb{R}^{(r+1)(s+1)}$. Since the class of all distributions of that type constitutes a family with strictly monotone likelihood ratios, it follows that the class of all level-α tests of (8.19) based upon $d^2(\hat{\gamma}/S, \mathbf{0})$ contains a uniformly most powerful element which rejects H if and only if $nd^2(\hat{\gamma}/S, \mathbf{0})/((r-1)(s-1))$ turns out to be less than or equal to the αth quantile of a F-distribution with the same numbers of degrees of freedom and noncentrality parameter $\lambda_{nc}^2 = n\varepsilon^2$. In view of the maximal invariance of the statistic $d^2(\hat{\gamma}/S, \mathbf{0})$ for the hypotheses (8.19) we can thus conclude that

$$\left\{ d^2(\hat{\gamma}/S, \mathbf{0}) < ((r-1)(s-1)/n)\, F_{(r-1)(s-1),(n-1)rs;\,\alpha}(n\varepsilon^2) \right\} \tag{8.21}$$

is *the critical region* of an UMPI level-α test for negligibility of interactions in a two-way ANOVA layout with rs cells. Of course, in order to render this statement true, the threefold subscribed symbol F must be defined by

$$F_{(r-1)(s-1),(n-1)rs;\,\alpha}(n\varepsilon^2) \equiv \text{lower } 100\alpha\text{-percentage point of}$$
$$\text{an } F\text{-distribution with } (r-1)(s-1),(n-1)rs \text{ degrees}$$
$$\text{of freedom and noncentrality parameter } n\varepsilon^2. \tag{8.22}$$

For the power of the test with rejection region (8.21) against any specific alternative with some given value, say ψ^2, of $d^2(\gamma/\sigma, \mathbf{0})$, we get a direct analogue to formula (7.12) referring to the noncentral F-test for equivalence of k homoskedastic Gaussian distributions as discussed in the previous chapter. More precisely speaking, if we denote the rejection probability of the test under any parameter constellation $(\mu, \alpha_1, \ldots, \alpha_r, \beta_1, \ldots, \beta_s, \gamma_{11}, \ldots, \gamma_{rs})$ such that $d^2(\gamma/\sigma, \mathbf{0}) = \psi^2$ by $\beta(\psi^2)$, then we can write

$$\beta(\psi^2) = P\big[\mathcal{F}_{(r-1)(s-1),(n-1)rs}(n\psi^2) < F_{(r-1)(s-1),(n-1)rs;l,\alpha}(n\varepsilon^2)\big] \tag{8.23}$$

with $\mathcal{F}_{(r-1)(s-1),(n-1)rs}(n\psi^2)$ representing a random variable whose distribution differs from that to be used for determining the critical constant only by changing the value of the noncentrality parameter from $n\varepsilon^2$ to $n\psi^2$.

Example 8.4

In a randomized clinical trial of the antimydriatic effects (to be brought about for the purpose of reversing scopolamine-induced pupil dilation at the end of cataract surgery) of acetylcholine and thymoxamine, a total of 228 eyes was subdivided into the following four treatment arms:

(1) placebo (pure solvent)

(2) acetylcholine

(3) thymoxamine

(4) acetylcholine + thymoxamine.

Randomization was strictly uniform so that $n = 57$ eyes were assigned to each of these treatment groups. The primary endpoint for assessing the efficacy of all treatments was pupillary constriction [mm] as measured 5 minutes after application. The following table summarizes the data obtained from this trial (as cellwise arithmetic means and standard deviations, respectively):

Table 8.8 *Arithmetic means and standard deviations (in parentheses) of pupillary restriction [mm] measured in the four arms of a clinical trial of the antimydriatic effects of acetylcholine and thymoxamine following a classical 2×2-design [n = 57 eyes treated in each group] (data from Pfeiffer et al., 1994)*

| | | Acetylcholine | |
		−	+
Thymox-	−	-0.0386 (.2433)	1.8561 (.6690)
amine	+	1.5281 (.7975)	3.4193 (.9801)

With these values, we calculate $\bar{X}_{1.} = 0.9088$, $\bar{X}_{.1} = 0.7448$, $\bar{X}_{2.} = 2.4737$, $\bar{X}_{.2} = 2.6377$, $\bar{X}_{..} = 1.6912$ yielding for the interaction parameters the estimates

$$\hat{\gamma}_{11} = -0.0386 - (0.9088 + 0.7448 - 1.6912) = -0.0009,$$

$\hat{\gamma}_{12} = -\hat{\gamma}_{11} = 0.0009$, $\hat{\gamma}_{21} = -\hat{\gamma}_{11} = 0.0009$ and $\hat{\gamma}_{22} = \hat{\gamma}_{11} = -0.0009$. Furthermore, using the parenthesized entries in Table 8.8, we find that the residual variance of the data set under analysis with respect to the unrestricted model (8.18) is $S^2 = (.2433^2 + .6690^2 + .7975^2 + .9801^2)/4 = .5258$. Thus, as estimated squared distance of γ/σ from the origin, we find here

$$d^2(\hat{\gamma}/S, \mathbf{0}) = 4 \cdot .0009^2/.5258 = 6.16 \cdot 10^{-6} \ .$$

Let us now suppose that the true interaction effects are to be considered negligible if γ/σ lies in a sphere of radius $\varepsilon = .25$ around $\mathbf{0}$ and that we want to perform the test at significance level $\alpha = .05$. Then, using the appropriate intrinsic SAS function, the critical upper bound which the estimated standardized distance of γ/σ from $\mathbf{0}$ has to be compared to according to (8.21), is computed to be

$$\frac{(r-1)(s-1)}{n} F_{(r-1)(s-1),(n-1)rs;\,\alpha}(n\varepsilon^2) = \frac{1}{57}\,\mathtt{finv}(.05,1,224,3.5625)$$

$$= \frac{1}{57} \cdot .125142 = .002195 \ .$$

Since this is clearly larger than the observed value of $d^2(\hat{\gamma}/S, \mathbf{0})$, the data of Table 8.8 allow us to reject the null hypothesis that there is a nonnegligible interaction between the antimydriatic effects of both substances. Although a common sample size of almost 60 for each treatment combination is unusually large for a multiarm trial performed in a rather specialized field, it is still much too small for ensuring that the power of the UMPI test exceeds 80% against the alternative that all interaction effects vanish. In fact, for $\psi^2 = 0$, evaluating the right-hand side of (8.23) by means of the SAS function $\mathtt{probf}$ yields under our present specifications

$$\beta(0) = P[\mathcal{F}_{1,224}(0) \leq 0.125142] = \mathtt{probf}(.125142,1,224) = .27614 \ .$$

Keeping α and ε fixed at $\alpha = .05$ and $\varepsilon = .25$, respectively, at least $n = 138$ observations per cell would be necessary for raising the power against the same type of alternative to 80% or more. With $\varepsilon = .50$, $n = 35$ would suffice for meeting the requirement $\beta(0) \geq .80$.

Generalization of the UMPI test for negligibility of interactions to nonbalanced designs

In an unbalanced two-way layout, the numbers n_{ij} of observations taken under the various treatment combinations are arbitrary natural numbers (discarding situations where some cells contain no data at all) allowed to be even pairwise different from each other. As holds generally true for analyses of classical linear models for multiway layouts, nonbalancedness induces complications both with regard to the computational techniques required for determining the test statistics and, still more important, interpretation of hypotheses.

From a computational perspective, the crucial change refers to the numerator of the (rescaled) F-statistic (8.20) which in the unbalanced case can no longer be written simply as the sum of squares of the best linear estimates of the γ_{ij} in the full model (8.18). In fact, $\bar{X}_{ij} - (\bar{X}_{i\cdot} + \bar{X}_{\cdot j} - \bar{X}_{\cdot\cdot})$ has to be replaced with $\bar{X}_{ij} - (\hat{\hat{\mu}} + \hat{\hat{\alpha}}_i + \hat{\hat{\beta}}_j)$ where $(\hat{\hat{\mu}}, \hat{\hat{\alpha}}_i, \hat{\hat{\beta}}_j)$ denotes the least squares estimate of (μ, α_i, β_j) in the interaction-constrained model $\mu_{ij} = \mu + \alpha_i + \beta_j$. With unbalanced data, the $\hat{\hat{\alpha}}_i$, $\hat{\hat{\beta}}_j$ and $\hat{\hat{\mu}}$ admit no explicit representation as linear functions of the cell means $\bar{X}_{ij}$ but must be determined by solving a system of linear equations whose coefficient matrix exhibits no closed-form inverse (for details see, e.g., Searle, 1987, § 4.9). Of course, instead of the ordinary we have to form the weighted sum of squares of the $\hat{\hat{\gamma}}_{ij} \equiv \bar{X}_{ij} - (\hat{\hat{\mu}} + \hat{\hat{\alpha}}_i + \hat{\hat{\beta}}_j)$ using weight-factors $n_{ij}/\bar{n}$ where

$$\bar{n} \equiv N/rs \equiv \frac{1}{rs} \sum_{i=1}^{r} \sum_{j=1}^{s} n_{ij} \ . \tag{8.24}$$

Making the dependence of the numerator of the test statistic on these weights explicit by adding the subscript **n** [symbolizing the so-called incidence-matrix $(n_{ij})_{(r,s)}$] to $d^2(\cdot\,,\cdot)$, we have to replace (8.20) in the unbalanced case with

$$d_{\mathbf{n}}^2(\hat{\hat{\gamma}}/S, \mathbf{0}) = \frac{\displaystyle\sum_{i=1}^{r} \sum_{j=1}^{s} (n_{ij}/\bar{n}) \big(\bar{X}_{ij} - (\hat{\hat{\mu}} + \hat{\hat{\alpha}}_i + \hat{\hat{\beta}}_j)\big)^2}{\displaystyle\sum_{i=1}^{r} \sum_{j=1}^{s} \sum_{k=1}^{n_{ij}} (X_{ijk} - \bar{X}_{ij})^2/(N - rs)} \ . \tag{8.25}$$

From a practical point of view, it makes almost no difference whether computation of the test statistic has to be based on formula (8.25) or can be simplified to (8.20). In fact, any well-designed program package for use in statistical applications contains a procedure for computing F-statistics for all hypotheses of interest in analyzing ANOVA higher-way layouts with arbitrary incidence matrices. Denoting the F-ratio for testing the null hypothesis of no interactions by $\mathcal{F}_{(r,s)}^{(\mathbf{n})}(\gamma|\mu, \alpha, \beta)$, we have just to read the value of the latter from the output list generated by running a suitable program (like **proc glm** in SAS) and multiply it by $(r-1)(s-1)/\bar{n}$ to obtain the observed value of $d_{\mathbf{n}}^2(\hat{\hat{\gamma}}/S, \mathbf{0})$ as defined in (8.25). Clearly, this suggests using

$$\left\{ d_{\mathbf{n}}^2(\hat{\hat{\gamma}}/S, \mathbf{0}) < \big((r - 1)(s - 1)/\bar{n}\big) \, F_{(r-1)(s-1), N-rs; \alpha}(\bar{n}\varepsilon^2) \right\} \ . \tag{8.26}$$

as the *rejection region* of the desired test for negligibility of interactions in the case of an arbitrary incidence matrix $\mathbf{n} \neq n\mathbf{1}_{(r,s)}$.

However, the hypotheses for which (8.26) gives a UMPI critical region can no longer be expressed in terms of a spherical neighbourhood of the origin in the space of the standardized true γ_{ij}. To see this, one has to examine the noncentrality parameter λ_{nc}^2 of the distribution of $\mathcal{F}_{(r,s)}^{(\mathbf{n})}(\gamma|\mu, \alpha, \beta) =$

$(\bar{n}/(r-1)(s-1))d_{\mathbf{n}}^2(\hat{\hat{\gamma}}/S, \mathbf{0})$ under an arbitrary parameter configuration with $\gamma \neq \mathbf{0}$. Discarding the factor $\bar{n}$, λ_{nc}^2 is obtained by substituting in the numerator of (8.25) every single observation X_{ijk} and hence every cell mean $\bar{X}_{ij}$ by its expectation μ_{ij}, and dividing the resulting expression by σ^2. Since $\hat{\hat{\gamma}}$ is a vector of linear functions, say $\hat{\hat{\mathbf{g}}}_{\mathbf{n}}(\bar{X}_{11}, \ldots, \bar{X}_{rs})$, of the cell means with coefficients determined by the n_{ij}, it follows that $\mathcal{F}_{(r,s)}^{(\mathbf{n})}(\gamma|\mu, \alpha, \beta)$ is noncentral F with $(r-1)(s-1), N-rs$ degrees of freedom and $\lambda_{nc}^2 = \bar{n}d_{\mathbf{n}}^2(\hat{\hat{\mathbf{g}}}_{\mathbf{n}}(\mu_{11}, \ldots, \mu_{rs})/\sigma, \mathbf{0})$ so that the hypotheses actually tested when using (8.26) as the critical region, are

$$H : d_{\mathbf{n}}^2(\hat{\hat{\mathbf{g}}}_{\mathbf{n}}(\mu_{11}, \ldots, \mu_{rs})/\sigma, \mathbf{0}) \geq \varepsilon^2$$

$$\text{versus} \quad K : d_{\mathbf{n}}^2(\hat{\hat{\mathbf{g}}}_{\mathbf{n}}(\mu_{11}, \ldots, \mu_{rs})/\sigma, \mathbf{0}) < \varepsilon^2 \qquad (8.27)$$

On the one hand, for any configuration $(\mu_{11}, \ldots, \mu_{rs}) \in \mathbb{R}^{rs}$ of true cell means satisfying the no-interaction model exactly, $d_{\mathbf{n}}^2(\hat{\hat{\mathbf{g}}}_{\mathbf{n}}(\mu_{11}, \ldots, \mu_{rs})/\sigma, \mathbf{0})$ vanishes and can thus be viewed as a generalized measure of distance between true and constraint model. On the other, the parameter sets corresponding to the hypotheses of (8.27) depend in a complicated way on the entries in the incidence matrix $\mathbf{n}$ and will be comparable in form to those considered in the balanced-data case only for small to moderate values of $(\max_{i,j} n_{ij}/\min_{i,j} n_{ij}) - 1$. In presence of gross differences between the cell frequencies, a more satisfactory solution to the problem of testing for negligibility of interactions might be obtained by keeping the hypotheses unchanged and constructing a large-sample test for (8.19) based on the asymptotic distribution of $\sqrt{N}(d^2(\hat{\gamma}/S, \mathbf{0}) - d^2(\gamma/\sigma, \mathbf{0}))$. Detailed comparisons of such an alternative approach with that based on (8.26) must be left as a topic for future research.

8.3.2 Establishing negligibility of carryover effects in the analysis of two-period crossover trials

In this subsection, we suppose that the data set under analysis stems from a standard two-period crossover trial involving two different treatments, say A and B. Trials of this type are very popular in various branches of clinical research and give in particular the standard case of a comparative bioavailability study to which the final chapter of this book is devoted in full length. The decisive feature of the two-period crossover design is that each experimental unit receives both treatments under comparison in temporal succession. Since there are of course two possible sequences in which the treatments can be administered the total sample of $N = m+n$ subjects is randomly split into sequence groups A/B and B/A, say. In the first of these groups, each subject receives treatment A at the beginning of the first period of the trial, and is switched to treatment B in a second period.

Usually, between the end of period 1 and the beginning of period 2, a sufficiently long washing-out period is scheduled. The only difference of the second sequence group B/A as compared to the first one is that the order of application of the treatments is reversed. It is furthermore assumed that the same univariate quantitative outcome measure is used in both periods to describe each subject's biological condition after administration of the respective treatment. A convenient notation is obtained by defining X_{ki} and Y_{kj} to be the outcome observed in period $k = 1, 2$ in the ith and the jth subject of sequence group A/B and B/A, respectively. Thus, a complete description of the layout is as follows:

Sequence Group	Period 1	Period 2
A/B	$X_{11}, \ldots, X_{1m}$	$X_{21}, \ldots, X_{2m}$
B/A	$Y_{11}, \ldots, Y_{1n}$	$Y_{21}, \ldots, Y_{2n}$

At first sight, such a design looks simply like a special case of a two-way ANOVA layout with both factors varying over just two levels. However, there is a marked difference deserving keen attention: In the crossover case, the observations from different cells are not mutually independent but form pairs within each row. In other words, the data set obtained from a two-period crossover trial consists of two unrelated samples of bivariate observations rather than 4 samples made up of one-dimensional variables. By far the most popular approach to analyzing the data of a standard crossover trial is based on a simple parametric model originally introduced by Grizzle (1965). Of course, it allows in particular for correlations within all pairs (X_{1i}, X_{2i}), (Y_{1j}, Y_{2j}) and can be written

$$X_{ki} = \mu_k + S_i^{(1)} + \varepsilon_{ki}^{(1)}, \quad i = 1, \ldots, m, \quad k = 1, 2, \tag{8.28a}$$

$$Y_{kj} = \nu_k + S_j^{(2)} + \varepsilon_{kj}^{(2)}, \quad j = 1, \ldots, n, \quad k = 1, 2, \tag{8.28b}$$

where all $S_i^{(1)}, S_j^{(2)}, \varepsilon_{ki}^{(1)}, \varepsilon_{kj}^{(2)}$ are mutually independent with,

$$S_i^{(1)}, \quad S_j^{(2)} \sim \mathcal{N}(0, \sigma_S^2) \tag{8.29}$$

and

$$\varepsilon_{1i}^{(1)}, \quad \varepsilon_{1j}^{(2)} \sim \mathcal{N}(0, \tau_1^2), \quad \varepsilon_{2i}^{(1)}, \varepsilon_{2j}^{(2)} \sim \mathcal{N}(0, \tau_2^2). \tag{8.30}$$

Usually, $S_i^{(1)}$ and $S_j^{(2)}$ is called the (random) effect of the ith and jth subject in sequence group A/B and B/A, respectively, σ_S^2 the between-subject variance, and τ_k^2 the within-subject variance for the kth period.

For the expected values μ_k, ν_k of the X_{ki}, Y_{kj}, Grizzle's model assumes that these can be additively decomposed into a overall mean ω, a "direct treatment effect" ϕ_A or ϕ_B, a period effect π_k, and for $k = 2$, a carryover effect denoted here $\lambda^{(1)} [\leftrightarrow A/B]$ and $\lambda^{(2)} [\leftrightarrow B/A]$, respectively. The corresponding model equations are

$$\mu_1 = \omega + \phi_A + \pi_1, \quad \mu_2 = \omega + \phi_B + \pi_2 + \lambda^{(1)}, \tag{8.31a}$$

$$\nu_1 = \omega + \phi_B + \pi_1, \quad \nu_2 = \omega + \phi_A + \pi_2 + \lambda^{(2)}. \tag{8.31b}$$

Clearly, the carryover effects reflect deviations from strict additivity of treatment and period effects and are thus another instance of interaction parameters. If they have some common value, say $\lambda^{(0)}$, they can be totally dropped from the above model equations since then $\omega + \lambda^{(1)}$ and $\omega + \lambda^{(2)}$ are simply relabelled versions of the same overall mean. Thus, with regard to the carryover effects in a two-period crossover setting, negligibility means equality except for irrelevant differences.

In authoritative expositions of inferential methods for the analysis of crossover trials (see, e.g., Jones and Kenward, 1989, in addition to Grizzle's pioneering paper of 1965), it is much more clearly understood than in the literature on classical ANOVA methods, that the primary aim of inference on interactions consists in ruling out the possibility that such effects must be taken into account. The standard argument which is usually presented in favour of this view is that otherwise none of the differential main effects $\phi_A - \phi_B$ and $\pi_1 - \pi_2$ admits unbiased estimation from the full data set. Nevertheless, also in this field, very little has changed over the years with regard to the usual practice of assessing the difference between both carryover effects: A preliminary test of the null hypothesis $\lambda^{(1)} = \lambda^{(2)}$ is carried out and a nonsignificant result considered sufficient to warrant the conclusion that the $\lambda^{(k)}$ can be discarded when assessing the main effects. As a tried way around the flaw that this test is obviously directed to the wrong side, Grizzle suggested to raise the nominal significance level to $\alpha = .10$, and this advice was adopted by Kenward and Jones.

Of course, it is our aim here to show how this makeshift solution of the problem of establishing approximate additivity of treatment and period effects in a crossover layout can be replaced with a rigorous inferential procedure. It will turn out that the problem can readily be reduced in such a way that its solution requires no new ideas but simply an application of some of the methods developed in Chapter 6. In order to see this let us recall the rationale behind the standard parametric test for the traditional two-sided problem $\lambda^{(1)} = \lambda^{(2)}$ vs. $\lambda^{(1)} \neq \lambda^{(2)}$. The initial step, from which the rest follows almost automatically, consists of forming for each subject the total response by summing up his responses to both treatments. Defining

$$X_i^+ = X_{1i} + X_{2i} \ \forall i = 1, \ldots, m, \quad Y_j^+ = Y_{1j} + Y_{2j} \ \forall j = 1, \ldots, n, \tag{8.32}$$

it is a straightforward exercise to verify by means of $(8.28) - (8.31)$ that the X_i^+ and Y_j^+ make up two independent samples from Gaussian distributions with common variance

$$\sigma_+^2 = 4\,\sigma_S^2 + \tau_1^2 + \tau_2^2 \tag{8.33}$$

and expected values $\mu_+ = E(X_i^+)$, $\nu_+ = E(Y_j^+)$ such that

$$\mu_+ - \nu_+ = \lambda^{(1)} - \lambda^{(2)}. \tag{8.34}$$

In view of (8.33) and (8.34), it is clearly appropriate to formulate the problem of establishing negligibility of carryover effects in the model due to Grizzle (1965) as the problem of testing

$$H_+ : |\mu_+ - \nu_+|/\sigma_+ \geq \varepsilon \text{ versus } K_+ : |\mu_+ - \nu_+|/\sigma_+ < \varepsilon \tag{8.35}$$

by means of the within-subject totals (8.32). Since the latter satisfy

$$X_i^+ \sim \mathcal{N}(\mu^+, \sigma_+^2) \; \forall\, i\,, \quad Y_j^+ \sim \mathcal{N}(\nu^+, \sigma_+^2) \; \forall\, j\,, \tag{8.36}$$

(8.35) is simply a special case of (6.2) $[\rightarrow$ p. 101]. Thus, there is a UMPI level-α test which rejects H_+ if and only if the absolute value of the ordinary two-sample statistic T_+, say, calculated with the X_i^+ and Y_j^+ as the raw data, turns out smaller than $\sqrt{F_{1,N-2;\,\alpha}(mn\varepsilon^2/N)}$ [for the definition of $F_{1,N-2;\,\alpha}$, recall (8.22)].

Example 8.5

It is instructive to compare the exact optimal test for (8.35) with the "inverted" two-sided t-test through applying both procedures to the same data set. Table 8.9 shows the results of a classical crossover trial of the efficacy of a certain oxygen gel $[\leftrightarrow (B)]$ in the improvement of dental plaque and gingival-inflammation, as compared with placebo $[\leftrightarrow (A)]$. The study was first reported by Zinner, Duany and Chilton (1979) and used at several places in the biostatistical literature for illustrating various techniques useful for the analysis of crossover trials (Brown, 1980; Jones and Kenward, 1989). The values displayed in the table represent improvements in a summary score of oral hygiene during each trial period.

Table 8.9 *Improvements in a summary score of oral hygiene observed in a crossover trial comparing a new oxygen gel (B) with placebo (A) (Data originally reported by Zinner, Duany and Chilton (1970); reproduced from Jones and Kenward (1989), with kind permission by Chapman and Hall, London.)*

Group A/B

i	1	2	3	4	5	6	7	8	9	10	11	12
X_{1i}	0.83	1.00	0.67	0.5	0.50	0.83	1.0	0.67	0.67	0.33	0.00	1.17
X_{2i}	1.83	2.17	1.67	1.5	2.33	1.83	0.5	0.33	0.50	0.67	0.83	1.33
X_i^+	2.66	3.17	2.34	2.0	2.83	2.66	1.5	1.00	1.17	1.00	0.83	2.50

	13	14	15	16	17	18	19	20	21	22	23	24
	0.00	0.50	0.33	0.33	0.50	1.00	0.00	0.5	-0.50	0.17	1.00	1.00
	0.67	1.83	1.50	1.50	1.17	1.67	1.33	1.5	2.83	2.33	1.33	1.67
	0.67	2.33	1.83	1.83	1.67	2.67	1.33	2.0	2.33	2.50	2.33	2.67

	25	26	27	28	29	30	31	32	33	34
	1.33	0.33	2	4.00	0.83	0.50	0.5	0.50	2.17	0.67
	0.67	0.83	1	0.17	1.67	1.33	1.5	1.67	1.33	1.17
	2.00	1.16	3	4.17	2.50	1.83	2.0	2.17	3.50	1.84

Group B/A

j	1	2	3	4	5	6	7	8	9	10	11	12
Y_{1j}	1.67	2.5	1.00	1.67	1.83	0.50	1.33	1.33	0.50	2.17	1.67	1.5
Y_{2j}	0.33	0.5	-0.17	0.50	0.50	0.33	0.67	0.00	0.17	0.83	0.33	0.0
Y_j^+	2.00	3.0	0.83	2.17	2.33	0.83	2.00	1.33	0.67	3.00	2.00	1.5

Table 8.9 *(continued)*

13	14	15	16	17	18	19	20	21	22	23	24
1.33	1.5	1.33	0.67	1.67	2.50	1.83	0.83	2.33	1.17	1.33	1.33
0.50	0.5	0.00	-0.17	0.50	0.67	0.00	0.67	0.17	0.50	0.00	0.83
1.83	2.0	1.33	0.50	2.17	3.17	1.83	1.50	2.50	1.67	1.33	2.16

25	26	27	28	29	30
0.33	2.17	1.00	0.33	1.17	0.5
1.33	1.17	0.33	1.00	0.17	0.5
1.66	3.34	1.33	1.33	1.34	1.0

As argued by Jones and Kenward (loc. cit., p. 39), the 28th subject of Group A/B should be removed as an outlier. With the remaining $N = 33 + 30$ within-subject totals, the t-statistic is computed to be

$$T_+ = \sqrt{\frac{33 \cdot 30}{63}} (2.0552 - 1.7883) / \left[(32 \cdot .699331^2 + 29 \cdot .730654^2)/61 \right]^{1/2}$$
$$= 1.4810.$$

In the conventional two-sided test, the associated p-value is .1438 so that the null hypothesis $\lambda^{(1)} = \lambda^{(2)}$ has to be accepted also at the 10%-level. According to Grizzle's rule there is thus no reason to suspect that the standard test for assessing the direct treatment and period effects might lead to invalid conclusions. Performing the t-test for equivalence of both distributions of within-subject totals instead, it seems appropriate to rely on a rather strict specification of the tolerance ε determining the hypotheses of (8.35). Following the recommendations put forward in §1.5 this amounts to setting $\varepsilon = .36$, and with that value of ε the critical constant of the UMPI test for (8.35) at level $\alpha = .05$ based on samples of size $m = 33$ and $n = 30$ is found to be (by means of the SAS intrinsic function for quantiles of arbitrary F-distributions)

$$\left[F_{1,61;\,.05}(33 \cdot 30 \cdot .36^2/63) \right]^{1/2} = \texttt{finv(.05,1,61,2.0366)**.05}$$
$$= 0.173292 \,.$$

Since the observed value of $|T_+|$ is far beyond this bound, our formal test for absence of relevant carryover effects does not lead to a positive decision in the case of the dental hygiene study of Zinner et al. Having a look at the power of the test, this result is far from being surprising: Even under the null alternative $\lambda^{(1)} = \lambda^{(2)}$, the rejection probability is as low as 13.7%, and in a balanced trial, 133 subjects in each sequence group would be required for raising the chance of detecting perfect additivity to 80%. From a different perspective, this result corroborates the conclusion drawn by Brown (1980) from his analysis of the efficiency of the carryover relative to a simple parallel-group design: The frequently invoked superiority of the former holds only in those cases where additivity of the main effects can be taken for granted a priori and need not be established by means of a valid preliminary test providing reasonable power to detect that the restriction $\lambda^{(1)} = \lambda^{(2)}$ is actually satisfied.

Alternative approaches

(i) *Assessing raw rather than standardized effects.* Sometimes, it might be preferable to measure the extent of the deviation from strict additivity of the main effects through the raw difference $\lambda^{(1)} - \lambda^{(2)}$ between the carryover effects. In such cases, it is reasonable to replace the testing problem (8.35) with

$$H'_+ : |\mu_+ - \nu_+| \geq \varepsilon' \quad \text{versus} \quad K'_+ : |\mu_+ - \nu_+| < \varepsilon' \tag{8.37}$$

and to apply the interval inclusion approach of §3.1 to the latter. A guidance for specifying the equivalence range $(-\varepsilon', \varepsilon')$ in this alternative formulation of the problem of testing for negligibility of the carryover effects can be found in Brown (1980): Considering the power of the traditional two-sided test, this author recommends to choose $\varepsilon' = \delta'/2$ with $\delta' > 0$ denoting the true difference one tries to detect in the standard test of equality of direct treatment effects.

Suppose the authors of the study considered in the above Example 8.5 eventually aimed at detecting an effect of $\delta' = 1.00$ of the oxygen gel as compared with placebo. Then, in the interval inclusion test at level $\alpha = .05$ for (8.37), rejection of H'_+ would require that $(-.50, .50) \supseteq (\bar{X}^+ - \bar{Y}^+ - t_{61;.95}\tilde{S}^+, \bar{X}^+ - \bar{Y}^+ + t_{61;.95}\tilde{S}^+)$, with $\tilde{S}^+$ denoting the standard error of $\bar{X}^+ - \bar{Y}^+$ as estimated from the pooled sample. Since $\tilde{S}^+$ can obviously be written $\tilde{S}^+ = |\bar{X}^+ - \bar{Y}^+|/|T^+|$ and we had $\bar{X}^+ = 2.0552$, $\bar{Y}^+ = 1.7883$, $T^+ = 1.4810$, the 95%-confidence bounds to $\mu_+ - \nu_+$ are computed to be $0.2668 \pm 1.67022 \cdot .2668/1.4810 = 0.2668 \pm .3009$. Thus, with $\varepsilon' = .50$ and at level $\alpha = .05$, the null hypothesis of a nonnegligible absolute difference between the carryover effects could not be rejected either.

(ii) *Testing for negligibility of the carryover effects without relying on parametric distributional assumptions.* In cases of doubt about the adequacy of the distributional assumptions (8.29), (8.30), it is generally advisable (cf. Jones and Kenward, 1989, § 2.8) to replace t-tests with their nonparametric counterparts. Of course, there is no reason for exempting the test for negligibility of the carryover effects from this recommendation. As we know from Chapter 6, there is a distribution-free analogue of the t-test for equivalence of two homoskedastic Gaussian distributions with respect to the standardized shift in location. With the computational tools presented in § 6.2, the Mann-Whitney test for equivalence of both distributions of within-subject totals is almost as easily carried out as the noncentral t-test. Specifying the equivalence range $(1/2 - \varepsilon_1', 1/2 + \varepsilon_2'') = (.40, .60)$ for the target functional $P[X_i^+ > Y_j^+]$ (which, according to the results of § 1.5, is approximately the same as requiring $|\mu_+ - \nu_+|/\sigma_+ < .36$ in the Gaussian case), we obtain by means of the *SAS* macro `mawi` with the data of Example 8.5:

$$W_+ = .59495, \ \hat{\sigma}[W_+] = .070076, \ C_{MW}(.05; .10, .10) = .17259 .$$

In view of $|W_+ - 1/2|/\hat{\sigma}[W_+] = 1.3550 > C_{MW}(.05; .10, .10)$, the decision is identical to that we were lead to take using the UMPI test at the same level for the parametric version of the problem.

CHAPTER 9

The assessment of bioequivalence

9.1 Introduction

Although the overwhelming majority of the existing literature on statistical tests for equivalence hypotheses refers to the analysis of comparative bioavailability trials (often also named bioequivalence trials, for the sake of brevity), the testing problems to be dealt with in the context of bioequivalence (BE) assessment are rather special in nature. This is because the regulatory authorities have set up strict guidelines for the planning and analysis of bioequivalence studies quite soon after this type of trial had begun to play an important role in pharmaceutics and clinical pharmacology. According to these rules, every bioequivalence study has to be conducted as a phase-I clinical trial which means that the subjects are healthy volunteers rather than patients suffering from a disease considered to be an indication for administering the drug under study. Furthermore, each subject has to be given several formulations of that drug in an experiment following a crossing-over scheme allowing for two different trial periods at least. The outcome measure to be used for characterizing the biological activity of the drug administered at the beginning of the respective period, has to be chosen from a very short list of pharmacokinetic parameters. The distributions of these outcome measures are of the continuous type throughout, modelled in the majority of cases in a fully parametric way, usually after logarithmic transformation of the primary measurements obtained during the trial.

A complete exposition covering all statistical facets of the planning and analysis of BE trials gives sufficient material for a monograph of its own (see Chow and Liu, 1992) so that we confine ourselves in this chapter to a discussion of the standard case of a bioequivalence trial involving two periods and as many different drug formulations. Actually, the restriction to this standard design is far from severe for practical purposes since real BE trials involving more than two periods and/or treatments are still a rare exception. Furthermore, even with regard to the 2×2 case, the controversy about the most appropriate statistical criterion for BE assessment is still very far from being settled and seems to be a never ending story within (bio-)statistical science. Not surprisingly, the major issue of the ongoing discussion refers to the conceptual level. In fact, from the mathematical and statistical perspective, it can be stated that there are very satisfactory solutions to an impressive manifold of problems put forward in this context. However, only a small number of them yield an intuitively plausible translation of the bio-medical question to be answered at the end of a BE trial into the formalism of decision making between statistical hypotheses. Thus, it can be argued that statistical BE assessment has developed into a field where more mathematically sophisticated solutions exist than problems worth the effort entailed in deriving solutions. In view of this situation, we prefer to concentrate on a careful discussion of the pros and cons of the most frequently applied approaches. Even within the scope of methods tailored for the analysis of BE trials following the standard design, we do not aim at a complete coverage of the existing literature. In return, the reader will find also some new ideas on the topic which lead beyond the solutions encouraged by the official guidelines or may even suggest questioning the adequacy of the rationale behind the latter.

The general frame of reference for the whole chapter is given by a conventional nonreplicated crossover design as had been considered from a totally different perspective in § 8.3.2. In the present context, the treatments under comparison are two drug products denoted "Test" (T) and "Reference" (R), adopting the usage almost universally followed in the field of BE assessment. Typically and most commonly, T is a generic drug to be approved for the market, and R a reference listed drug containing chemically identical active ingredients. The total sample of subjects recruited to a standard BE trial consists of N healthy volunteers randomly assigned to one of the two possible sequence groups T/R and R/T. Although the randomization is usually performed under the restriction of generating a strictly balanced layout, by technical difficulties it might happen that a few subjects have gotten lost from one or the other group due to providing incomplete or otherwise insufficient pharmacokinetic data. Thus, we allow for arbitrary sample sizes m ($\leftrightarrow T/R$) and n ($\leftrightarrow R/T$) in both sequence groups.

The basic data set consists of two vectors per subject whose components give the ordinates of the concentration-time profile recorded in both periods of the trial. (In the majority of BE studies, the concentration of the active ingredient of interest is measured in the blood plasma or serum.) Figure 9.1 shows a schematic example of such a pair of observed concentration-time profiles. Instead of analyzing the individual profiles as multivariate data, they are usually reduced in a preliminary step to a single real value by calculating one of the following pharmacokinetic characteristics:

- area under the profile as a whole (AUC)
- maximum concentration ($C_{\max}$)
- time at which the peak concentration $C_{\max}$ was measured ($t_{\max}$).

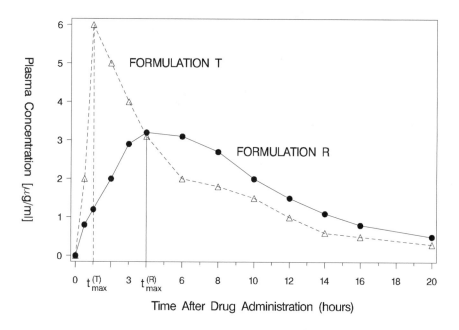

Figure 9.1 *Example of a pair of concentration-time profiles observed in a given subject during both periods of a standard bioequivalence trial. (Redrawn from Rodda, 1990, with kind permission by Marcel Dekker, Inc.)*

Commonly, AUC and $C_{\max}$ are considered as alternative estimates of the extent of the absorption process induced in a trial subject, whereas $t_{\max}$ is interpreted as measuring its rate. All three pharmacokinetic parameters are accepted as a reasonable choice for selecting a reference measure of bioavailability to be used as the endpoint variable in both periods and all subjects enrolled in the trial.

The data set eventually to be analyzed for the purpose of BE assessment consists of two independent samples $(X_{11}, X_{21}), \ldots, (X_{1m}, X_{2m}), (Y_{11}, Y_{21}), \ldots, (Y_{1n}, Y_{2n})$ of pairs of one-dimensional random variables such that

$$X_{ki} = \text{bioavailability measured in the } i\text{th subject } (i = 1, \ldots, m)$$
$$\text{of sequence group } T/R \text{ during the } k\text{th period } (k = 1, 2);$$
$$Y_{kj} = \text{bioavailability measured in the } j\text{th subject } (j = 1, \ldots, n)$$
$$\text{of sequence group } R/T \text{ during the } k\text{th period } (k = 1, 2).$$

In order to ensure at least approximate normality of the distributions of these variables, it is generally recommended (see FDA/CDER, 2001, § VI.A) to determine their values by taking logarithms of the bioavailabilities computed from the individual concentration-time profiles. Thus, if the AUC has been selected as the measure of bioavailability of interest, then we have $X_{11} = \log(A_{11}), Y_{11} = \log(B_{11})$ with A_{11} and B_{11} denoting the area under the profile obtained in Period 1 in the 1st subject of group T/R and R/T, respectively, and so on.

If not explicitly stated otherwise, we assume throughout (following once more the current official guidance for conducting in vivo BE studies) that the log-bioavailabilities X_{ki}, Y_{kj} satisfy the basic parametric model for the analysis of 2×2 crossover trials [see (8.28)-(8.31)] with the following slight modifications: The within-subject variability (usually interpreted as reflecting measurement error) is this time allowed to depend on treatment rather than period so that we let

$$Var\left[\varepsilon_{1i}^{(1)}\right] = Var\left[\varepsilon_{2j}^{(2)}\right] \equiv \sigma_{eT}^2 \tag{9.1a}$$

and

$$Var\left[\varepsilon_{2i}^{(1)}\right] = Var\left[\varepsilon_{1j}^{(2)}\right] \equiv \sigma_{eR}^2 \tag{9.1b}$$

for all $i = 1, \ldots, m$ and $j = 1, \ldots, n$. Furthermore, the direct treatment effects are now called formulation effects and written ϕ_T, ϕ_R instead of ϕ_A, ϕ_B. Except for § 9.5, we adopt the conventional view that in analyzing a properly conducted BE trial, nonexistence of carryover effects can be taken for granted a priori, due to a careful procedure of eliminating the residual activity of the drug administered in the initial period during the washing-out interval. Of course, having renamed the treatment effects, this leads to the simplified model equations

$$E(X_{1i}) = \mu_1 = \omega + \phi_T + \pi_1, \quad E(X_{2i}) = \mu_2 = \omega + \phi_R + \pi_2$$
$$(i = 1, \ldots, m) \tag{9.2a}$$

$$E(Y_{1j}) = \nu_1 = \omega + \phi_R + \pi_1, \quad E(Y_{2j}) = \nu_2 = \omega + \phi_T + \pi_2$$
$$(j = 1, \ldots, n). \tag{9.2b}$$

In a broad sense, it is clear what bioequivalence of the two drug formulations means: sufficient similarity of the distributions of bioavailabilities measured after administration of T and R, respectively. However, there are obviously many ways of making this idea precise in terms of a hypothesis to be established by means of some suitable test of significance. The still most frequently used criterion focusses on the difference $\phi_T - \phi_R$ of formulation effects. In the guidelines and the biostatistical literature on BE assessment, testing procedures allowing to decide whether or not a criterion of this type is satisfied, are called tests for "average bioequivalence". Due to their overwhelming importance for biostatistical practice, the best established approaches to the assessment of average BE are discussed in the first of the core sections of this chapter. A totally different philosophy underlies the methods presented in § 9.3: "Individual bioequivalence" in the "probability-based" sense requires that in the underlying population, there is a sufficiently high proportion of subjects such that the bioavailabilities induced by T and R in the same individual are identical except for some pharmacologically irrelevant difference. Methods of testing for "population bioequivalence", which will be discussed in §9.4, aim at establishing that the distributions of bioavailabilities associated with T and R, are similar *both* with respect to location and variability. Finally, in §9.5 we argue that any marked difference between the *joint* distribution of the (X_{1i}, X_{2i}) and that of the (Y_{1j}, Y_{2j}) is at variance with equivalence of both drug formulations with respect to the given measure of bioavailability. Accordingly, the testing procedure derived in this final section, are bivariate analogues of the univariate two-sample tests for continuous data discussed in Chapter 6.

9.2 Methods of testing for average bioequivalence

9.2.1 Equivalence with respect to nonstandardized mean bioavailabilities

The traditional approach to BE assessment recommended even in the most recent official guidelines on statistical methods for the analysis of comparative bioavailability trials (FDA/CDER, 2001) as a standard procedure, focusses on the raw formulation effects ϕ_T, ϕ_R as appearing in the model equations (9.2). In the simplest version of the concept, average BE is defined to be satisfied if and only if the true value of $\phi_T - \phi_R$ lies in a sufficiently small neighbourhood of zero. By the so-called $80 - 125\%$ convention, the radius of this neighbourhood is specified

$$\delta_{\circ} = \log(5/4) = .2231 \,, \tag{9.3}$$

which can be motivated as follows: Suppose the period effects can also be dropped from the model equations (which, according to experience, holds true for the majority of real BE studies), and the within-subject variance is the same under both treatments (which is a standard assumption in the classical model for the 2×2 crossover). Then, the distribution of the non-logarithmic bioavailability induced by formulation T and R is log-normal with parameters $\omega + \phi_T$, $\sigma_S^2 + \sigma_e^2$ and $\omega + \phi_R$, $\sigma_S^2 + \sigma_e^2$, respectively. Hence (cf. Johnson, Kotz and Balakrishnan, 1994, p. 212), the expected values, say μ_T^* and μ_R^*, of these distributions are given by $\mu_T^* = \exp\{\omega + \phi_T + (\sigma_S^2 + \sigma_e^2)/2\}$, $\mu_R^* = \exp\{\omega + \phi_R + (\sigma_S^2 + \sigma_e^2)/2\}$, so that their ratio is $\mu_T^*/\mu_R^* = \exp\{\phi_T - \phi_R\}$. This shows that under the additional restrictions made explicit above, the condition $|\phi_T - \phi_R| < \log(5/4)$ is the same as $4/5 < \mu_T^*/\mu_R^* < 5/4$, and it has become part of good pharmaceutical practice to consider the latter sufficient for neglecting the differences in the response to both formulations of the drug.

Keeping the specification (9.3) in mind, assessment of average BE in the usual sense requires that we are able to perform a valid test of

$$H : |\phi_T - \phi_R| \geq \delta_\circ \quad \text{versus} \quad K : |\phi_T - \phi_R| < \delta_\circ \, . \qquad (9.4)$$

In order to see how such a test can be constructed, it is helpful to re-call the standard parametric procedure of testing the conventional null hypothesis $\phi_T = \phi_R$ in a 2×2 crossover design satisfying strict addi-tivity of direct treatment and period effects. The basic step enabling an easy derivation of such a test consists in reducing the bioavailabilities (X_{1i}, X_{2i}), (Y_{1j}, Y_{2j}) observed in the successive trial periods, to within-subject differences measuring the change in response level from Period 1 to Period 2 (to be computed in that order throughout, irrespective of the sequence group to which a given subject has been assigned). Denoting this difference by X_i^- ($\leftrightarrow$ Group T/R) and Y_j^- ($\leftrightarrow$ Group R/T), respectively, we have

$$X_i^- = X_{1i} - X_{2i} \; \forall \, i = 1, \ldots, m, \;\; Y_j^- = Y_{1j} - Y_{2j} \; \forall \, j = 1, \ldots, n, \quad (9.5)$$

and it readily follows from (9.1) and (9.2) that

$$X_i^- \sim \mathcal{N}(\phi_T - \phi_R + \pi_1 - \pi_2, \, \sigma^2) \; \forall \, i = 1, \ldots, m, \qquad (9.6\text{a})$$

$$Y_j^- \sim \mathcal{N}(\phi_R - \phi_T + \pi_1 - \pi_2, \, \sigma^2) \; \forall \, j = 1, \ldots, n, \qquad (9.6\text{b})$$

with

$$\sigma^2 = \sigma_{eT}^2 + \sigma_{eR}^2 \, . \qquad (9.7)$$

Clearly, (9.6) implies that the within-subject differences X_i^- and Y_j^- sat-isfy the assumptions of the ordinary two-sample t-test where the shift in location of both Gaussian distributions admits the representation

$$\mu_- - \nu_- \equiv E(X_i^-) - E(Y_j^-) = 2(\phi_T - \phi_R) \, . \qquad (9.8)$$

Thus, treating the X_i^- and Y_j^- as the raw data, (9.4) is nothing but a special instance of the problem of testing for equivalence of two homoskedastic Gaussian distributions with respect to the absolute shift in location. As we know from § 3.1, the simplest solution of an equivalence testing problem of that kind is through an application of the principle of confidence interval inclusion.

For a concise description of the corresponding decision rule, it is conve-nient to introduce the following notation making explicit that all statistics involved have to be computed from the inter-period differences defined by (9.5):

$$\bar{X}^- = (1/m) \sum_{i=1}^{m} X_i^- \, , \;\; \bar{Y}^- = (1/n) \sum_{j=1}^{n} Y_j^- \, ;$$

$$\tilde{S}^- = \left[\left(\left(\sum_{i=1}^{m} (X_i^- - \bar{X}^-)^2 + \sum_{j=1}^{n} (Y_j^- - \bar{Y}^-)^2 \right) \Big/ (m+n-2) \right) \left(\frac{1}{m} + \frac{1}{n} \right) \right]^{1/2} \, .$$

In terms of these symbols, a pair of confidence bounds for $\phi_T - \phi_R$ of the same one-sided level $1 - \alpha$ reads

$$(1/2) \cdot (\bar{X}^- - \bar{Y}^- \mp \tilde{S}^- \, t_{N-2;\,1-\alpha}) \qquad (9.9)$$

with $N = m + n$ and $t_{N-2;\,1-\alpha}$ denoting the $(1 - \alpha)$-quantile of a central t-distribution with $N - 2$ degrees of freedom. Correspondingly, the level-α interval inclusion test of (9.4) is given by the decision rule:

Reject average bioinequivalence if and only if it turns

out that $|\bar{X}^- - \bar{Y}^-| < 2\delta_\circ - \tilde{S}^- \, t_{N-2;\,1-\alpha}$. $\qquad (9.10)$

Except for relying on confidence bounds of one-sided level $1 - \alpha$ rather than $1 - \alpha/2$, this solution to the problem of average BE assessment has been proposed as early as in the seminal paper of Westlake (1972). Although the underlying criterion for the equivalence of two normal distributions with the same variance can be criticized for missing a crucial point (as will be explained in § 9.2.2), the method is still strongly recommended in the guidelines as a standard procedure. One of the undisputed advantages of the decision rule (9.10) is computational simplicity. Unfortunately, this advantage is more or less cancelled out by the fact that exact power computations are rather complicated requiring numerical integration even if the null alternative $\phi_T = \phi_R$ is selected. The power of the interval inclusion test (9.10) for average BE against an arbitrary specific alternative $|\phi_T - \phi_R| = \delta < \delta_\circ$ can easily be shown to admit the representation

$POW_{\delta_\circ}(\delta, \sigma) =$

$$\int_0^{v(\delta_\circ/\sigma;\, m,n,\alpha)} \left[\Phi\left(\sqrt{\frac{mn}{N}}\, 2(\delta_\circ - \delta)/\sigma - vt_\alpha^* \right) - \Phi\left(-\sqrt{\frac{mn}{N}} \cdot \right. \right.$$

$$\left. \left. 2(\delta_\circ + \delta)/\sigma + vt_\alpha^* \right) \right] \sqrt{N-2}\; g_{N-2}\left(\sqrt{N-2}\,v\right) dv\,, \quad (9.11)$$

where

$$t_\alpha^* = t_{N-2;\,1-\alpha}, \quad v(\delta_\circ/\sigma; m, n, \alpha) = \sqrt{mn/N}\, 2(\delta_\circ/\sigma)/t_\alpha^*\,, \qquad (9.12)$$

and $g_{N-2}(\cdot)$ stands for the density function of a so-called χ-distribution with $N - 2$ degrees of freedom. By the usual definition (cf. Johnson, Kotz and Balakrishnan, 1994, p. 417), the latter is explicitly given as

$$g_{N-2}(u) = 2^{2-N/2}\, e^{-u^2/2} \cdot u^{N-3}/\Gamma\left(N/2 - 1\right), \quad u > 0\,. \qquad (9.13)$$

Numerical evaluation of the integral (9.11) can be carried out by means of the same technique recommended earlier [see § 3.2] for exact computation of marginal posterior probabilities for equivalence ranges. An *SAS* macro which enables its user to determine the power of the interval inclusion test

(9.10) with higher accuracy than required for virtually all practical applications can be found at http://www.zi-mannheim.de/wktsheq/pow_abe. The program allows for arbitrary specifications of the nominal significance level α, the sample sizes m, n in both sequence groups, and the parameters $\delta \in \mathbb{R}_+ \cup \{0\}$, $\sigma \in \mathbb{R}_+$. Since δ can in particular be chosen as any point in $[\delta_0, \infty)$, the procedure can also be used for studying the exact size of the test (9.10).

Example 9.1

We illustrate the standard procedure of testing for average BE by applying it to the areas under the serum-concentration curves from time 0 to the last time with measurable concentration obtained in a bioequivalence study whose results have been available at the FDA web-site since December 1997, on a file named gen10.txt. Although the original trial aimed primarily at detecting a possible gender-by-treatment interaction, the data are analyzed here as in a conventional comparative bioavailability study. Table 9.1 displays the log-AUC's observed in each subject during both periods, together with the inter-period differences.

Computing the empirical means and variances with the entries in the bottom lines of the two parts of the above table gives:

$$\bar{X}^- = -0.06058; \quad S^2_{X^-} = .0277288;$$
$$\bar{Y}^- = -0.04515; \quad S^2_{Y^-} = .0336990.$$

Using these values of the sample variances, the pooled estimate of the standard error of $\bar{X}^- - \bar{Y}^-$ is obtained as

$$\tilde{S}^- = \left[(11 \cdot .0277288 + 12 \cdot .0336990)/23\right]^{1/2} \cdot [1/12 + 1/13]^{1/2}$$
$$= .070306.$$

Since the 95th percentile of the central t-distribution with $N - 2 = 23$ degrees of freedom is $t_{23;\,.95} = 1.713872$, the critical upper bound to $|\bar{X}^- - \bar{Y}^-|$ to be used in the interval inclusion test for average BE at level $\alpha = 5\%$ is computed to be:

$$2\log(5/4) - .070306 \cdot 1.713872 = .102648.$$

With the observed values of the sample means, we have $|\bar{X}^- - \bar{Y}^-| = .015430$, so that applying rejection rule (9.10) leads to a decision in favour of average BE.

Taking the observed value of $\tilde{S}^-/\sqrt{1/m + 1/n}$ for the true value of the population standard deviation σ of the difference between single within-subject differences gives $\sigma = .175624$, and under this assumption, the exact power of the test against $\delta = \delta_0/2$ and $\delta = 0$ turns out (running program pow_abe) to be .92415 and .99993, respectively. If the true value of σ is assumed to be twice as large, i.e., .351249, these power values drop to .45679 and .84831, respectively.

Table 9.1 *Logarithmically transformed AUC-values and inter-period differences computed from the FDA (1997) sample bioequivalence data set gen10*

Sequence Group T/R

i	1	2	3	4	5	6	7	8
X_{1i}	4.639	4.093	4.222	4.549	4.241	4.279	4.309	4.436
X_{2i}	4.501	4.353	4.353	4.580	4.064	4.618	4.380	4.565
X_i^-	0.138	-0.260	-0.131	-0.031	0.177	-0.339	-0.071	-0.129

	9	10	11	12
	4.572	4.546	3.882	4.561
	4.492	4.577	4.121	4.452
	0.080	-0.031	-0.239	0.109

Sequence Group R/T

j	1	2	3	4	5	6	7	8
Y_{1j}	4.746	4.521	4.009	4.818	4.040	4.099	4.140	4.369
Y_{2j}	4.560	4.486	3.953	5.001	4.114	4.511	3.816	4.363
Y_j^-	0.186	0.035	0.056	-0.183	-0.074	-0.412	0.324	0.006

	9	10	11	12	13
	4.445	4.714	4.018	4.145	4.449
	4.598	4.831	4.199	4.129	4.539
	-0.153	-0.117	-0.181	0.016	-0.090

Modifications and extensions

The interval inclusion test (9.10) has been considered by many authors from very different perspectives. Mandallaz and Mau (1981) showed that it admits a representation as a Bayesian testing procedure with respect to an noninformative reference prior for (μ^-, ν^-, σ), and Schuirmann (1987) pointed out its equivalence with a "combination" of two one-sided t-tests with shifted common boundary of the hypotheses [see also §3.1]. From a mathematical point of view, it is perhaps its most striking property (becoming immediately obvious from (9.11), (9.12)) that, given any value of the (absolute) difference $\delta = \phi_T - \phi_R$ between the true formulation effects, its rejection probability converges to zero as $\sigma \to \infty$, implying that there are specific alternatives against which the power is much smaller than the significance level α.

Various attempts have been made to reduce or even totally eliminate this lack of unbiasedness of the standard procedure of testing for average BE. Anderson and Hauck (1983) proposed to use the rejection region

$$\left\{ F_{N-2}^T((|\bar{D}^-| - 2\delta_\circ)/\tilde{S}^-) - F_{N-2}^T((-|\bar{D}^-| - 2\delta_\circ)/\tilde{S}^-) < \alpha \right\}, \quad (9.14)$$

where $F_{N-2}^T(\cdot)$ denotes the cdf of a central t-distribution with $N-2$ degrees of freedom and $\bar{D}^- \equiv \bar{X}^- - \bar{Y}^-$. The level and power properties of (9.14) were extensively studied by Frick (1987) and Müller-Cohrs (1988) using numerical methods. First of all, the results obtained from these investigations show that the modification suggested by Anderson and Hauck leads to an anticonservative solution of the problem of testing for average BE which is not surprising. In fact, the function $F_{N-2}^T(\cdot)$ is positive everywhere on $\mathbb{R}$ so that (9.14) is a proper superset of $\left\{ F_{N-2}^T((|\bar{D}^-| - 2\delta_\circ)/\tilde{S}^-) < \alpha \right\} = \left\{ (|\bar{D}^-| - 2\delta_\circ)/\tilde{S}^- < (F_{N-2}^T)^{-1}(\alpha) \right\} = \left\{ |\bar{D}^-| < 2\delta_\circ + \tilde{S}^- t_{N-2;\,\alpha} \right\} = \left\{ |\bar{D}^-| < 2\delta_\circ - \tilde{S}^- t_{N-2;\,1-\alpha} \right\}$ and thus of the critical region of the interval inclusion test which is well known to have exact size α. Aligning both tests with respect to size, the Anderson-Hauck procedure has better power against alternatives it detects with probability 60% at most. However, it still fails to be unbiased, but the bias is not as extreme as that of the interval inclusion test: For fixed $\delta \in [0, \delta_\circ)$, the power of the Anderson-Hauck test against the alternative (δ, σ) converges to the nominal level rather than zero, as $\sigma \to \infty$. Munk (1993) proposed a "mixture" of both tests defined by the rule that (9.10) has to be used for values of $\tilde{S}^-$ falling short of some cut-off value k^* (depending on the target significance level α and the number $N-2$ of degrees of freedom), and (9.14) with corrected nominal level $\alpha^* < \alpha$ for $\tilde{S}^- > k^*$.

Finally, the testing problem (9.4) admits also of constructing a critical region which is strictly unbiased. This has been shown by Brown, Hwang and Munk (1997) adapting Hodges and Lehmann's (1954) approach to deriving an unbiased test for the dual problem to be written $H' : |\phi_T - \phi_R| \leq \delta_o$ vs. $K' : |\phi_T - \phi_R| > \delta_o$ in the present context. Unfortunately, the form of the unbiased critical region exhibits still more counterintuitive features than that of Anderson and Hauck's test. In fact, as a function of the realized value $\tilde{s}^-$ of $\tilde{S}^-$, the width of its horizontal sections is not only nonmonotonic, but even jagged. Like (9.14), the unbiased critical region contains a large subregion of points in the $(\bar{d}^-, \tilde{s}^-)$-plane whose distance from the vertical axis is larger than the theoretical equivalence limit to the target parameter $2|\delta|$ (see Figure 9.2), notwithstanding the fact that $\bar{D}^-$ is the natural estimator of 2δ. Since the gain in power which can be achieved when using such curiously shaped critical regions instead of the triangular region corresponding to (9.10) seems not really relevant from a practical point of view, it is not surprising that neither of the modifications to the interval inclusion test mentioned above made its way in the routine of BE assessment.

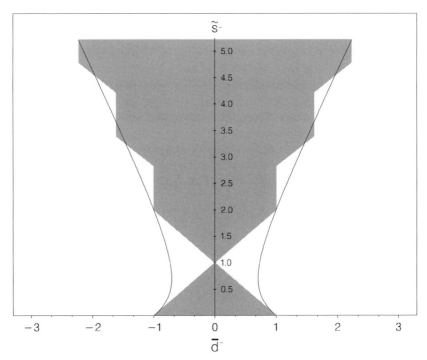

Figure 9.2 *Critical region of the interval inclusion test (lower triangular part of shaded region), the level-corrected Anderson-Hauck test (——) and the unbiased test (shaded region as a whole) for (9.4) with $2\delta_o$ replaced by unity and $N - 2 = 1$. [Exact size of all three regions: $\alpha = .25$.] (Redrawn from Brown, Hwang and Munk, 1997, with kind permission by the International Mathematical Institute.)*

As pointed out by Hauschke, Steinijans and Hothorn (1996), the problem of testing for average BE on the basis of the inter-period (log-)differences X_i^- and Y_j^- differs fundamentally from an ordinary two-sample t-test setting with regard to the possibility of justifying the assumption of homoskedasticity. In fact, in the vast majority of real applications, it is reasonable to suppose that the within-subject variability, if different from period to period at all, depends only on treatment as such and not on treatment order, which implies by (9.7) that we have $Var(X_i^-) = Var(Y_j^-)$ even for grossly different treatment-specific variances σ_{eT}^2 and σ_{eR}^2. If one thinks it necessary to allow for heteroskedasticity of both distributions under comparison anyway, then it suggests itself to apply to (9.10) and (9.14) the same modifications which lead from the classical to a heteroskedasticity-corrected two-sample t-test. Adopting Welch's (1938) approximate solution to the ordinary Behrens-Fisher problem, this means that we have to replace $\tilde{S}^-$ and $F_{N-2}^T(\cdot)$ with $\tilde{S}_*^- \equiv \left[\frac{1}{m}S_{X^-}^2 + \frac{1}{n}S_{Y^-}^2\right]^{1/2}$ and $F_{\hat{\nu}}^T(\cdot)$, respectively, where $S_{X^-}^2, S_{Y^-}^2$ denote the two sample variances, and $\hat{\nu}$ stands for the corrected (random) number of degrees of freedom to be determined from

$$\frac{1}{\hat{\nu}} = \left(\frac{S_{X^-}^2}{S_{X^-}^2 + (m/n)S_{Y^-}^2}\right)^2 \frac{1}{m-1} + \left(\frac{(m/n)S_{Y^-}^2}{S_{X^-}^2 + (m/n)S_{Y^-}^2}\right)^2 \cdot \frac{1}{n-1}.$$

The resulting modification of the critical region proposed by Anderson and Hauck has been studied by Dannenberg, Dette and Munk (1994) with respect to size and power. The simulation results obtained by these authors show in particular that the Welch-corrected Anderson-Hauck test exhibits a similar (slight) tendency towards anticonservatism as the original version (9.14) in the homoskedastic case. Of course, the simplest means of reducing or even eliminating this tendency is to apply Welch's correction to the double t-test.

A problem still easier to handle than heteroskedasticity but much more important for real applications, is nonnormality of the distributions of the inter-period differences X_i^-, Y_j^-. Clearly, the classical parametric confidence limits $(\bar{X}^- - \bar{Y}^-) \mp \tilde{S}^- t_{N-2;1-\alpha}$ which the standard test (9.10) for average BE is based upon, can be replaced with any other pair of confidence bounds of one-sided level $1 - \alpha$ each for the shift in location of two continuous distributions of identical shape. As is well known from the nonparametrics literature (see Lehmann, 1975, §2.6), confidence bounds which are fully distribution-free in the two-sample shift model are given by suitable order statistics for the mn-dimensional vector of all differences $X_i^- - Y_j^-$ between observations from different samples. As was already mentioned in §6.2, this distribution-free variant of the interval inclusion rule (9.10) has been recommended for assessment of average BE in several contributions to pharmaceutical and clinical pharmacology journals (among others, see Hauschke, Steinijans and Diletti, 1990; Hauck et al., 1997).

9.2.2 Testing for scaled average bioequivalence

For a correct interpretation of the meaning of a positive result of the standard test for average BE as well as any of its variants, it is indispensable to note the following basic fact: According to the alternative hypothesis to be established in the parametric model, it makes no difference whether some sufficiently small value, say .10, of the difference $E(X_i^-) - E(Y_j^-)$ between the true means of the normal distributions under consideration, goes with a common (theoretical) standard deviation σ of .001 or 1000. Presumably, not many statisticians will disagree with the conclusion we came to in our general discussion $[\rightarrow \S 1.4]$ of sensible and less reasonable parametrizations of equivalence testing problems, that this conception of similarity between normal distributions is hardly tenable. If one tries to trace back the literature on statistical methods of assessing what is nowadays called average BE, one finds that except for notational variations, hypotheses formulation (9.4) was taken as definitively given already in the earliest pertinent contributions. So there is strong indication that it was not the idea of statisticians to measure the distance between two homoskedastic Gaussian distributions on the basis of the absolute means only. In the early seventies when biostatisticians first started research on methods for analyzing BE studies (Westlake, 1972; Metzler, 1974), questioning the adequacy of that measure would have amounted to challenging a well-established tradition within the pharmaceutical sciences including clinical pharmacology.

Reformulating the problem of testing for average BE as

$$\tilde{H} : 2|\phi_T - \phi_R|/\sigma \geq \varepsilon \text{ versus } \tilde{K} : 2|\phi_T - \phi_R|/\sigma < \varepsilon \qquad (9.15)$$

gives several important advantages over the traditional formulation (9.4). First of all, in view of (9.7) and (9.8), the alternative hypothesis now specifies that the ratio of the shift in location of the two Gaussian distributions under comparison over their common standard deviation be sufficiently small. Thus, the underlying measure of distance is scale-free and accommodates to the obvious fact that two normal distributions with common variance σ^2 and given absolute difference .10 of their expected values are indistinguishable for all practical purposes if $\sigma = 1000$, whereas for $\sigma = .001$, the regions bounded by their density curves are almost perfectly disjoint. Furthermore, the arguments supporting a certain numerical specification of the tolerance ε do not depend on the special context of bioequivalence assessment, and for (9.15) there exists an exact unbiased test satisfying a strong optimality criterion and admitting power calculations in terms of a function which is predefined in advanced statistical packages and can thus be taken as giving explicit expressions. All tools required for carrying out the corresponding alternative test for (scaled) average BE as well as for planning a trial to be analyzed by means of it, have been provided in $\S 6.1$. Thus, except for calculating the actual numerical values of the test statistic and the critical constant, nothing new comes into play if we base the analysis of a standard bioequivalence study like that considered in Example 9.1, on the two-sample t-test for equivalence.

Example 9.1 (continued)

Suppose the entries in the bottom rows of Table 9.1 are the realized values of $N = 12 + 13 = 25$ mutually independent random variables distributed as in (9.6), and we want to perform the UMPI test of §6.1 at level $\alpha = .05$ in order to prove statistically that the underlying normal distributions are equivalent in the sense of satisfying $|\mu_- - \nu_-| = 2|\phi_T - \phi_R| < \varepsilon$ with $\varepsilon = .74$ [← Table 1.1, (v)]. Then, by (6.6), we have to compare the absolute value of the two-sample t-statistic, say T^-, computed from the X_i^- and Y_j^-, to a critical upper bound obtained as

$$\tilde{C}_{.05;12,13}(.74) = \left[F_{1,23;\,.05}\big((12 \cdot 13/25) \cdot .74^2\big) \right]^{1/2}$$

$$= \left[\texttt{finv(.05,1,23,3.417024)} \right]^{1/2}$$

$$= \sqrt{.111742} = .334278 \,,$$

using the *SAS* function for quantiles of noncentral F-distributions. On the other hand, we had $\bar{X}^- = -0.06058$, $\bar{Y}^- = -0.04515$ and $\tilde{S}^- = 0.070306$, so that the observed value of the t-statistic is $T^- = -0.015430/0.070306 = -0.219469$. Thus, the data shown in Table 9.1 lead to a positive decision in the test for scaled average bioequivalence as well [at the 5% level, and with equivalence range $(-.74/2, .74/2)$ for $\phi_T - \phi_R$].

Discussion

(i) Generally, there is no reason to expect that assessing scaled average BE will lead to the same qualitative decision as any of the procedures being available for testing of equivalence with respect to the absolute means. In particular, it is not unusual that with a given data set, the test for scaled average BE has to accept inequivalence although raw average BE can be established even by means of the simple interval inclusion rule (9.10). At first sight, one might suspect that this is a contradiction to the asserted optimality of the t-test for equivalence. Actually, this would be true only if for some $\varepsilon > 0$, the null hypothesis of (9.15) implied that of (9.4) which is obviously not the case. By the same reason, power comparisons between tests for average BE in the ordinary sense and scaled average BE are pointless in any case.

(ii) Researchers in the pharmaceutical sciences often base their reservation about applying the scaled criterion of average BE on the argument that the exact value of the population variance σ^2 of the inter-period (log-)differences is unknown to the experimenter. This would be a serious point only if transforming a given equivalence range for the absolute mean difference was the only way of coming to a consensus about what can be considered an adequate numerical specification of the equivalence limit to the standardized difference of means of two normal distributions with the same variance. Actually, as was explained in Chapter 1, nothing prevents from treating $|\mu_- - \nu_-|/\sigma$ as the primary distance measure admitting direct specification of an equivalence limit without taking into consideration any other function of the three unknown parameters μ_-, ν_- and σ^2 involved in the problem. In addition, as is the case with any well-designed study to be eventually analyzed by means of hypotheses testing methods, planning of a BE trial also involves calculation of minimally required sample sizes, and it follows from equation (9.11) that this presupposes knowledge of σ^2 even if the standard test for unscaled average BE shall be used. Long-term experience shows that despite a high variability of the bioavailabilities measured in the individual periods of a BE trial, the standard deviation of the inter-period differences between the bioavailabilities observed in the same subject is typically smaller than the equivalence limit $2\delta_\circ = .4462$ to be specified for $E(X_i^-) - E(Y_j^-)$ according to the guidelines of the regulatory authorities. Accordingly, a positive result of a test for unscaled average BE in the majority of cases ensures at best that the shift in location of the two normal distributions under comparison does not substantially exceed their common standard deviation. Thus, it seems not unfair to state that from a statistical point of view, the condition satisfied by two drug formulations proven bioequivalent with respect unscaled averages is often remarkably weak.

(iii) Another objection which frequently has been raised against the use of $|\mu^- - \nu^-|/\sigma = 2|\phi_T - \phi_R|/\sigma$ as the basic distance measure for assessment of average BE is that an experimenter who deliberately "inflates" the variability of the observed bioavailabilities by careless handling of the measurement procedure, will be "rewarded" by enabling him to meet the criterion of BE even for a comparatively large value of $|\phi_T - \phi_R|$. A good deal of skepticism seems in order about the soundness of this argument as well. First of all, it is not clear how an imagined experimenter who adopts the strategy in mind, can protect himself from increasing the shift in location of the distributions at the same time. Even if he succeeds in this latter respect, one cannot but admit that virtually all inferential procedures are liable to biases induced by manipulation of the conditions under which the primary observations are taken. To put it differently, methods of statistical inference are made for extracting the maximum information from data collected by people who are willing to adhere to the principles of good

scientific practice, rather than for providing protection against fraud
and doctoring of data.

9.3 Individual bioequivalence: criteria and testing procedures

9.3.1 Introduction

The introduction of the concept of individual bioequivalence by Anderson
and Hauck (1990) and Wellek (1990; 1993a) was the beginning of a process
which, although overdue already at that time, is still going on and aims at
emancipating bioequivalence assessment from taking into account only the
first two moments of the distributions of the inter-period (log-) differences
X_i^- and Y_j^-. The idea behind the concept in its original version is simple
enough, and its logical basis is easily grasped even by people exclusively
interested in the pharmacological and clinical issues connected with bioequivalence testing: Even perfect coincidence of $\mu_- = E(X_i^-)$ and $\nu_- =
E(Y_j^-)$ by no means admits the conclusion that the proportion of individ-
uals whose responses to both drug formulations exhibit the pharmacologically desirable degree of similarity, is sufficiently large. But precisely this
has to be guaranteed in order to justify declaring the two formulations of
the drug equivalent in the sense of allowing to switch from one to the other
in the same individual without altering the response to a relevant extent
(cf. Chen, 1997, p. 7).

The question of how this notion can be translated into a statistical hypothesis admits a straightforward answer if we restrict the model for the
2×2 crossover design we have to consider when analyzing a standard BE
trial, by assuming that the period effects also coincide and can thus be
dropped from the expressions for the four cell means. Actually, this additional assumption is not as oversimplistic as it might seem at first sight.
First of all, the proportion of real BE trials leading to a rejection of the null
hypothesis $\pi_1 = \pi_2$ in a suitable test of significance, is extremely low (con-
firming a general statement of Chow and Liu, 1992, p. 49). Moreover, there
is no problem to positively establish approximate equality of both period
effects by means of a preliminary t-test for equivalence of the distribution
of the X_i^- to that of the $-Y_j^-$ with respect to their standardized means.
Thus, for practical purposes, it entails only a minor loss in generality to
assume that through defining

$$Z_i = X_i^- , \; i = 1, \ldots, m; \; Z_{i+j} = -Y_j^- , \; j = 1, \ldots, n \qquad (9.16)$$

and

$$\zeta = \phi_T - \phi_R , \qquad (9.17)$$

$Z_1, \ldots, Z_N$ becomes a single homogeneous sample of size $N = m + n$ with

$$Z_l \sim \mathcal{N}(\zeta, \sigma^2) \; \forall \, l = 1, \ldots, N , \; \zeta \in \mathbb{R}, \, \sigma^2 > 0 . \qquad (9.18)$$

In view of (9.16), (9.5) and the definition of the X_{ki}, Y_{kj} as logarithms of the selected measure of bioavailability, nonexistence of period effects clearly ensures that $|\exp\{Z_l\} - 1|$ measures the dissimilarity of the responses to both drug formulations observed in the same subject making up the lth element of the pooled sample. Now, according to basic standards of clinical pharmacology, we can expect that switching over from one formulation of the drug to the other will not change its potential therapeutic effect induced in the lth individual as long as the intraindividual bioavailability ratio $\exp\{Z_l\}$ remains within the limits set by the $80-125\,\%$ rule. More generally, i.e., without restricting attention to a particular specification of the range considered acceptable for an individual bioavailability ratio, a natural formalization of the basic concept of individual BE is obtained by requiring that

$$P[(1+\varepsilon)^{-1} < \exp\{Z_l\} < (1+\varepsilon)] > \pi^* \tag{9.19}$$

where ε denotes a positive constant determining the tolerance for intraindividual differences in response levels, and π^* stands for the smallest value acceptable for the probability of observing bioequivalent responses in a randomly selected individual. The term "probability-based individual bioequivalence" (abbreviated to PBIBE in the sequel) has been used in the literature since the mid-nineties in order to distinguish (9.19) from an alternative condition proposed by Sheiner (1992) and Schall and Luus (1993) as a criterion of individual BE. This so-called moment-based criterion of individual BE is not discussed here because it presupposes that replicate crossover designs be used (for more details see FDA/CDER, 2001).

In the parametric model given by (9.18), the probability of observing bioequivalent responses at the individual level can obviously be written

$$P[(1+\varepsilon)^{-1} < \exp\{Z_l\} < (1+\varepsilon)] = \pi_\varepsilon(\zeta, \sigma)\,, \tag{9.20}$$

provided we define

$$\pi_\varepsilon(\zeta, \sigma) = \Phi\left(\frac{\log(1+\varepsilon) - \zeta}{\sigma}\right) - \Phi\left(\frac{-\log(1+\varepsilon) - \zeta}{\sigma}\right)\,. \tag{9.21}$$

In §9.3.2, we will treat $P[(1+\varepsilon)^{-1} < \exp\{Z_l\} < (1+\varepsilon)]$ as a functional allowed to depend on the cdf of the Z_l in an arbitrary way. The corresponding distribution-free test for PBIBE is based on a simple counting statistic and can thus be expected to leave a large margin for improvements in power when we assume that the expression on the left-hand side of (9.19) admits the representation (9.21). Although the problem of testing for a sufficiently large value of the parametric function $\pi_\varepsilon(\zeta, \sigma)$ looks fairly simple, a satisfactory solution is difficult to find by means of classical methods. In §9.3.3, a Bayesian construction is proposed instead which can be shown by numerical methods to maintain the ordinary frequentist significance level

without being overly conservative and to yield gains in power of up to 30 %
as compared to the distribution-free procedure.

9.3.2 Distribution-free approach to testing for probability-based individual bioequivalence

If establishing the validity of (9.19) is accepted as a reasonable objective
of bioequivalence assessment, we need a procedure for testing

$$H_\varepsilon^{(1)} : p_\varepsilon \leq \pi^* \quad \text{versus} \quad K_\varepsilon^{(1)} : p_\varepsilon > \pi^* \,, \tag{9.22}$$

where p_ε symbolizes the probability of the event $\{ (1+\varepsilon)^{-1} < \exp\{Z_l\} < (1+\varepsilon) \} = \{ |Z_l| < \log(1+\varepsilon) \}$ under an arbitrary cdf $F_Z(\cdot)$, say, of the
observed individual log-bioavailability ratios. Provided $F_Z(\cdot)$ is continuous,
the (one-sided) testing problem (9.22) admits an easy solution exhibiting
attractive theoretical properties. To see this, let us introduce the statistic

$$N_+ \equiv \#\Big\{ l \in \{1, \ldots, N\} \,\big|\, |Z_l| < \log(1+\varepsilon) \Big\} \tag{9.23}$$

which simply counts the number of subjects in the sample who exhibit
a relative bioavailability lying within the tolerated range. Of course, the
distribution of N_+ is $\mathcal{B}(N, p_\varepsilon)$ [binomial with parameters N, p_ε]. Hence, it
is natural to decide between the hypotheses of (9.22) by carrying out in
terms of N_+ the UMP level-α test of the null hypothesis $p \leq \pi^*$ about the
unknown parameter of a binomial distribution generated by repeating the
same Bernoulli experiment independently N times. Clearly, this leads to
the decision rule

$$\begin{cases} \text{Rejection of } H_\varepsilon^{(1)} & N_+ > k_N^*(\alpha) \\[2mm] \text{Rejection of } H_\varepsilon^{(1)} \text{ with} & \text{if } \quad N_+ = k_N^*(\alpha)\,, \\ \text{probability } \gamma_N^*(\alpha) & \\[2mm] \text{Acceptance of } H_\varepsilon^{(1)} & N_+ < k_N^*(\alpha) \end{cases} \tag{9.24}$$

where the critical constants have to be determined from

$$k_N^*(\alpha) = \min\Big\{ k \in \mathbb{N}_0 \,\Big|\, \sum_{j=k+1}^{N} b(j; N, \pi^*) \leq \alpha \Big\}\,, \tag{9.25}$$

$$\gamma_N^*(\alpha) = \Big(\alpha - \sum_{j=k_N^*(\alpha)+1}^{N} b(j; N, \pi^*) \Big) \Big/ b\big(k_N^*(\alpha); N, \pi^*\big)\,, \tag{9.26}$$

with $b(\,\cdot\,; N, \pi^*)$ as the probability mass function of $\mathcal{B}(N, \pi^*)$. Obviously,
(9.24) is simply a variant of the one-sided sign test which implies in particular that it is completely distribution-free. Since the hypotheses $H_\varepsilon^{(1)}$ and
$K_\varepsilon^{(1)}$ refer to the class of *all* continuous distributions of the individual observations Z_l, mimicking Lehmann's (1986, pp. 106-107) proof of the UMP

property of the ordinary sign test, (9.24) can be shown to be uniformly most powerful among all level-α tests of the nonparametric version of the null hypothesis of individual bio-inequivalence in the probability-based sense.

Under the acronym TIER (for Testing Individual Equivalence Ratios) coined by Anderson and Hauck (1990), the conservative, nonrandomized version of the procedure (9.24) gained some popularity for a time. Clearly, its most conspicuous practical advantage is extreme simplicity. In fact, neither for determining the critical constants nor the exact power against some specific alternative $p_\varepsilon \in (\pi^*, 1)$, other computational devices than an extensive table or a program for the binomial distribution function are required. Therefore, presentation of an extra example illustrating the practical use of the method is dispensable here.

With regard to its conceptual basis, the simple criterion (9.19) of PBIBE has rightly been criticized by several authors for potentially using a lower bound to the probability of observing equivalent bioavailabilities in a randomly selected subject which may be unattainable even in a study comparing the reference formulation to itself. A reasonable way around this potential difficulty recommended in the literature (see Schall, 1995, (2.3)) consists of replacing π^* by a bound scaled by relating it to a reliable estimate of the probability of finding the condition $|Z_l| < \log(1+\varepsilon)$ satisfied in a pseudo-trial of two identical drug products. In the parametric submodel (9.18), this probability is clearly given by $\pi_\varepsilon(0, \sigma) = 2\,\Phi(\log(1 + \varepsilon)/\sigma) - 1$ so that it seems natural to scale the bound π^* of (9.19) by replacing it with the number

$$\pi_{sc}^* \equiv \pi^* \cdot \left(2\,\Phi(\log(1 + \varepsilon)/\sigma^*) - 1\right), \qquad (9.27)$$

where σ^* denotes some realistic value of the population standard deviation σ of log-bioavailability ratios measured for the drug product under investigation. In contrast to the basic measurements taken in the individual period of a BE trial, σ^2 does not depend on the between-subject variance component σ_S^2 [recall (8.29)] but reflects the technical and analytical precision of the measurement process as such. Thus, σ^2 is a substance-specific rather than biological constant, and a comparatively stable estimate might be obtained by pooling the point estimates over a variety of trials of the same or chemically related agents. Experience shows that in a BE trial performed in strict adherence to the established technical standards, the observed standard deviation of the Z_l often remains below $.20$. Using this as σ^* and $.75$ as the unscaled bound to $P[|Z_l| < \log(1 + \varepsilon)]$ yields for $\varepsilon = .25$:

$$\pi_{sc}^* = .75 \cdot \left(2\,\Phi(.2231/.2000) - 1\right) = .75 \cdot .7353 \approx .55\,.$$

A more sophisticated approach to scaling the criterion of PBIBE is available in the Bayesian framework developed in the next subsection.

9.3.3 An improved parametric test for probability-based individual bioequivalence

In this subsection, we consider the parametric version of the problem of testing for PBIBE which arises from replacing in (9.22) the functional p_ε with $\pi_\varepsilon(\zeta, \sigma)$ as defined in (9.21). In other words, we now put forward the problem of testing

$$\tilde{H}_\varepsilon^{(1)} : \pi_\varepsilon(\zeta, \sigma) \leq \pi^* \quad \text{versus} \quad \tilde{K}_\varepsilon^{(1)} : \pi_\varepsilon(\zeta, \sigma) > \pi^* \qquad (9.28)$$

by means of a sample $Z_1, \ldots, Z_N$ of independent observations from $\mathcal{N}(\zeta, \sigma^2)$.

Our construction of a Bayesian test for (9.28) will be based on the usual (see Box and Tiao, 1973, p. 92) reference prior for the expectation ζ and the standard deviation σ of the underlying Gaussian distribution. This means that a priori we treat the true value of the population parameter (ζ, σ) as the realization of a random variable $(\boldsymbol{\zeta}, \boldsymbol{\sigma})$, say, inducing an improper probability distribution defined by the following density with respect to Lebesgue measure on $\mathbb{R}^2$:

$$\varrho(\zeta, \sigma) = \begin{cases} \sigma^{-1} & -\infty < \zeta < \infty, \ \sigma > 0 \\ & \text{for} \\ 0 & -\infty < \zeta < \infty, \ \sigma \leq 0 \end{cases} . \qquad (9.29)$$

The corresponding posterior density of $(\boldsymbol{\zeta}, \boldsymbol{\sigma})$ given the realized values $(\bar{z}, s)$ of the sufficient statistics $\bar{Z} = \sum_{i=1}^N Z_i/N$, $S = \left[(N-1)^{-1} \sum_{i=1}^N (Z_i - \bar{Z})^2\right]^{1/2}$, is well known (cf. Box and Tiao, loc. cit., pp. 93-6) to be given as

$$\varrho_{(\bar{z}, s)}(\zeta, \sigma) = \\ \left(\sqrt{N}/\sigma\right) \varphi\left(\sqrt{N}(\zeta - \bar{z})/\sigma\right) \sqrt{N-1}\,(s/\sigma^2)\,g_{N-1}\left(\sqrt{N-1}\,s/\sigma\right) \quad (9.30)$$

where $\varphi(\cdot)$ denotes the standard normal density and $g_{N-1}(\cdot)$ the density of a χ-distribution with $N-1$ degrees of freedom $[\to (9.13)$ with N augmented by 1].

Now, an algorithm for computing the posterior probability of the (alternative) hypothesis of (9.28) is obtained by exploiting the following basic facts:

(i) For arbitrarily fixed $\sigma > 0$, the set of values of ζ satisfying $\tilde{K}_\varepsilon^{(1)}$ admits the representation

$$\{\zeta \in \mathbb{R} \mid \pi_\varepsilon(\zeta, \sigma) > \pi^*\} = \left(-\sigma\,q(\tilde{\varepsilon}/\sigma, \pi^*), \ \sigma\,q(\tilde{\varepsilon}/\sigma, \pi^*)\right), \qquad (9.31)$$

where $\tilde{\varepsilon} = \log(1 + \varepsilon)$ and $q(\tilde{\varepsilon}/\sigma, \pi^*)$ has to be determined by solving the equation

$$\Phi(\tilde{\varepsilon}/\sigma - \psi) - \Phi(-\tilde{\varepsilon}/\sigma - \psi) = \pi^*, \quad \psi > 0. \qquad (9.32)$$

(ii) The solution of (9.32) exists and is uniquely determined for all σ falling below an upper bound σ_ε^*, say, defined by

$$\sigma_\varepsilon^* = \tilde{\varepsilon}/\Phi^{-1}((1 + \pi^*)/2). \tag{9.33}$$

[In view of Theorem A.1.5 (iii), this follows immediately from the fact that the left-hand side of (9.32) coincides with the power function of a test with critical region $\{-\tilde{\varepsilon}/\sigma < U < \tilde{\varepsilon}/\sigma\}$, where $U \sim \mathcal{N}(\psi, 1)$.]

(iii) Combining (i) and (ii) with (9.30) shows that the posterior probability of the alternative hypothesis $\{\pi_\varepsilon(\zeta, \sigma) > \pi^*\}$ of (9.28) can be written as

$$
P_{(\bar{z},s)}\Big[\pi_\varepsilon(\zeta, \sigma) > \pi^*\Big] = \int_0^{\sigma_\varepsilon^*} \bigg(\Big[\Phi\big(\sqrt{N}\,(q(\tilde{\varepsilon}/\sigma, \pi^*) - \\
\bar{z}/\sigma)\big) - \Phi\big(\sqrt{N}\,(-q(\tilde{\varepsilon}/\sigma, \pi^*) - \bar{z}/\sigma)\big)\Big] \cdot \\
\sqrt{N-1}\,(s/\sigma^2)g_{N-1}\big(\sqrt{N-1}\,s/\sigma\big) \bigg) d\sigma. \tag{9.34}
$$

The integral on the right-hand side of (9.34) can be evaluated with very high numerical accuracy by means of Gauss-Legendre quadrature. Since computation of individual values of the function $\sigma \mapsto q(\tilde{\varepsilon}/\sigma, \pi^*)$ on the basis of (9.32) is very fast and the cumulative standard normal distribution function $\Phi(\cdot)$ is predefined in any programming environment to be taken into consideration for the present purpose, the degree of the polynomial determining the abscissas can once more be chosen as large as 96.

A *SAS* implementation of the algorithm described above for the computation of the posterior probability of $\tilde{K}_\varepsilon^{(1)}$ given an arbitrary realization $(\bar{z}, s)$ of the sufficient statistic $(\bar{Z}, S)$, can be found at http://www.zi-mannheim.de/wktsheq under the program name po_pbibe. Using this computational tool, it is no problem to perform the Bayesian test with respect to the reference prior (9.29). For definiteness, its rejection region reads

$$\Big\{(\bar{z}, s) \in \mathbb{R} \times \mathbb{R}_+ \,\Big|\, P_{(\bar{z},s)}\Big[\pi_\varepsilon(\zeta, \sigma) > \pi^*\Big] > 1 - \alpha\Big\}. \tag{9.35}$$

For the specific case $\alpha = .05$, $\varepsilon = .25$, $\pi^* = .75$, and sample size $N = 20$, the corresponding set in the sample space of $(\bar{Z}, S)$ is displayed as the filled portion of the graph shown in Figure 9.3. Roughly speaking, it looks like a vertically compressed image of the region bounded by the upper solid curve which is the geometric representation of the alternative hypothesis under consideration. Since $(\bar{z}, s)$ is the observed value of the natural estimator for (ζ, σ), it is clear that no test which is valid with respect to the significance level, can have a rejection region being larger than the subset of the parameter space specified by the alternative hypothesis one wishes to establish. Hence, the form of the Bayesian rejection region seems very reasonable.

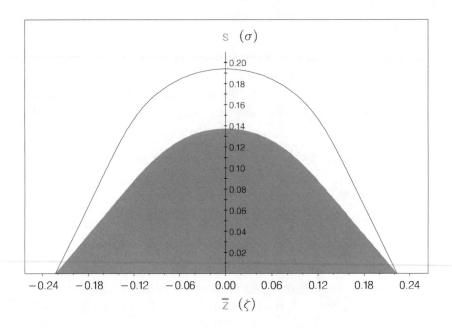

Figure 9.3 *Rejection region of the Bayesian test at (nominal) level* $\alpha = .05$ *for PBIBE, for* $\varepsilon = .25$, $\pi^* = .75$ *and* $N = 20$. *[Upper solid line: Boundary of the parameter subspace specified by the alternative hypothesis.] (From Wellek, 2000a, with kind permission by Wiley-VCH.)*

Numerical study of size and power of the Bayesian critical region

The following result (rigorously proven in Wellek, 2000a) forms the basis of an algorithm for computing exact rejection probabilities of the Bayesian test with rejection region (9.35).

(a) For any fixed point s_o in the sample space of the statistic S, there exists a nonnegative real number denoted $\bar{z}^*_{\alpha\varepsilon}(s_o)$ in the sequel, such that

$$\left\{ \bar{z} \in \mathbb{R} \,\middle|\, P_{(\bar{z}, s_o)}\!\left[\pi_\varepsilon(\zeta, \sigma) > \pi^*\right] > 1 - \alpha \right\} =$$
$$\left(- \bar{z}^*_{\alpha,\varepsilon}(s_o),\, \bar{z}^*_{\alpha\varepsilon}(s_o) \right) . \qquad (9.36)$$

Thus, all horizontal sections of the rejection region (9.35) are symmetric intervals on the real line.

(b) The number $\bar{z}^*_{\alpha\varepsilon}(s_\circ)$ is either zero [so that the corresponding section of (9.35) is empty], or it is uniquely determined by the equation

$$P_{(\bar{z},s_\circ)}\Big[\pi_\varepsilon(\boldsymbol{\zeta},\boldsymbol{\sigma}) > \pi^*\Big] = 1 - \alpha, \quad \bar{z} \in \mathbb{R}_+. \tag{9.37}$$

(c) There exists a positive real number $s^*_{\alpha,\varepsilon}$ [depending, like $\bar{z}^*_{\alpha\varepsilon}(s_\circ)$, not only on α and ε, but also on N and π^*] such that we have

$$\big\{s \in \mathbb{R}_+ | \bar{z}^*_{\alpha,\varepsilon}(s) > 0\big\} = \big[0, s^*_{\alpha,\varepsilon}\big). \tag{9.38}$$

Let now $\beta^*_{\alpha,\varepsilon}(\zeta,\sigma)$ denote the rejection probability of the Bayesian test under any parameter constellation $(\zeta,\sigma) \in \mathbb{R} \times \mathbb{R}_+$. In view of the independence of the two components of the sufficient statistic $(\bar{Z}, S)$, applying (a) – (c) yields the following integral representation of $\beta^*_{\alpha,\varepsilon}(\zeta,\sigma)$:

$$\beta^*_{\alpha,\varepsilon}(\zeta,\sigma) = \int_0^{s^*_{\alpha,\varepsilon}} \Big[\Phi\Big(\sqrt{N}\,(\bar{z}^*_\alpha(s) - \zeta)/\sigma\Big) -$$
$$\Phi\Big(\sqrt{N}\,(-\bar{z}^*_\alpha(s) - \zeta)/\sigma\Big)\Big]\,(\sqrt{N-1}\,/\sigma)\,g_{N-1}(s\,\sqrt{N-1}/\sigma)\,ds \tag{9.39}$$

where $g_{N-1}(\cdot)$ again stands for the density function of the square root of a variable following a central χ^2-distribution with $N-1$ degrees of freedom. The formal structure of the integrand appearing on the right-hand side of this equation is similar to that of the function to be integrated in order to compute the posterior probability of the alternative hypothesis of (9.28) by means of (9.34). Hence, in evaluating (9.39), 96 point Gauss-Legendre integration works as well as it does in computing the posterior probability of $\tilde{K}^{(1)}_\varepsilon$ given an arbitrary realization of $(\bar{Z}, S)$.

Table 9.2 shows the results of applying formula (9.39) to various parameter constellations (ζ,σ) lying on the common boundary of the hypotheses (9.28) for $\varepsilon = .25, \pi^* = .75$, the nominal significance level $\alpha = .05$, and three different sample sizes whose order of magnitude ranges from "small" $(N = 20)$ through "moderate" $(N = 50)$ to "large" $(N = 100)$. For true standard deviations σ being smaller than or equal to .10, the differences between $\beta^*_{\alpha,\varepsilon}(\zeta,\sigma)$ and the nominal α are clearly negligible, and even for the largest values of σ to be taken into consideration for purposes of assessing the level properties of the Bayesian test, the differences nowhere go in the wrong, e.g., anticonservative direction.

Table 9.2 *Exact rejection probabilities of the Bayesian test for PBIBE on the common boundary of the hypotheses* $[\alpha = .05, \quad \pi^* = .75, \quad \varepsilon = .25 \ (\leftrightarrow \tilde{\varepsilon} = .2231)]$ *(From Wellek, 2000a, with kind permission by Wiley-VCH)*

ζ	σ	N	$\beta^*_{\alpha,\varepsilon}(\zeta,\sigma)$
.2164	.01	20	.050 000
.2164	.01	50	.050 009
.2164	.01	100	.049 758
.1894	.05	20	.050 000
.1894	.05	50	.050 000
.1894	.05	100	.050 000
.1557	.10	20	.048 438
.1557	.10	50	.049 401
.1557	.10	100	.049 659
.1163	.15	20	.035 674
.1163	.15	50	.040 441
.1163	.15	100	.043 053
.0709	.18	20	.028 230
.0709	.18	50	.034 270
.0709	.18	100	.038 209

Of course, (9.39) allows also numerically exact computation of the power of the Bayesian test against arbitrary specific alternatives $(\zeta,\sigma) \in \tilde{K}^{(1)}_\varepsilon$. Since computing the rejection probabilities of the distribution-free procedure of testing for PBIBE under arbitrary values of $p_\varepsilon \in (0,1]$ is an elementary matter, we are able to systematically assess the gain in efficiency achievable from using the Bayesian test based on (9.35) instead of the so-called TIER procedure (9.24). Although the randomized version of the latter is of theoretical interest only, Table 9.3 compares the rejection probabilities of both the nonrandomized and the optimal version with that of the Bayesian test for all specific alternatives selected. Otherwise, we would not be in a position to discriminate true gains in power achieved by using the parametric test, from "spurious" improvements vanishing if the conventional 5% level is replaced with a level "natural" for the counting statistic $N_\varepsilon = \# \left\{ l \in \{1,\ldots N\} \,\middle|\, |Z_l| < \log(1+\varepsilon) \right\}$.

Table 9.3 *Exact rejection probabilities of the Bayesian test and both versions of TIER against various specific alternatives, for the case $\alpha = .05$, $\pi^* = .75$, and $\varepsilon = .25$ (From Wellek, 2000a, with kind permission by Wiley-VCH)*

ζ	σ	$\pi_\varepsilon(\zeta,\sigma)$	N	Bayes	TIER nonrandom.	TIER random.
.16423	.07	.80	20	.14423	.06918	.12171
.16423	.07	.80	50	.25380	.19041	.20238
.16423	.07	.80	100	.41369	.27119	.31550
.12127	.12	.80	20	.12532	.06918	.12171
.12127	.12	.80	50	.23833	.19041	.20238
.12127	.12	.80	100	.40096	.27119	.31550
.03745	.17	.80	20	.08508	.06918	.12171
.03745	.17	.80	50	.19513	.19041	.20238
.03745	.17	.80	100	.36831	.27119	.31550
.17132	.05	.85	20	.34955	.17556	.26355
.17132	.05	.85	50	.68261	.51875	.53404
.17132	.05	.85	100	.92453	.76328	.79930
.11937	.10	.85	20	.33178	.17556	.26355
.11937	.10	.85	50	.67423	.51875	.53404
.11937	.10	.85	100	.92231	.76328	.79930
.03891	.15	.85	20	.23753	.17556	.26355
.03891	.15	.85	50	.61062	.51875	.53404
.03891	.15	.85	100	.91057	.76328	.79930
.15907	.05	.90	20	.67436	.39175	.50117
.15907	.05	.90	50	.97097	.87785	.88444
.15907	.05	.90	100	.99977	.98999	.99264
.09456	.10	.90	20	.63842	.39175	.50117
.09456	.10	.90	50	.96741	.87785	.88444
.09456	.10	.90	100	.99974	.98999	.99264
.01338	.135	.90	20	.52538	.39175	.50117
.01338	.135	.90	50	.95347	.87785	.88444
.01338	.135	.90	100	.99970	.98999	.99264

Overall the results displayed in Table 9.3 admit the following conclusions:

- The Bayesian test dominates the nonrandomized TIER uniformly on the selected grid of points in $\tilde{K}_\varepsilon^{(1)}$. In many cases, the difference between the two power functions has an order of magnitude making further comments on the practical relevance of the improvement dispensable.

- Even as compared to the randomized version of TIER, the Bayesian test comes out as clearly superior because for the few constellations with a negative sign of the difference, the distance between the power functions is practically negligible.

Generalizations

1. Scaling of the criterion of PBIBE. The Bayesian framework admits the possibility of letting the factor to be used for scaling the bound π^* to the probability of obtaining a bioequivalent individual response, depend on the actual value of the standard deviation σ of the log-bioavailability ratios Z_l. As explained on p. 223, the natural candidate for a function of σ whose values give suitable weight factors to π^*, is $\sigma \to \pi_\varepsilon(0, \sigma)$, so that we propose to modify the condition $\pi_\varepsilon(\zeta, \sigma) > \pi^*$ for PBIBE by requiring that $\pi_\varepsilon(\zeta, \sigma) > \pi^* \cdot \pi_\varepsilon(0, \sigma)$. This leads to replacing (9.28) with

$$\tilde{\tilde{H}}_\varepsilon^{(1)} : \frac{\pi_\varepsilon(\zeta, \sigma)}{\pi_\varepsilon(0, \sigma)} \leq \pi^* \quad \text{versus} \quad \tilde{\tilde{K}}_\varepsilon^{(1)} : \frac{\pi_\varepsilon(\zeta, \sigma)}{\pi_\varepsilon(0, \sigma)} > \pi^* . \tag{9.40}$$

As shown in the graphical representation of Figure 9.4, incorporation of that kind of scaling induces a radical change to the shape of the equivalence region specified by the alternative hypothesis to be established by means of the data. In contrast to $\tilde{K}_\varepsilon^{(1)}$ of (9.28) [$\to$ outer contour plotted in Fig. 9.3], $\tilde{\tilde{K}}_\varepsilon^{(1)}$ corresponds to a region in the (ζ, σ)-plane being unbounded in upward direction such that the width of the horizontal sections increases to infinity as $\sigma \to \infty$. This implies in particular, that for whatever large a shift in the mean away from zero, scaled PBIBE in the sense of (9.40) is satisfied for any sufficiently extreme degree of variability. If the latter property is considered undesirable, it might make sense to combine the Bayesian test for $\tilde{\tilde{K}}_\varepsilon^{(1)}$ whose rejection region is shown in Figure 9.4 as well [again for $\alpha = .05$, $\varepsilon = .25$, $N = 20$, and a lower bound to the target parametric function of .75], with a test for reasonably low variability, as described in the following subsection in connection with a disaggregate test for population bioequivalence.

2. Accommodating nonnegligible period effects. If the period effects cannot be neglected (which is, as mentioned earlier, quite exceptional in bioequivalence trials), the difference (9.17) between the direct formulation effects can be written $\zeta = \zeta_1 - \zeta_2$ where ζ_1 and ζ_2 denote the expectations of two normal distributions with common (unknown) variance σ_*^2 from which independent samples $Z_1^{[1]}, \ldots, Z_m^{[1]}$ and $Z_1^{[2]}, \ldots, Z_n^{[2]}$ have been taken. Clearly, we have just to put $Z_i^{[1]} = X_i^-/2$, $Z_j^{[2]} = Y_j^-/2$, and observe that the standard deviation σ we are interested in according to (9.21) is now given by $\sigma = 2\sigma_*$.

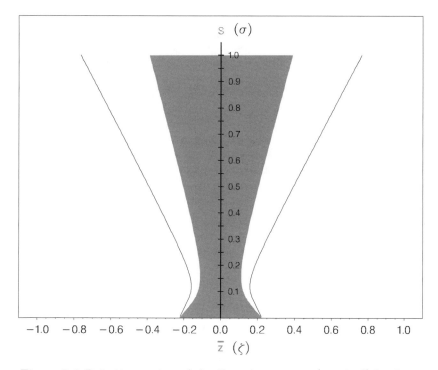

Figure 9.4 *Rejection region of the Bayesian test at (nominal) level* $\alpha =$ *.05 for scaled PBIBE in the sense of (9.40), for* $\varepsilon = .25$, $\pi^* = .75$ *and* $N = 20$. *[Outer solid line: Boundary of the parameter subspace specified by the alternative hypothesis. (From Wellek, 2000a, with kind permission by Wiley-VCH.)]*

Now, the posterior distribution of (ζ, σ_*) given the observed values of $\bar{Z}^{[1]} - \bar{Z}^{[2]}$ and $S_* = \left[(m + n - 2)^{-1} \left(SQ_Z^{[1]} + SQ_Z^{[2]} \right) \right]^{1/2}$ $\left[\text{with } SQ_Z^{[1]} \text{ and } SQ_Z^{[2]} \text{ as the corrected sum of squares for the } Z_i^{[1]} \text{ and the } Z_j^{[2]}, \text{ respectively} \right]$ has the same form as in the paired t-test setting considered in the body of this paper. In fact, as shown in § 2.5.1 of Box and Tiao (1973), the posterior density of (ζ, σ_*) with respect to the reference prior with (improper) density $(\zeta_1, \zeta_2, \sigma_*) \mapsto \sigma_*^{-1}$ on $\mathbb{R}^2 \times \mathbb{R}_+$, is given by:

$$\varrho_{(\hat{\zeta}, s_*)}(\zeta, \sigma_*) = \sqrt{mn/N}\,(1/\sigma_*)\,\varphi\left(\sqrt{mn/N}(\zeta - \hat{\zeta})/\sigma_*\right) \cdot$$
$$\sqrt{N - 2}\,(s_*/\sigma_*^2)\,g_{N-2}\left(\sqrt{N - 2}\,s_*/\sigma_*\right) \qquad (9.41)$$

where $g_{N-2}(\cdot)$ has to be defined as in (9.13). Hence, except for minor modifications, the algorithms described above can also be used for computing posterior probabilities of the alternative hypotheses of (9.28) and (9.40), as well as exact rejection probabilities of the associated Bayesian tests for (scaled) PBIBE with data from bioequivalence trials involving nonnegligible period effects.

Example 9.2

For illustration, we use the data set analyzed by means of a nonparametric procedure for the assessment of scaled average BE in Wellek (1996). It has been obtained from a standard comparative bioavailability study of a generic (T) and the original manufacturer's formulation (R) of the calcium blocking agent nifedipine. As is so often the case in practice of bioequivalence assessment, the total sample size has been rather small $(N = 20)$. The complete listing of the raw data is given in Table 9.4.

Although the primary analysis performed in the reference cited above used an approach allowing for unequal period effects $\pi_1 \neq \pi_2$, the natural estimator $(1/2)(\bar{X}^- + \bar{Y}^-)$ of $\pi_1 - \pi_2$ (see, e.g., Jones and Kenward, 1989, § 2.3) turns out to be rather small [-.0028] as compared to its standard error [.0357]. Hence there seems little harm in assuming that switching from the first period to the second per se does not change the average bioavailability of the active agent under study. This leads to treating the values of $\log(AUC_1/AUC_2)$ from the subjects in sequence group T/R and those of $\log(AUC_2/AUC_1)$ from the subjects randomized to R/T, as a single sample of size $N = 20$ from the same Gaussian distribution $\mathcal{N}(\zeta, \sigma^2)$. The values of the sufficient statistics are readily computed to be $\bar{Z} = -.05168$ and $S = .15559$, respectively.

Setting the nominal significance level α equal to the conventional value 5%, the tolerance ε determining the equivalence range for an intra-subject bioavailability ratio to .25, and the lower bound for ordinary and scaled PBIBE to .75, we are able to apply both versions of the Bayesian decision rule simply by means of the graphical devices provided by Figure 9.3 and 9.4. On the one hand, the observed point $(-.05168, .15559)$ fails to be included in the rejection region displayed in Figure 9.3 whose vertex is located below $s = .14$. Accordingly, in the Bayesian test for nonscaled PBIBE as specified by the alternative hypothesis $\tilde{K}_\varepsilon^{(1)}$ of (9.28), the data

Table 9.4 *Results of a bioequivalence trial of two for-*
mulations of the calcium-blocking agent nifedipine (From
Wellek, 1996, with kind permission by Wiley-VCH)

Subject ID (l)	AUC_1	AUC_2	SEQ	Z_l
1	106.9	112.9	T/R	-0.05461
2	131.3	124.4	T/R	0.05398
3	81.4	89.5	T/R	-0.09486
4	154.7	134.9	T/R	0.13695
5	111.2	108.3	T/R	0.02643
6	85.8	94.0	T/R	-0.09128
7	295.2	418.6	T/R	-0.34926
8	217.0	207.0	T/R	0.04718
9	252.3	239.3	T/R	0.05290
10	157.9	207.3	T/R	-0.27221
11	217.3	195.2	R/T	-0.10725
12	174.4	122.7	R/T	-0.35161
13	155.8	188.2	R/T	0.18893
14	299.5	309.2	R/T	0.03187
15	157.6	153.5	R/T	-0.02636
16	121.4	104.7	R/T	-0.14799
17	143.9	119.3	R/T	-0.18748
18	157.0	146.8	R/T	-0.06717
19	114.5	138.2	R/T	0.18813
20	71.0	70.3	R/T	-0.00991

shown in Table 9.4 do not allow a positive decision. On the other hand, $(-.05168, .15559)$ is obviously an inner point of the left half of the grey filled region shown in Figure 9.4 so that the Bayesian test for scaled PBIBE decides in favour of the alternative $\tilde{K}_\varepsilon^{(1)}$ [$\to$ (9.40)] with the same data. Interestingly, such a qualitative discrepancy between the final decisions to be taken also occurs if, in assessing the above data set, the conventional test (9.10) for average bioequivalence is contrasted with the t-test for scaled average bioequivalence (Wellek, 1991): At the 5% level, average bioequivalence in the sense of the well-known $80 - 125\%$ criterion can be established, but scaled average bioequivalence cannot, even if a shift by up to a whole common standard deviation is defined compatible with equivalence of two homoskedastic Gaussian distributions.

9.4 Approaches to defining and establishing population bioequivalence

9.4.1 Introduction

With regard to coherence of terminology, the concept of population bioequivalence which has attained considerable popularity within in the pertinent literature since the last 10 years, is hardly a fortunate choice. As a matter of fact, every inferential method of BE assessment aims at establishing a certain statement about the populations from which the subjects participating in the actual trial have been recruited by means of random selection. So the term population bioequivalence, which was originally coined by Anderson and Hauck (1990) and technically elaborated by Schall and Luus (1993), reveals almost nothing about the specific content of the concept it denotes. Nevertheless, after the preparations made in §9.1, its technical content can readily be made precise. The idea is to require of bioequivalent drug formulations that the marginal distributions associated with the treatments in the two sequence groups be sufficiently similar both with respect to the treatment-related component of the mean, and total variability. Under the standard model for the 2×2 crossover design, the variances of the X_{ki} and the Y_{kj} depend only on treatment and are given by

$$Var(X_{1i}) = Var(Y_{2j}) = \sigma_S^2 + \sigma_{eT}^2 \equiv \sigma_{TT}^2, \qquad (9.42a)$$

$$Var(X_{2i}) = Var(Y_{1j}) = \sigma_S^2 + \sigma_{eR}^2 \equiv \sigma_{TR}^2. \qquad (9.42b)$$

In the existing literature (see, e.g., Schall and Luus, 1993; Holder and Hsuan, 1993), as well as in the guidelines of the regulatory agencies (FDA/CDER, 2001), so-called aggregate criteria of population BE have been preferred up to now. Instead of aiming to establish sufficient similarity both of ϕ_T to ϕ_R and of σ_{TT}^2 to σ_{TR}^2, such an aggregate approach relies on a single real-valued function of all four parameters to be compared to some prespecified upper bound. As a so-called reference-scaled version of such an aggregate criterion, the most recent FDA guidance for BE trials recommends

$$\theta_P = \frac{(\phi_T - \phi_R)^2 + (\sigma_{TT}^2 - \sigma_{TR}^2)}{\sigma_{TR}^2}. \qquad (9.43)$$

There are several reasons to question whether it really makes sense to aggregate the moments under comparison exactly in the way leading to (9.43).

(i) Except for the scale-factor $1/\sigma_{TR}^2$, the parametric function to be assessed according to (9.43) combines a Euclidean distance (viz., that between the formulation effects) with an ordinary signed difference. The commonly referenced argument (see Schall and Luus, loc. cit.) for the use of this combination is based on the equation $E[(Y_T - Y_R)^2 -$

$(Y_R - Y_{R'})^2] = (\phi_T - \phi_R)^2 + \sigma_{TT}^2 - \sigma_{TR}^2$. However, the latter presupposes that all three observed (log)-bioavailabilities Y_T, Y_R and $Y_{R'}$ are taken from different subjects whereas in a real bioequivalence trial the drug formulations are administered consecutively to each individual.

(ii) In principle, scaling the primary distance measure has much to recommend it, provided there exists an intrinsic relationship between the parametric function to be scaled and the parameter with respect to which standardization is done. However, the incommensurability of the two terms making up the numerator of (9.43) raises a question as to whether a single parameter can give an appropriate reference for both and hence for their sum. In fact, under the basic parametric model for two-period crossover BE studies [$\rightarrow$ (8.28), (8.29), (9.1), (9.2)], the optimal estimator for $\phi_T - \phi_R$ has a sampling variance which is proportional to the sum of the two intra-subject variances σ_{eT}^2 and σ_{eR}^2. Hence, a suitably scaled measure for the distance between the formulations with respect to average log-bioavailability is given by

$$\eta^2 = \frac{(\phi_T - \phi_R)^2}{\sigma^2} \tag{9.44}$$

where

$$\sigma^2 = \sigma_{eT}^2 + \sigma_{eR}^2 . \tag{9.45}$$

On the other hand, the adequacy of $1/\sigma_{TR}^2$ as a scaling factor for the second term in the numerator of the parametric function introduced in (9.43) is obvious. Hence, it is natural to require of population-bioequivalent drug formulations that both η^2 and

$$\Lambda = \sigma_{TT}^2/\sigma_{TR}^2 - 1 \tag{9.46}$$

should be sufficiently small.

In order to circumvent the problems pointed out above, Wellek (2000b) proposed a disaggregate scaled criterion of population BE which requires that the two inequalities

$$(\phi_T - \phi_R)^2/(\sigma_{WT}^2 + \sigma_{WR}^2) < \varepsilon_\phi^* \tag{9.47a}$$

and

$$\sigma_{TT}^2/\sigma_{TR}^2 < 1 + \varepsilon_\sigma^* \tag{9.47b}$$

must be satisfied *simultaneously*, for suitably chosen constants $\varepsilon_\phi^*, \varepsilon_\sigma^* > 0$. A formal inferential procedure for assessing population BE in this latter sense consists of performing a valid test of

$$H_\cup : H_\phi \vee H_\sigma \quad \text{versus} \quad K_\cap : K_\phi \wedge K_\sigma \tag{9.48}$$

where the elementary testing problems involved read in explicit formulation

$H_\phi : (\phi_T - \phi_R)^2/(\sigma_{WT}^2 + \sigma_{WR}^2) \geq \varepsilon_\phi^*$ vs.

$$K_\phi : (\phi_T - \phi_R)^2/(\sigma_{WT}^2 + \sigma_{WR}^2) < \varepsilon_\phi^* \qquad (9.48\text{a})$$

and

$$H_\sigma : \sigma_{TT}^2/\sigma_{TR}^2 \geq 1 + \varepsilon_\sigma^* \quad \text{vs.} \quad K_\sigma : \sigma_{TT}^2/\sigma_{TR}^2 < 1 + \varepsilon_\sigma^* . \qquad (9.48\text{b})$$

Exploiting the intersection-union principle formulated and proven in §7.1, testing of (9.48) reduces to performing a valid test for each of the elementary problems. But in view of (9.45), except for renaming the equivalence bound to $|\phi_T - \phi_R|/\sigma$, (9.48a) is the same as the problem of testing for scaled average BE in the sense of §9.2.2. Hence, all that is really left to do for constructing a test for establishing the proposed disaggregate criterion of population BE, is to derive a solution for the one-sided testing problem (9.48b). This will be the topic of §9.4.2. In §9.4.3, the rejection region of the complete disaggregate testing procedure will be presented, and its use illustrated by reanalyzing the BE trial considered in Example 9.1 of §9.2.1. The section will be concluded by presenting simulation results on the power of the disaggregate test, and the sample sizes required for attaining given power against selected specific alternatives, respectively.

9.4.2 A testing procedure for establishing one-sided bioequivalence with respect to total variability

The basic idea behind the construction of an exact level-α test for (9.48b) to be described in this subsection, goes back as far as to the thirties (Pitman, 1939; Morgan, 1939) and was exploited in a slightly modified version by Liu and Chow (1992) as well as Guilbaud (1993) for deriving tests for one-sided equivalence with respect to intra-subject rather than total variability of the pharmacokinetic measure of interest.

As before [recall p. 207], let us denote the log-bioavailabilities observed during the kth period in a subject randomized to sequence group T/R and R/T by X_{ki} and Y_{kj}, respectively. Furthermore, for any fixed positive number ω let

$$U_{1i}^\omega = X_{1i} + \omega X_{2i} \quad , \quad U_{2i}^\omega = (1/\omega)X_{1i} - X_{2i} \quad , \quad i = 1, ..., m, \qquad (9.49\text{a})$$

and

$$V_{1j}^\omega = Y_{2j} + \omega Y_{1j} \quad , \quad V_{2j}^\omega = (1/\omega)Y_{2j} - Y_{1j} \quad , \quad j = 1, ..., n. \qquad (9.49\text{b})$$

Then, it follows from (8.28), (8.29) (9.1) and (9.2) that the pairs $(U_{1i}^\omega, U_{2i}^\omega)$ and $(V_{1j}^\omega, V_{2j}^\omega)$ form samples from two bivariate normal distributions with possibly different mean vectors but the same covariance matrix. Hence, in particular the correlation within any pair of U^ω's is the same as within any pair of V^ω's, and the common correlation coefficient ρ_ω, say, is easily computed to be

$$\rho_\omega = \frac{\sigma_{TT}^2 - \omega^2\,\sigma_{TR}^2}{\sqrt{(\sigma_{TT}^2 + \omega^2\,\sigma_{TR}^2)^2 - 4\omega^2\sigma_S^4}} \ . \tag{9.50}$$

In view of the possible heterogeneity of the distributions of the $(U_{1i}^\omega, U_{2i}^\omega)$ and the $(V_{1j}^\omega, V_{2j}^\omega)$ with respect to the means, ρ_ω cannot be estimated by the empirical correlation coefficient for the pooled sample consisting of all $(U_{1i}^\omega, U_{2i}^\omega)$ and $(V_{1j}^\omega, V_{2j}^\omega)$ together. Instead, pooling has to be done for the sample moments which have to be computed first separately for the $(U_{1i}^\omega, U_{2i}^\omega)$ and the $(V_{1j}^\omega, V_{2j}^\omega)$ which leads to the estimator

$$R_\omega = \left[\left(SSX^{(1)} + SSY^{(2)}\right) - \omega^2\left(SSX^{(2)} + SSY^{(1)}\right)\right] \Big/$$
$$\left[\left(\left(SSX^{(1)} + SSY^{(2)}\right) + \omega^2\left(SSX^{(2)} + SSY^{(1)}\right)\right)^2\right.$$
$$\left. -4\omega^2\left(SPX + SPY\right)^2\right]^{1/2} . \tag{9.51}$$

In this formula, $SSX^{(k)}$ and $SSY^{(k)}$ stands for the (corrected) sum of squares of the X_{ki} and Y_{kj} $(k = 1,2)$, respectively. Similarly, SPX and SPY have to be defined as $\sum_{i=1}^{m}(X_{1i} - \bar{X}_1)(X_{2i} - \bar{X}_2)$ and $\sum_{j=1}^{n}(Y_{1j} - \bar{Y}_1)(Y_{2j} - \bar{Y}_2)$ where $\bar{X}_k = \sum_{i=1}^{m} X_{ki}/m$ and $\bar{Y}_k = \sum_{j=1}^{n} Y_{kj}/n$ $(k = 1,2)$, respectively.

The appropriateness of R_ω with $\omega = \sqrt{1 + \varepsilon_\sigma^*}$ as a test statistic for (9.48b) follows from the following properties:

(i) If ω equals the true value of the ratio σ_{TT}/σ_{TR} of total standard deviations, then R_ω has the same distribution as the empirical correlation coefficient for a single sample of size $m + n - 1$ from a bivariate normal distribution with diagonal covariance matrix. Equivalently, this means that for $\omega = \sigma_{TT}/\sigma_{TR}$, the distribution of

$$T_\omega = \sqrt{m + n - 3}\, R_\omega/\sqrt{1 - R_\omega^2} \tag{9.52}$$

is central t with $m + n - 3$ degrees freedom.

(ii) For fixed sums of squares $SSX^{(k)}, SSY^{(k)}$ $(k = 1,2)$ and sums of products SPX, SPY, and arbitrary $\omega_1, \omega_2 > 0$, there holds the relation

$$\omega_1 \le \omega_2 \implies T_{\omega_1} \ge T_{\omega_2} \ . \tag{9.53}$$

Property (i) is plausible from the obvious fact that ρ_ω vanishes for $\omega = \sigma_{TT}/\sigma_{TR}$ and that R_ω is by definition the empirical correlation coefficient pooled over two independent samples from bivariate normal distributions with the same theoretical correlation ρ_ω (a rigorous proof can be given by means of Theorems 7.3.2 and 7.6.1 of Anderson, 1984). The other property

(ii) can be established by examining the derivative with respect to ω of the expression on the right-hand side of (9.51). Combining both properties shows that the decision rule

$$\text{Reject } H_\sigma \text{ if and only if } T_{\sqrt{1+\varepsilon_\sigma^*}} < t_{m+n-3;\,\alpha} \qquad (9.54)$$

defines an unbiased test of exact level α for (9.48b). Of course, this statement holds under the customary notational convention for central t-quantiles according to which $t_{\nu;\,\gamma}$ symbolizes the lower 100γth percentile of a central t-distribution with ν degrees of freedom (for any $0 < \gamma < 1$).

9.4.3 Complete disaggregate testing procedure and illustrating example

Bearing equation (9.44) in mind, it becomes immediately clear that putting $\varepsilon = 2\sqrt{\varepsilon_\phi^*}$ makes the alternative hypothesis $\tilde{K}$ of (9.15) coincide with the first condition required by our aggregate criterion of population BE. Thus, the testing sub-problem (9.48a) admits an optimal solution which is obtained by applying the critical region (6.6) of the two-sample t-test for equivalence with $\varepsilon = 2\sqrt{\varepsilon_\phi^*}$ and the within subject differences X_i^- and Y_j^- as the primary observations. This gives the rejection region

$$\left\{ |\bar{X}^- - \bar{Y}^-|/\tilde{S}^- < \tilde{C}_{\alpha;m,n}\left(2\sqrt{\varepsilon_\phi^*}\right) \right\} \qquad (9.55)$$

where $\bar{X}^-$, $\bar{Y}^-$ and $\tilde{S}^-$ have to computed in the way explained on p. 210. Now, according to the intersection-union principle, we have to combine (9.55) and (9.54) into the aggregated decision rule:

Reject lack of population BE if and only if there holds both

$$|\bar{X}^- - \bar{Y}^-|/\tilde{S}^- < \tilde{C}_{\alpha;m,n}\left(2\sqrt{\varepsilon_\phi^*}\right) \quad \text{and}$$

$$\sqrt{m+n-3}\,R_{\sqrt{1+\varepsilon_\sigma^*}} \Big/ \sqrt{1 - R^2_{\sqrt{1+\varepsilon_\sigma^*}}} < t_{m+n-3,\,\alpha}\,. \qquad (9.56)$$

Example 9.1 (continued)

We illustrate the use of the aggregate decision rule (9.56) by applying it to the same data set that has been analyzed in §9.2 by means of the interval inclusion test for average BE and the two-sample t-test for scaled average BE. Table 9.1 [$\to$ p. 213] displays the raw data in a format well suited to carrying out almost all necessary computational steps by means of a simple pocket calculator. To begin with the first component problem H_ϕ vs. K_ϕ [$\to$ (9.48a)], we already know from §9.2.2 that for $\varepsilon_\phi^* = (.74/2)^2 = .1369$, the UMPI test rejects at the 5%-level. Thus, there remains to extend the analysis of the data set by carrying out the test for one-sided equivalence of the total variabilities derived in §9.4.2.

The raw input data for computing the test statistic (9.52) are the entries in the middle rows of Table 9.1. Calculating the sums of squares and products appearing on the right-hand side of equation (9.51) with these values gives:

$$SSX^{(1)} = 0.5814, \quad SSX^{(2)} = 0.3503, \quad SPX = 0.3133;$$

$$SSY^{(1)} = 1.0280, \quad SSY^{(2)} = 1.3879, \quad SPY = 1.0059.$$

If we specify the constant determining the upper equivalence limit in the hypotheses (9.48b) $\varepsilon_\sigma^* = 1.00$, by plugging in into (9.51) it follows that $R_{\sqrt{1+\varepsilon_\sigma^*}} = -.2715$. The corresponding value of the t-statistic (9.52) is $T_{\sqrt{1+\varepsilon_\sigma^*}} = -1.3229$. Since the lower 5 percentage point of a central t-distribution with $m + n - 3 = 22$ degrees of freedom is -1.7171, (9.54) implies that the null hypothesis H_σ of a relevant increase of the total variability associated with the test formulation of the drug, cannot be rejected. Hence, relying on the specifications $\varepsilon_\sigma = 1.00$ and $\alpha = .05$, one-sided equivalence with respect to total variability cannot be established, and as a final consequence it has to be stated that the data of Table 9.1 do not contain sufficient evidence in support of population BE in the sense of the disaggregate criterion underlying (9.48).

For comparison, we mention that an application of the aggregate criterion of population BE suggested in the current FDA/CDER guidance to the same data leads to an identical qualitative conclusion. In fact, the point estimate of the parametric function (9.43) is obtained to be $\hat{\theta}_P = .4293$, and taking $B = 100,000$ bootstrap samples from the observed empirical distributions gave a (bias-corrected) upper 95%-confidence bound of 1.0609 for θ_P which is actually quite large.

9.4.4 Some results on power and sample sizes

If Π denotes the power of any statistical test obtained by means of the intersection-union principle against an arbitrarily selected specific alternative and each elementary test ϕ_ν ($\nu = 1, ..., q$) [cf. (7.3)] has rejection probability Π_ν under the same parameter constellation, then an application of the elementary Bonferroni inequality yields the relationship

$$\Pi \geq 1 - \sum_{\nu=1}^{q} (1 - \Pi_\nu) . \tag{9.57}$$

Using the expression appearing on the right-hand side of this inequality as a first order approximation to the power of the compound test can be recommended only for settings in which for any $\nu_1 \neq \nu_2$, the acceptance regions of subtests $\phi_{\nu 1}$ and $\phi_{\nu 2}$ correspond to almost disjoint events. Furthermore, the approximation based on (9.57) is of real use for practice only if the power of each component test is a quantity easily accessible by direct computational techniques.

Among the two individual tests making up our decision procedure for the assessment of disaggregate population BE, the first one admits exact power calculations as shown in § 6.1. In contrast to the two-sample t-statistic, the correlation coefficient $R_{\sqrt{1+\varepsilon_\sigma^*}}$ used for assessing possible differences between drug formulations in total variability, has a rather complicated distribution, and exact computation of nonnull rejection probabilities of the corresponding test would require numerical integration in several dimensions. Hence, in the case being our concern here, even the right-hand side of (9.57) cannot be evaluated exactly without recourse to advanced and time-consuming numerical methods. In view of this, the power of the test for one-sided equivalence with respect to total variability as well as that of the complete disaggregate testing procedure was investigated by means of Monte Carlo simulation.

Table 9.5 *Rejection probabilities of the t-test for scaled average bio-equivalence ($\leftrightarrow \Pi_1$), the test for one-sided equivalence with respect to total variability ($\leftrightarrow \Pi_2$) and the disaggregate test for PBE as a whole ($\leftrightarrow \Pi$) [Except for Π_1, all probabilities are based on simulation, with 100,000 replications per experiment] (Partially reproduced from Wellek, 2000b, with kind permission by John Wiley & Sons, Inc.)*

m	n	$\tilde{\varepsilon}_\phi$ [†]	ε_σ^*	σ_{TR}^2/σ_S^2	Π_1	Π_2	Π
12	12	0.74	1.00	2.00	.24453	.57116	.13881
12	12	1.00	1.00	2.00	.57214	.57015	.32245
12	12	1.00	2.00	3.00	.57214	.84551	.48139
12	12	1.40	2.25	3.00	.90558	.88555	.80123
12	12	1.00	2.00	5.00	.57214	.82286	.47036
12	12	1.00	1.50	5.00	.57214	.69319	.39415
18	18	0.74	1.00	2.00	.44688	.74091	.32827
18	18	1.00	1.00	2.00	.81196	.74109	.60117
18	18	1.00	1.00	3.00	.81196	.67928	.55122
18	18	1.00	2.00	3.00	.81196	.95286	.77391
18	18	1.00	2.00	5.00	.81196	.94106	.76486
24	24	0.74	1.00	2.00	.63693	.84767	.53882
24	24	1.00	1.00	2.00	.92162	.84957	.78173
24	24	1.00	1.00	3.00	.92162	.79226	.72912
24	24	1.00	2.00	3.00	.92162	.98714	.91064
24	24	1.00	2.00	5.00	.92162	.98215	.90421
24	24	1.00	0.50	2.00	.92162	.47040	.43184

[†] equivalence limit for $2(\phi_T - \phi_R)/\sqrt{\sigma_{WT}^2 + \sigma_{WR}^2}$

All simulation results shown in Table 9.5 refer to the 5% level and to balanced designs with equal numbers of subjects assigned to both sequence groups. As the only specific alternative of interest, perfect coincidence of the marginal distributions corresponding to the drug formulations, i.e., $\phi_T = \phi_R$ and $\sigma_{TT}^2 = \sigma_{TR}^2$ is assumed. Inspecting the numerical material displayed in the table leads to the following major conclusions:

- The minimum sample size required to guarantee a reasonable overall power Π of the disaggregate testing procedure (9.56), is a complicated function both of the equivalence limits $\tilde{\varepsilon}_\phi, 1 + \varepsilon_\sigma^*$, and the ratio σ_{TR}^2/σ_S^2 between the total and the inter-subject variance.

- For fixed sample sizes m, n and given upper equivalence limit $1 + \varepsilon_\sigma^*$ for $\sigma_{TT}^2/\sigma_{TR}^2$, the power Π_2 of the test for equivalence in total variability decreases in σ_{TR}^2/σ_S^2.

- The approximation to the overall power Π based on (9.57) is poor if the power of at least one of the two subtests is smaller than .70. However, if both Π_1 and Π_2 are larger than .80, the approximation is remarkably accurate.

9.4.5 Discussion

Technically, there is no problem to obtain a left-sided analogue of the test (9.54) for noninferiority with respect to total variability and to combine it with the right-sided version by means of the intersection-union principle into a test for equivalence in the strict, i.e., two-sided sense (for an unbiased test for two-sided equivalence with respect to intra-subject variability which is uniformly more powerful than the corresponding double one-sided test see Wang, 1997). However, reducing bioequivalence assessment with respect to variability to a one-sided testing problem of the form (9.48b) seems conceptually much more adequate than working with the two-sided version of that testing problem. To be sure, it is obvious that "hyperavailability" of a drug formulation under assessment in the sense of an increased population average may cause serious problems in patients treated with the drug. But it is hard to see any reason why a relevantly reduced variability of the pharmacokinetic measure of interest should be considered an undesirable property of a drug formulation which its potential consumer must be protected against. Hence, for purposes of establishing population bioequivalence, it seems fully sufficient indeed to give convincing evidence for the truth of (9.48a) and (9.48b) whereas the double two-sided criterion $(\phi_T - \phi_R)^2/(\sigma_{WT}^2 + \sigma_{WR}^2) < \varepsilon_\phi^*, 1 - \varepsilon_\sigma^* < \sigma_{TT}^2/\sigma_{TR}^2 < 1 + \varepsilon_\sigma^{**}$ with $\varepsilon_\sigma^* < 1$ seems unnecessarily restrictive. This restrictiveness entails a rather drastic loss in the power of the associated testing procedure. For instance, replacing the equivalence region $0 < \sigma_{TT}/\sigma_{TR} < 2.00$ by $0.50 < \sigma_{TT}/\sigma_{TR} < 2.00$ in the situation covered by line 14 of Table 9.5 would imply that the power of the second subtest and of the overall testing procedure drops from .7923 and .7291 to .5866 and .5392, respectively.

Finally, it seems worth noticing that for both elementary tests we did combine to form our disaggregate procedure, suitable nonparametric or distribution-free analogues are available. A distribution-free procedure for testing a hypothesis which coincides with that of (9.48a) in the standard parametric model is obtained by applying the Mann-Whitney test for equivalence discussed in § 6.2 to the within-subject differences X_i^- and Y_j^-. Furthermore, nonparametric tests for one-sided equivalence with respect to intra-subject variability are provided in Section 2 of Liu and Chow (1992). The latter can readily be adopted for the problem of testing for one-sided equivalence with respect to total variability.

9.5 Bioequivalence assessment as a problem of comparing bivariate distributions

Although the same basic model is used for describing the *primary* observations, i.e., the log-bioavailabilities observed in the individual periods of the trial [recall p. 207], the view taken in this final subsection of the problem of BE assessment differs radically from all approaches treated up to now since no reduction of the pairs $(X_{1i}, X_{2i}), (Y_{1j}, Y_{2j})$ to univariate quantities will be carried out. The reason for this change of perspective is so elementary that one may ask why it has been totally ignored in the existing literature on the topic: If both formulations of the drug under study are actually identical, $(Y_{11}, Y_{21}), \ldots, (Y_{1n}, Y_{2n})$ must be just a replicate sample from the *same* bivariate distribution from which the random sample $(X_{11}, X_{21}), \ldots, (X_{1m}, X_{2m})$ making up the data set for sequence group T-R, has been taken. Thus, for identical formulations, we must in particular have $E(X_{1i}, X_{2i}) = E(Y_{1j}, Y_{2j})$ (for arbitrary $i \in \{1, \ldots, m\}$, $j \in \{1, \ldots, n\}$) which is incompatible with a nonzero difference both of the direct treatment and the carryover effects. In fact, if (9.2) is replaced with (8.31) [with (ϕ_A, ϕ_B) being renamed (ϕ_T, ϕ_R)], then we have $E(X_{1i}) - E(Y_{1j}) = \phi_T - \phi_R$, $E(X_{2i}) - E(Y_{2j}) = (\phi_R - \phi_T) + (\lambda^{(1)} - \lambda^{(2)})$ so that $\phi_T \neq \phi_R \Rightarrow E(X_{1i}) \neq E(Y_{1j})$ and $(\phi_T = \phi_R, \lambda^{(1)} \neq \lambda^{(2)}) \Rightarrow E(X_{2i}) \neq E(Y_{2j})$. As a clear conclusion of this simple argument, we can state that inequality of carryover effects is a specific form of inequivalence rather than a violation of the conditions for the validity of a suitable BE assessment procedure using the data from both periods of the trial. (Essentially the same fact has been pointed out from a nonequivalence perspective by Jones and Kenward, 1989, p. 41.) Thus, in what follows we adopt the view that assessment of BE requires comparison of the distributions underlying the pairs (X_{1i}, X_{2i}) and (Y_{1j}, Y_{2j}).

Assuming the usual parametric model in the simplified version with treatment-independent within-subject variances, we have

$$(X_{1i}, X_{2i}) \sim \mathcal{N}\big((\mu_1, \mu_2), \boldsymbol{\Sigma}\big), \quad (Y_{1j}, Y_{2j}) \sim \mathcal{N}\big((\nu_1, \nu_2), \boldsymbol{\Sigma}\big), \quad (9.58)$$

where the elements of the common covariance matrix $\boldsymbol{\Sigma}$ are given by

$$\sigma_1^2 = \sigma_S^2 + \sigma_e^2, \quad \sigma_{12} = \sigma_{21} = \sigma_S^2, \quad \sigma_2^2 = \sigma_S^2 + \sigma_e^2. \quad (9.59)$$

In the sequel, except symmetry and nonsingularity, no additional restriction on $\boldsymbol{\Sigma}$ will be needed. So we let its elements be arbitrary real numbers satisfying $\sigma_1^2, \sigma_2^2 > 0$ and $\sigma_1^2 \sigma_2^2 > \sigma_{12}^2$. A suitable measure of dissimilarity between the two bivariate Gaussian distributions of (9.58) is Mahalanobis' distance as defined in any textbook on classical multivariate statistics (see, e.g., Anderson, 1984, §6.4). In the bivariate case, it can be written

$$\Delta^2(\boldsymbol{\mu}, \boldsymbol{\nu}; \boldsymbol{\Sigma}) =$$
$$\frac{(\mu_1 - \nu_1)^2 \sigma_2^2 - 2\sigma_{12}(\mu_1 - \nu_1)(\mu_2 - \nu_2) + (\mu_2 - \nu_2)^2 \sigma_1^2}{\sigma_1^2 \sigma_2^2 - \sigma_{12}^2}. \quad (9.60)$$

Now it seems natural to require of bioequivalent drug formulations that the Mahalanobis distance between the bivariate Gaussian distributions underlying the nonreduced data set obtained in both sequence groups, be smaller than some specified positive bound, say $\Delta_\circ^2$. Following this idea, bioequivalence assessment consists in performing a valid test of significance for the problem

$$H_b : \Delta^2(\boldsymbol{\mu}, \boldsymbol{\nu}; \boldsymbol{\Sigma}) \geq \Delta_\circ^2 \text{ versus } K_b : \Delta^2(\boldsymbol{\mu}, \boldsymbol{\nu}; \boldsymbol{\Sigma}) < \Delta_\circ^2. \quad (9.61)$$

It is interesting to have a closer look at the geometric shape of the region in the parameter space which corresponds to the alternative hypothesis of (9.61). Under the restricted covariance structure (9.59) arising from the standard model for BE trials, K_b can easily be shown to hold true if and only if we have

$$\left[\left(\frac{(\phi_T - \phi_R) + (\lambda^{(2)} - \lambda^{(1)})/2}{\sigma_e/\sqrt{2}} \right)^2 + \right.$$
$$\left. \left(\frac{\lambda^{(2)} - \lambda^{(1)}}{2\sqrt{\sigma_S^2 + \sigma_e^2/2}} \right)^2 \right]^{1/2} < \Delta_\circ. \quad (9.62)$$

Obviously, (9.62) defines a circular disk of radius $\Delta_\circ$ around zero in a suitable two-dimensional space. The most important feature of this space is that it refers to a two-dimensional parameter whose Euclidean distance from the origin increases both with $|\phi_T - \phi_R|$ and $|\lambda^{(1)} - \lambda^{(2)}|$. Moreover, the circular disk corresponding to (9.62) provides a good approximation to the equivalence region specified by K_b even in cases where two different within-subject variances σ_{eT}^2 and σ_{eR}^2 have to be taken into account. In order to see this, it suffices to note that (9.62) reflects the independence of the natural estimators of $(\phi_T - \phi_R) + (\lambda^{(2)} - \lambda^{(1)})/2$ and $(\lambda^{(2)} - \lambda^{(1)})/2$ implied by $\sigma_{eT}^2 = \sigma_{eR}^2$. But in the general case, the square of the same correlation is easily computed to be $\dfrac{(\sigma_{eT} - \sigma_{eR})^2(\sigma_{eT} + \sigma_{eR})^2}{(\sigma_{eT}^2 + \sigma_{eR}^2)(4\sigma_S^2 + \sigma_{eT}^2 + \sigma_{eR}^2)}$ which is typically still close to zero since the within-subject variances will be much smaller than the between-subject variance.

An optimal test for (9.61) can be based on the well-known two-sample Hotelling T^2-statistic. It can be represented as a normalized plug-in estimator of the Mahalanobis distance $\Delta^2(\boldsymbol{\mu}, \boldsymbol{\nu}; \boldsymbol{\Sigma})$ obtained by replacing on the right-hand side of (9.60) the μ_k and ν_k with the respective sample means and each element of $\boldsymbol{\Sigma}$ with the homologous entry in the pooled sample covariance matrix $\mathbf{S} = \begin{pmatrix} S_1^2 & S_{12} \\ S_{12} & S_2^2 \end{pmatrix}$ defined in the usual way, i.e., as

$$
\mathbf{S} = \frac{1}{N-2}\left[\sum_{i=1}^{m}\big((X_{1i}, X_{2i}) - (\bar{X}_1, \bar{X}_2)\big)\big((X_{1i}, X_{2i}) - (\bar{X}_1, \bar{X}_2)\big)'\right.
$$
$$
\left. + \sum_{j=1}^{n}\big((Y_{1j}, Y_{2j}) - (\bar{Y}_1, \bar{Y}_2)\big)\big((Y_{1j}, Y_{2j}) - (\bar{Y}_1, \bar{Y}_2)\big)'\right]. \tag{9.63}
$$

Carrying out these substitutions and using mn/N as normalizing factor yields

$$
T^2 = \frac{mn}{N(S_1^2 S_2^2 - S_{12}^2)}\Big[(\bar{X}_1 - \bar{Y}_1)^2 S_2^2 -
$$
$$
2S_{12}^2(\bar{X}_1 - \bar{Y}_1)(\bar{X}_2 - \bar{Y}_2) + (\bar{X}_2 - \bar{Y}_2)^2 S_1^2\Big]. \tag{9.64}
$$

The distribution of T^2 is well-known (see, e.g., Anderson, 1984, §5.2.2) to be given by

$$
T^2 (N - 3)/\big(2(N - 2)\big) \overset{d}{=} \mathcal{F}_{2,N-3}(mn\delta^2/N) \tag{9.65}
$$

under arbitrary $(\boldsymbol{\mu}, \boldsymbol{\nu}, \boldsymbol{\Sigma})$ such that $\Delta^2(\boldsymbol{\mu}, \boldsymbol{\nu}, \boldsymbol{\Sigma}) = \delta^2 > 0$, where $\mathcal{F}_{2,N-3}(\psi^2)$ denotes a random variable following an F-distribution with $2, N-3$ degrees of freedom and noncentrality parameter $\psi^2 \geq 0$. Hence, the critical region of an exact level-α test for (9.61) can be written

$$
\Big\{T^2 < 2\big((N - 2)/(N - 3)\big) F_{2,N-3;\,\alpha}(mn\Delta_\circ^2/N)\Big\}. \tag{9.66}
$$

The power of this T^2-test (9.66) for equivalence against any specific alternative $(\boldsymbol{\mu}, \boldsymbol{\nu}, \boldsymbol{\Sigma})$ with $\Delta^2(\boldsymbol{\mu}, \boldsymbol{\nu}, \boldsymbol{\Sigma}) = \Delta_a^2 \in [0, \Delta_\circ^2)$ admits the explicit representation

$$
\beta(\Delta_a^2) = F_{2,N-3;\,mn\Delta_a^2/N}\big(F_{2,N-3;\,\alpha}(mn\Delta_\circ^2/N)\big) \tag{9.67}
$$

where $F_{2,N-3;\,\psi^2}(\cdot)$ stands for the cdf of $\mathcal{F}_{2,N-3}(mn\Delta_a^2/N)$.

Like its univariate counterpart [cf. §6.1], the T^2-test for equivalence of two bivariate Gaussian distributions with common covariance structure exhibits a number of noticeable mathematical properties. First of all, it is unbiased at the prespecified nominal significance level $\alpha \in (0,1)$. Moreover, it is uniformly most powerful among all level-α tests for (9.61) which remain invariant under a large group of linear transformations of the sample space generated by several subgroups. The most important of these transformations are of the form

$$(X_{1i}, X_{2i}) \mapsto (a_1, a_2) + (X_{1i}, X_{2i}) \cdot \boldsymbol{B}, \, i = 1, \ldots, m,$$
$$(Y_{1j}, Y_{2j}) \mapsto (a_1, a_2) + (Y_{1j}, Y_{2j}) \cdot \boldsymbol{B}, \, j = 1, \ldots, n,$$

with $(a_1, a_2) \in \mathbb{R}^2$ and $\boldsymbol{B}$ as an arbitrary nonsingular 2×2 matrix.

Of course, without the assumption of homoskedasticity and bivariate normality of the distributions under comparison, it cannot even taken for granted that the rejection region (9.66) has size α, which raises the question of robustness against departures from one or the other of these assumptions. Separate simulation studies were conducted to assess the impact of nonnormality and heteroskedasticity on size and power to detect exact coincidence of both mean vectors. Table 9.6 shows the simulated rejection probabilities under constellations with non-Gaussian forms of the distributions, and first and second moments defining a point in the parameter space lying on the common boundary of the hypotheses and at the most extreme specific alternative, respectively.

Table 9.6 *Simulation results on the sensitivity of the T^2-test for (bio-)equivalence against nonnormality of distributions*

m	n	σ_S^2	σ_e^2	Distributional Shape	Reject. Prob. at $\Delta^2 = \Delta$	Power at $\Delta^2 = 0$
10	10	*	*	Gaussian	.0500[†]	.3581[†]
"	"	.165	.020	Logistic	.0487	.3546
"	"	.20	.10	" "	.0416	.3535
"	"	.165	.020	Exponential	.0428	.3375
"	"	.20	.10	" "	.0416	.3349
15	15	*	*	Gaussian	.0500[†]	.5840[†]
"	"	.165	.020	Logistic	.0496	.5793
"	"	.20	.10	" "	.0480	.5793
"	"	.165	.020	Exponential	.0451	.5741
"	"	.20	.10	" "	.0431	.5737

[†] Exact values, depending on all parameters only through Δ^2

The distributional forms appearing in the fifth column refer to the marginal distributions of linearly transformed pairs $(D_i^{(1)}, Z_i^{(1)})$ [$\leftrightarrow$ group T/R,

$(D_j^{(2)}, Z_j^{(2)})$ [$\leftrightarrow$ group R/T] with uncorrelated components. In the homoskedastic case $\sigma_{eT}^2 = \sigma_{eR}^2$, such transforms are readily obtained by setting $D_i^{(1)} = X_{1i} - X_{2i}$, $Z_i^{(1)} = X_{1i} + X_{2i}$ and $D_j^{(2)} = Y_{1j} - Y_{2j}$, $Z_j^{(2)} = Y_{1j} + Y_{2j}$, respectively. Clearly, the invariance properties of the T^2-test imply that it makes no difference whether the (X_{1i}, X_{2i}), (Y_{1j}, Y_{2j}) or the $(D_i^{(1)}, Z_i^{(1)})$, $(D_j^{(2)}, Z_j^{(2)})$ are treated as the primary data. Table 9.7 shows analogous simulation results for bivariate Behrens-Fisher situations. For generating the data for the Monte Carlo experiments performed for the purpose of studying the influence of heteroskedasticity on the size of the critical region (9.66), Mahalanobis' distance was computed with respect to the average $\boldsymbol{\Sigma}^{(0)} = (1/2)(\boldsymbol{\Sigma}^{(1)} + \boldsymbol{\Sigma}^{(2)})$ of both group-specific covariance matrices, and the mean vectors $\boldsymbol{\mu}$, $\boldsymbol{\nu}$ were specified in a way ensuring that $\Delta^2(\boldsymbol{\mu}, \boldsymbol{\nu}; \boldsymbol{\Sigma}^{(0)})$ attains the bound $\Delta_\circ^2$ set to equivalent homoskedastic Gaussian distributions under the original alternative hypothesis K_b.

Both series of simulation experiments refer to a nominal significance level of 5% and an equivalence bound $\Delta_\circ^2$ of unity. All rejection probabilities shown in the tables are estimates based on 40,000 replications of the respective Monte Carlo experiment. The insights provided by the results into both aspects of the robustness problem arising in the present context are as clear-cut as encouraging:

- Both kinds of deviations from the original model affect mainly the size of the test.

- The differences found between the nominal level and the true rejection probabilities on the boundary of the region of nonequivalence point to the overconservative direction.

- Given the size of both samples, overconservatism is more marked under heteroskedasticity than deviations from the Gaussian form of the marginal distributions.

Table 9.7 *Simulation results on the sensitivity of the T^2-test for (bio-) equivalence against heteroskedasticity*

m	n	σ_S^2	σ_{eT}^2	σ_{eR}^2	Reject. Prob. under $\Delta^2(\boldsymbol{\mu},\boldsymbol{\nu}; \boldsymbol{\Sigma}^{(0)\dagger)}) = \Delta_\circ^2$	Power against $\boldsymbol{\mu} = \boldsymbol{\nu}$
10	10	.165	.005	.020	.0406	.3578
"	"	.20	.05	.20	.0325	.3588
15	15	.165	.005	.020	.0361	.5810
"	"	.20	.05	.20	.0277	.5823
20	20	.165	.005	.020	.0344	.7539
"	"	.20	.05	.20	.0264	.7532

$^\dagger)\,\boldsymbol{\Sigma}^{(0)} \equiv (1/2)(\boldsymbol{\Sigma}^{(1)} + \boldsymbol{\Sigma}^{(2)})$

Example 9.3

As an illustration of the bivariate approach to testing for scaled average BE, we apply it to the log-bioavailabilities shown in Table 9.8. With these

Table 9.8 *Logarithmically transformed AUC's measured in both pe-*
riods of a standard bioequivalence trial of two other formulations of
nifedipine [different from those referred to in Example 9.2]

Sequence Group T/R

i	1	2	3	4	5	6
X_{1i}	5.32833	4.60833	4.61290	4.85399	4.82933	4.61250
X_{2i}	4.91018	4.98835	4.53084	5.00148	4.88278	4.68550

7	8	9	10
4.89988	4.48080	6.00856	4.58419
4.83594	4.43013	5.72340	4.63451

Sequence Group R/T

j	1	2	3	4	5	6
Y_{1j}	4.97670	5.79190	5.37921	5.11251	5.29075	4.64138
Y_{2j}	5.32219	5.51966	5.17163	4.98796	5.31198	4.34402

7	8	9	10
4.52988	4.70318	5.35740	5.13770
4.79501	4.50227	5.56355	5.17898

data, the sample means and pooled estimates of the covariance and both variances are calculated

$$\bar{X}_1 = 4.8819 \quad , \quad \bar{X}_2 = 4.8623 \; ;$$
$$\bar{Y}_1 = 5.0921 \quad , \quad \bar{Y}_2 = 5.0697 \; ;$$
$$S_1^2 = 0.1839 \quad , \quad S_2^2 = 0.1490 \; ; \; S_{12} = 0.1405$$

Plugging in these values in Equation (9.64) yields

$$T^2 = \frac{100}{20(.1839 \cdot .1490 - .1405^2)} \Big[(4.8819 - 5.0921)^2 \cdot$$
$$.1490 - 2 \cdot .1405 \cdot (4.8819 - 5.0921) \cdot (4.8623 - 5.0697)$$
$$+ (4.8623 - 5.0697)^2 \cdot .1839 \Big] = 1.4643 \,.$$

On the other hand, specifying $\Delta_\circ = 1$ and using the SAS intrinsic function finv for computing the noncentral F-quantile required for determining the critical upper bound to T^2, we obtain the latter as

$$2 \frac{N-2}{N-3} F_{2,N-3;\,\alpha}(mn\Delta_\circ^2/N) = 2 \cdot \frac{18}{17} \text{ finv}(.05,2,17,5.00)$$
$$= 2.1176 \cdot 0.4551 = 0.9637 \,,$$

provided of course, that the test has to be carried out at the usual level $\alpha = 5\%$. Since the observed value of T^2 clearly fails to remain under this bound, we have to accept the null hypothesis H_b of (9.61) with the present data, despite the fact that $\Delta_\circ$ has been chosen to be much larger than recommended earlier [$\rightarrow$ §1.5] for the univariate version of the same test.

It is of considerable interest to note that this negative result is almost exclusively due to a comparatively large estimated difference between the carryover effects, whereas estimating the difference of treatment effects gives a standardized value being as small as .0272. Thus, the data set shown in Table 9.7 is an instance of the possibility that the bivariate and the conventional univariate approach to testing for (scaled) average BE may lead to opposite conclusions. With regard to contributions to the existing literature dealing with the problem of BE assessment from a point of view declared explicitly to be multivariate in nature (see Chinchilli and Elswick, 1997), it is important to note that a different kind of multivariateness is intended there. In fact, these authors propose to avoid reduction of the serum-concentration profile to simple univariate measures of bioavailability like AUC and $C_{\max}$ by using a measure of distance between the profiles obtained from the same subject which integrates the distances at all relevant points on the time axis.

Basic theoretical results

A.1 UMP Tests for equivalence problems in STP₃ families

A.1.1 Definition. Let $(p_\theta(\cdot))_{\theta \in \Theta}$ be a family of real-valued functions with common domain $\mathcal{X}$. Suppose that both $\mathcal{X}$ and the parameter space Θ is some simply ordered set. Moreover, for arbitrary $n = 1, 2, \ldots$, let $\mathcal{X}^{(n)}$ and $\Theta^{(n)}$ denote the set of all increasingly ordered n-tuples of pairwise different points in $\mathcal{X}$ and Θ, respectively, and define

$$\Delta_n \begin{pmatrix} x_1, \ldots, x_n \\ \theta_1, \ldots, \theta_n \end{pmatrix} \equiv \det \begin{pmatrix} p_{\theta_1}(x_1) & \cdots & p_{\theta_1}(x_n) \\ \vdots & \ddots & \vdots \\ p_{\theta_n}(x_1) & \cdots & p_{\theta_n}(x_n) \end{pmatrix} \tag{A.1}$$

for arbitrary $(x_1, \ldots, x_n) \in \mathcal{X}^{(n)}$, $(\theta_1, \ldots, \theta_n) \in \Theta^{(n)}$. Then, the family $(p_\theta(\cdot))_{\theta \in \Theta}$ is said to be strictly totally positive of order $r \geq 1$ (abbreviated to STP$_r$) if for each $n = 1, \ldots, r$ we have that

$$\Delta_n \begin{pmatrix} x_1, \ldots, x_n \\ \theta_1, \ldots, \theta_n \end{pmatrix} > 0 \ \forall \, ((x_1, \ldots, x_n), (\theta_1, \ldots, \theta_n)) \in \mathcal{X}^{(n)} \times \Theta^{(n)}. \tag{A.2}$$

If (A.2) holds true for every $n \in \mathbb{N}$, the family $(p_\theta(\cdot))_{\theta \in \Theta}$ is called strictly totally positive of order ∞ (STP$_\infty$).

Important special STP$_\infty$ families of probability densities on $\mathbb{R}$

A.1.2 Lemma. Let $\mathcal{X}$ be a Borelian set in $\mathbb{R}^1$, $\mu(\cdot)$ a σ-finite measure on $\mathcal{X}$, and $(P_\theta)_{\theta \in \Theta}$ a family of probability distributions on $\mathcal{X}$ such that Θ is a nondegenerate interval on the real line and for each $\theta \in \Theta$, a μ-density of P_θ is given by

$$p_\theta(x) = c(\theta) \exp\{\theta x\} h(x), \quad x \in \mathcal{X}, \tag{A.3}$$

with $c(\cdot) : \Theta \to \mathbb{R}_+$ and h as a Borel-measurable transformation from $\mathcal{X}$ to $\mathbb{R}_+$ [$\leftrightarrow$ one-parameter exponential family in x and θ]. Then, $(p_\theta(\cdot))_{\theta \in \Theta}$ is STP$_\infty$.

Proof. → Karlin (1968, p. 19). ∎

A.1.3 Lemma. For arbitrary $\nu \in \mathbb{N}$ and $\theta \in \mathbb{R}$ let $p_\theta(\,\cdot\,; \nu)$ be the density (with respect to Lebesgue measure) of a noncentral t-distribution with ν degrees of freedom and noncentrality parameter θ. Then it follows that $(p_\theta(\,\cdot\,; \nu))_{\theta \in \mathbb{R}}$ is STP_∞.

Proof. $\rightarrow$ Karlin [1968, §4(ii)].   ∎

A.1.4 Lemma. For any $(\nu_1, \nu_2) \in \mathbb{N}^2$, let V denote a random variable whose distribution is central F with ν_1 and ν_2 degrees of freedom. Furthermore, let $h_\varrho(\cdot)$ be the density function of $\varrho \cdot V$ where ϱ denotes any positive real number. Then, the family $(h_\varrho(\cdot))_{\varrho > 0}$ (occasionally called family of stretched F-densities with ν_1, ν_2 degrees of freedom – see, e.g., Witting, 1985, p. 217) is STP_∞.

Proof. Let (U_1, U_2) be an independent pair of random variables such that $\nu_1 U_1$ and $\nu_2 U_2$ has a central χ^2-distribution with ν_1 and ν_2 degrees of freedom, respectively. Moreover, define for any $(a, b) \in \mathbb{R}_+^2$ $\tilde{g}_{\nu_1}(a; b) \equiv b\, g_{\nu_1}(ab)$, $\tilde{g}_{\nu_2}(a; b) \equiv b\, g_{\nu_2}(ab)$ with $g_{\nu_1}(\cdot)$ and $g_{\nu_2}(\cdot)$ as the density function of U_1 and U_2, respectively. Clearly, for any $b > 0$, the density function of $b^{-1} \cdot U_1$ and $b^{-1} \cdot U_2$ is then given by $\tilde{g}_{\nu_1}(\,\cdot\,; b)$ and $\tilde{g}_{\nu_2}(\,\cdot\,; b)$ respectively.

By definition of V, we have hat $\varrho V \overset{d}{=} U_1/(\varrho^{-1} \cdot U_2)$. Hence, applying the well-known formula for the density of the product of two independent random variables of the absolutely continuous type (see, e.g., Kingman and Taylor, 1973, p. 299, Ex. 11.5.3), we can write for any $z \in \mathbb{R}_+$:

$$h_\varrho(z) = \int_0^\infty y\, g_{\nu_1}(yz)\, \tilde{g}_{\nu_2}(y; \varrho)\, dy = \int_0^\infty \tilde{g}_{\nu_1}(z; y)\, \tilde{g}_{\nu_2}(y; \varrho)\, dy. \quad (A.4)$$

As shown by Witting (1985, Theorem 2.33 a) the families $(\tilde{g}_{\nu_1}(\,\cdot\,; y))_{y > 0}$ and $(\tilde{g}_{\nu_2}(\,\cdot\,; \varrho))_{\varrho > 0}$ both exhibit the structure assumed in A.1.2 and are thus STP_∞. Hence, we can apply the composition theorem for pairs of strictly (totally) positive families (Karlin, 1968, p. 17) with $X = Z = Y = (0, \infty)$, $r = s = 1$, $K(z, y) = \tilde{g}_{\nu_1}(z; y)$, $L(y, \varrho) = \tilde{g}_{\nu_2}(y; \varrho)$, $\sigma = \lambda\big|_{(0,\infty)\,\mathcal{B}}$ yielding the proposed result.   ∎

Existence and basic properties of UMP tests for equivalence in STP$_3$ families of distributions

A.1.5 Theorem. Let α be an arbitrary real number in $(0\,,1)$, $\mathcal{X}$ a non-degenerate interval in $\mathbb{R}$, $\mathcal{B}_\mathcal{X}$ the Borelian σ-algebra on $\mathcal{X}$, μ a σ-finite measure on $\mathcal{B}_\mathcal{X}$ whose support contains at least two different points, and $(p_\theta(\cdot))_{\theta \in \Theta}$ an STP$_3$ family of μ-densities on $\mathcal{X}$ with Θ exhibiting the form of some nondegenerate interval on the real line as well. Assume further that the function $(x, \theta) \mapsto p_\theta(x)$ is continuous in both of its arguments, and that some fixed pair (θ_1, θ_2) of points in Θ with $\theta_1 < \theta_2$ is given. Then, the following statements hold true:

(i) For the problem $H : \theta \in \Theta \setminus (\theta_1, \theta_2)$ versus $K : \theta \in (\theta_1, \theta_2)$ there exists a UMP level-α test $\phi : \mathcal{X} \to [0, 1]$ given by

$$\phi(x) = \begin{cases} 1 & x \in (C_1, C_2) \\ \gamma_i & \text{for} \quad x = C_i, \ i = 1, 2 \ , \\ 0 & x \in \mathcal{X} \setminus [C_1, C_2] \end{cases} \tag{A.5}$$

where $C_i \in \mathcal{X}, \ i = 1, 2, \ C_1 \leq C_2$ and

$$E_{\theta_i}\phi(X) \equiv \int \phi \, p_{\theta_i} d\mu = \alpha \ \text{for} \quad i = 1, 2. \tag{A.6}$$

(ii) This ϕ minimizes the rejection probability $E_\theta \phi(X)$ uniformly in $\theta \in \Theta \setminus [\theta_1, \theta_2]$ among all tests which satisfy (A.6).

(iii) If the cardinality of the set which the dominating measure μ is concentrated upon, is greater than 2, then there exists a point $\theta_\circ \in (\theta_1, \theta_2)$ such that the power function $\theta \mapsto E_\theta \phi(X)$ of the UMP test is monotonically in- and decreasing on $(-\infty, \theta_\circ] \cap \Theta$ and $[\theta_\circ, \infty) \cap \Theta$, respectively.

Proof. A proof a weaker version of the theorem restricted to the special case that the underlying family of distributions exhibits the form (A.3), can be found in Lehmann (1986, Ch. 3.7). Proving the same result in full generality as repeatedly used in the present book, is left to the reader of Lehmann's book as an exercise worked out by Kallenberg et al. (1984, pp. 54–58). ∎

Simplified computation of the UMP test for equivalence under symmetry restrictions

A.1.6 Lemma. Under the assumptions and notational conventions of Theorem A.1.5, let the limits of the equivalence range for θ be chosen as $\theta_1 = -\varepsilon$, $\theta_2 = \varepsilon$, with arbitrarily fixed $\varepsilon > 0$. Suppose further that under $\theta = \varepsilon$ the random variable which the hypotheses H and K refer to, has the same distribution as $-X$ under $\theta = -\varepsilon$. Then, a UMP level-α test for $H : \theta \in \Theta \setminus (-\varepsilon, \varepsilon)$ versus $K : \theta \in (-\varepsilon, \varepsilon)$ is given by

$$\phi(x) = \begin{cases} 1 & |x| < C \\ \gamma & \text{if} \quad |x| = C \\ 0 & |x| > C \end{cases}, \tag{A.7}$$

where

$$C = \max\left\{ x \in [0, \infty) \,\Big|\, P_\varepsilon[|X| < x] \le \alpha \right\} \tag{A.8}$$

and

$$\gamma = \begin{cases} \dfrac{\alpha - P_\varepsilon[|X| < C]}{P_\varepsilon[|X| = C]} & P_\varepsilon[|X| = C] > 0 \\ \\ 0 & P_\varepsilon[|X| = C] = 0 \end{cases} \quad \text{for} \tag{A.9}$$

Proof. In view of (A.7) and (A.6), it suffices to show that

$$P_{-\varepsilon}[|X| < C] + \gamma P_{-\varepsilon}[|X| = C] = \alpha = P_\varepsilon[|X| < C] + \gamma P_\varepsilon[|X| = C].$$

The validity of the second of the above equalities is obvious since (A.8) and (A.9) simply give the solution to the equation $P_\varepsilon[|X| < x] + q P_\varepsilon[|X| = x] = \alpha$, $0 \le x < \infty$, $0 \le q < 1$. Furthermore, the assumption of the equality of the distribution of $-X$ with respect to $P_{-\varepsilon}$ and that of X with respect to P_ε trivially implies that we have $P_{-\varepsilon}[|X| \in B_+] = P_\varepsilon[|X| \in B_+]\ \forall\, B_+ \in \mathcal{B}_{[0,\infty)}$. Putting $B_+ = [0, C)$ and $B_+ = \{C\}$, respectively, this yields $P_{-\varepsilon}[|X| < C] + \gamma P_{-\varepsilon}[|X| = C] = P_\varepsilon[|X| < C] + \gamma P_\varepsilon[|X| = C]$, as required. ∎

A.1.7 Corollary. Suppose the assumptions of Theorem A.1.5 are satisfied, and there exist isotonic continuous mappings $T : \mathcal{X} \to \mathbb{R}$, $h : \Theta \to \mathbb{R}$ such that $Z \equiv h(\Theta)$ is an interval symmetric about zero and the distribution of $-T(X)$ under $h^{-1}(-\zeta)$ is the same as that of $T(X)$ under $h^{-1}(\zeta)$ for each $\zeta \in Z$. Furthermore, let $\theta_1 = h^{-1}(-\zeta_\circ)$, $\theta_2 = h^{-1}(\zeta_\circ)$ for some $\zeta_\circ \in Z \cap \mathbb{R}_+$, and define

$$t^* = \max\left\{t \in [0,\infty) \,\Big|\, P_{\theta_2}[|T(X)| < t] \leq \alpha\right\}, \tag{A.10}$$

$$C_1 = T^{-1}(-t^*), \quad C_2 = T^{-1}(t^*), \tag{A.11}$$

$$\gamma^* = \begin{cases} \dfrac{\alpha - P_{\theta_2}[|T(X)| < t^*]}{P_{\theta_2}[|T(X)| = t^*]} & P_{\theta_2}[|T(X)| = t^*] > 0 \\[2ex] \quad\quad 0 & P_{\theta_2}[|T(X)| = t^*] = 0 \end{cases} \quad \text{for} \quad , \tag{A.12}$$

$$\phi(x) = \begin{cases} 1 & C_1 < x < C_2 \\ \gamma^* & \text{if} \quad x \in \{C_1, C_2\} \\ 0 & x \in \mathcal{X} \setminus [C_1, C_2] \end{cases} . \tag{A.13}$$

Then, ϕ is a UMP level-α test for $H : \theta \in \Theta \setminus (\theta_1, \theta_2)$ versus $K : \theta \in (\theta_1, \theta_2)$. If we consider the rejection probability ϕ as a function of $\zeta = h(\theta)$, the latter is symmetric about $\zeta = 0$ and increases (decreases) on the left (right) of zero.

Proof. Continuity and isotony of the mapping h and injectivity of the transformation T imply that the problem H versus K originally put forward is the same as that of testing $H^* : \zeta \in Z \setminus (-\zeta_\circ, \zeta_\circ)$ versus $K^* : \zeta \in (-\zeta_\circ, \zeta_\circ)$ in the family of distributions of $T(X)$.

For brevity, let us denote $P^{T(X)}_{h^{-1}(\zeta)}$, i.e., the distribution of $T(X)$ under $\theta = h^{-1}(\zeta)$, by P^*_ζ, and the image $T(\mu)$ of the basic measure μ under the transformation T by μ^*. Then, it is readily verified by means of the transformation theorem for μ-integrals (see, e.g., Halmos, 1974, p. 163) that a density of P^*_ζ with respect to μ^* is given by $p^*_\zeta = p_{h^{-1}(\zeta)} \circ T^{-1}$. Since, by assumption, both T and h are continuous and isotonic, it is clear that $(p^*_\zeta)_{\zeta \in Z}$ shares with $(p_\theta)_{\theta \in \Theta}$ the property of being an STP$_3$ family satisfying the continuity conditions of Theorem A.1.5. Thus, all prerequisites are fulfilled for an application of the above Lemma A.1.6 with $(T(X), \zeta, \zeta_\circ)$ instead of (X, θ, ε). Accordingly, we can conclude that a UMP level-α test ϕ^* for H^* versus K^* is obtained by computing the critical constants t^*, γ^* from

$$t^* = \max\left\{t \in [0,\infty) \,\Big|\, P^*_{\zeta_\circ}[|T(X)| < t] \leq \alpha\right\}, \tag{A.8*}$$

$$\gamma^* = \begin{cases} \dfrac{\alpha - P^*_{\zeta_\circ}[|T(X)| < t^*]}{P^*_{\zeta_\circ}[|T(X)| = t^*]} & P^*_{\zeta_\circ}[|T(X)| = t^*] > 0 \\[2ex] \quad\quad 0 & P^*_{\zeta_\circ}[|T(X)| = t^*] = 0 \end{cases} \quad \text{for} \quad , \tag{A.9*}$$

and defining ϕ^* by

$$\phi^*(t) \quad = \quad \begin{cases} 1 & |t| < t^* \\ \gamma^* & \text{for} \quad |t| = t^* \\ 0 & |t| > t^* \end{cases} . \tag{A.7*}$$

In view of $P^*_{\zeta_0} \equiv P^{T(X)}_{h^{-1}(\zeta_0)} = P^{T(X)}_{\theta_2}$, we obviously have (A.8*) $\Leftrightarrow$ (A.10) and (A.9*) $\Leftrightarrow$ (A.12). Moreover, the assumptions made on the transformation T ensure that there holds $\phi(x) = \phi^*(T(x)) \ \forall x \in \mathcal{X}$ with ϕ and (C_1, C_2) defined as in (A.13) and (A.11), respectively. Hence ϕ is obtained by representing the UMP level-α test ϕ^* for H^* vs. K^* as a function of x rather than t which in view of the equivalence of the testing problems (H, K) and (H^*, K^*) implies that ϕ is indeed UMP among all level-α tests for the former.

Thus, it only remains to show that the function $\zeta \mapsto E_{h^{-1}(\zeta)}\phi(X)$ is symmetric about zero and exhibits the monotonicity properties stated in the second part of the corollary. By $\phi = \phi^* \circ T$, $P^*_\zeta = T\big(P_{h^{-1}(\zeta)}\big)$, we may write for arbitrary $\zeta \in Z$:

$$E_{h^{-1}(\zeta)}\phi(X) \equiv \int \phi \, dP_{h^{-1}(\zeta)} = \int \phi^* \circ T \, dP_{h^{-1}(\zeta)} = \int \phi^* \, dP^*_\zeta . \tag{A.14}$$

By construction, ϕ^* is a UMP level-α test for $H^* : \zeta \in Z \backslash (-\zeta_0, \zeta_0)$ versus $K^* : \zeta \in (-\zeta_0, \zeta_0)$ with ζ as the parameter of a family of distributions which satisfies the conditions of Theorem A.1.5. By part (iii) of A.1.5, it thus follows that the interval $(-\zeta_0, \zeta_0)$ contains some point ζ^*_0 such that the function $\zeta \mapsto \int \phi^* dP^*_\zeta$ in- and decreases strictly on $Z \cap (-\infty, \zeta^*_0]$ and $Z \cap [\zeta^*_0, \infty)$, respectively.

From (A..7*), it is obvious that we may write $\phi^*(T(x)) = \psi^*(|T(x)|)$ $\forall x \in \mathcal{X}$ with $\psi^* \equiv I_{[0, C^*)} + \gamma^* I_{\{C^*\}}$. Hence, we can replace the middle of the equations (A.14) with

$$E_{h^{-1}(\zeta)}\phi(X) = \int \psi^* \, d\Big(|T|(P_{h^{-1}(\zeta)})\Big) . \tag{A.15}$$

The assumption $(-T)\big(P_{h^{-1}(-\zeta)}\big) = T\big(P_{h^{-1}(\zeta)}\big)$ clearly implies that the measure which respect to which the integral on the right-hand side of (A.15) has to be taken, coincides with $|T|(P_{h^{-1}(-\zeta)})$, so that we have $E_{h^{-1}(-\zeta)}\phi(X) = E_{h^{-1}(\zeta)}\phi(X) \ \forall \zeta \in Z$ which establishes the asserted symmetry of the power function $\zeta \mapsto E_{h^{-1}(\zeta)}\phi(X)$. But a function which is symmetric about zero can only attain a strict global maximum, if the latter is attained at 0. ∎

A.2 UMPU equivalence tests in multiparameter exponential families

A.2.1 Definition. Let $(\mathcal{X}, \mathcal{B}_\mathcal{X})$ be a measurable space, μ a σ-finite measure on $(\mathcal{X}, \mathcal{B}_\mathcal{X})$, $\Theta \subseteq \mathbb{R}$, $\Omega \subseteq \mathbb{R}^k$, $k \in \mathbb{N}$. Suppose further that for each $(\theta, \boldsymbol{\vartheta}) = (\theta, \vartheta_1, \ldots, \vartheta_k) \in \Theta \times \Omega$, $P_{\theta, \boldsymbol{\vartheta}}$ is a probability distribution on $\mathbf{X}$ having a μ-density of the form

$$p_{\theta, \boldsymbol{\vartheta}}(x) = c(\theta, \boldsymbol{\vartheta}) \exp\left\{\theta\, T(x) + \sum_{j=1}^k \vartheta_j\, S_j(x)\right\}, \quad x \in \mathcal{X}, \qquad (\text{A.16})$$

with $c(\theta, \boldsymbol{\vartheta}) \in \mathbb{R}_+ \; \forall (\theta, \; \boldsymbol{\vartheta})$ and $T(\cdot), S_1(\cdot), \ldots, S_k(\cdot)$ as $\mathcal{B}_\mathcal{X}$-measurable transformations from $\mathcal{X}$ to $\mathbb{R}$. Then, $\left(P_{\theta, \boldsymbol{\vartheta}}\right)_{(\theta, \boldsymbol{\vartheta}) \in \Theta \times \Omega}$ is called a $(k+1)$-parameter exponential family in $(\theta, \vartheta_1, \ldots, \vartheta_k)$ and $(T, S_1, \ldots, S_k)$.

A.2.2 Theorem. In the situation described by the above definition, let Θ and Ω be a nondegenerate interval in $\mathbb{R}^1$ and $\mathbb{R}^k$, respectively, and (θ_1, θ_2) a pair of points in Θ satisfying $\theta_1 < \theta_2$. Then, at any level $\alpha \in (0, 1)$, there exists a uniformly most powerful unbiased (UMPU) test $x \mapsto \phi\big(T(x), \boldsymbol{S}(x)\big)$ for

$$H : (\theta, \boldsymbol{\vartheta}) \in \big(\Theta \setminus (\theta_1, \theta_2)\big) \times \Omega \quad \text{versus} \quad K : (\theta, \boldsymbol{\vartheta}) \in (\theta_1, \theta_2) \times \Omega \; . \; (\text{A.17})$$

Given the value $\boldsymbol{s}$ of the statistic $\boldsymbol{S} \equiv (S_1, \ldots, S_k) : \mathcal{X} \to \mathbb{R}^k$, $\phi(\,\cdot\,, \boldsymbol{s}) : T(\mathcal{X}) \to [0, 1]$ is obtained by constructing by means of Theorem A.1.5 a UMP level-α test for the problem $H_{\boldsymbol{s}} : \theta \in \Theta \setminus (\theta_1, \theta_2)$ versus $K_{\boldsymbol{s}} : \theta \in (\theta_1, \theta_2)$ concerning the family $\left(P_\theta^{T(X)|\boldsymbol{s}}\right)_{\theta \in \Theta}$ of conditional distributions of $T(X)$ given $\{\boldsymbol{S} = \boldsymbol{s}\}$.

Proof. See Lehmann (1986, Ch. 4.4). ∎

A.3 A sufficient condition for the asymptotic validity of tests for equivalence

A.3.1 Definition. For each $N \in \mathbb{N}$, let $X^{(N)} = (X_1, \ldots, X_N)$ be a vector of p-dimensional ($p \in \mathbb{N}$) random variables on a common probability space $(\Omega, \mathcal{A}, P)$. Suppose the distribution of $X^{(N)}$ is determined by a fixed number $k \geq 1$ (independent of N) of p-dimensional distribution functions $F_1, \ldots, F_k$ in the following way:

$$
\begin{aligned}
X_1, \ldots, X_{n_1(N)} &\sim F_1 \\
X_{n_1(N)+1}, \ldots, X_{n_2(N)} &\sim F_2 \\
\vdots \qquad\qquad &\ \ \vdots \ \ \vdots \\
X_{n_{k-1}(N)+1}, \ldots, X_{n_k(N)} &\sim F_k \,,
\end{aligned}
$$

where $n_1(N) + \ldots + n_k(N) = N$. Furthermore, let $\theta(\cdot)$ denote some functional on the underlying space of cdf's, $\mathcal{H}$ the class of all vectors $\boldsymbol{F} = (F_1, \ldots, F_k)$ of cdf's satisfying the null hypotheses $H : \theta(\boldsymbol{F}) \in \Theta \setminus (\theta_1, \theta_2)$, and $P_{\boldsymbol{F}}^{(N)}$ the common distribution of $(X_1, \ldots, X_N)$ under $\boldsymbol{F}$.

A test $\phi_N : \mathbb{R}^{pN} \to [0, 1]$ is said to be asymptotically valid at level $\alpha \in (0, 1)$ for H if we have

$$
\limsup_{N \to \infty} E_{\boldsymbol{F}}(\phi_N) \leq \alpha \quad \forall \ \boldsymbol{F} \in \mathcal{H} \tag{A.18}
$$

where

$$
E_{\boldsymbol{F}}^{(N)}(\phi_N) \equiv \int \phi_N(x_1, \ldots, x_N) \, dP_{\boldsymbol{F}}^{(N)}(x_1, \ldots, x_N) \,. \tag{A.19}
$$

A.3.2 Lemma. For any $s > 0$ denote

$$
c_\alpha^{\theta_1, \theta_2}(s) = C_\alpha\big(s\,(\theta_2 - \theta_1)/2\big) \tag{A.20}
$$

with $C_\alpha(\psi)$ as the square root of the α-quantile of a χ^2-distribution with a single degree of freedom and noncentrality parameter $\psi^2 > 0$. Then

$$
c_\alpha^{\theta_1, \theta_2}(s) - s\,(\theta_2 - \theta_1)/2 \to u_\alpha \quad \text{as} \ \ s \to \infty \tag{A.21}
$$

provided that $u_\alpha = \Phi^{-1}(\alpha)$.

Proof. $\to$ Wellek (1996, p. 707). ∎

A.3.3 Lemma. For each natural number N let S_N be a positive random variable on some probability space $(\Omega, \mathcal{A}, P_N)$ such that $S_N \overset{P_N}{\to} c$ as $N \to \infty$ for some $c \in (0, \infty)$, $q(\cdot)$ a function from $(0, \infty)$ into $\mathbb{R}$ converging to some $y^* \in \mathbb{R}$ as $s \to \infty$, and (a_N) a sequence of positive real numbers with $a_N \to +\infty$ as $N \to \infty$. Then, we can conclude that

$$q(a_N S_N) \overset{P_N}{\to} y^* \quad \text{as} \quad N \to \infty \ . \tag{A.22}$$

Proof. $\to$ Wellek (1996, p. 707). ∎

A.3.4 Theorem. Let $\left(X^{(N)}\right)_{N \in \mathbb{N}}$ be as specified in A.3.1 with $\mathcal{F}$ as the underlying class of k-tuples of distribution functions, and assume that for each $N \in \mathbb{N}$, a test statistic T_N on the sample space of $X^{(N)}$ is given such that we have

$$\frac{\sqrt{N}(T_N - \theta(\boldsymbol{F}))}{\sigma(\boldsymbol{F})} \overset{\mathcal{L}}{\to} Z \sim \mathcal{N}(0, 1) \quad \text{as} \quad N \to \infty \ \forall \boldsymbol{F} \in \mathcal{F} \tag{A.23}$$

for suitable functionals $\theta(\cdot) : \mathcal{F} \to \mathbb{R}$ and $\sigma(\cdot) : \mathcal{F} \to \mathbb{R}_+$. Suppose further, that $(\hat{\sigma}_N)_{N \in \mathbb{N}}$ is a consistent estimator of $\sigma(\boldsymbol{F})$ for each $\boldsymbol{F} \in \mathcal{F}$, and $c_\alpha^{\theta_1, \theta_2}(\cdot)$ is as in (A.20). If we then define

$$\phi_N\left(X^{(N)}\right) = \begin{cases} 1 & \sqrt{N}|T_N - \theta_\circ|/\hat{\sigma}_N < c_\alpha^{\theta_1, \theta_2}\left(\sqrt{N}/\hat{\sigma}_N\right) \\ & \text{for} \\ 0 & \sqrt{N}|T_N - \theta_\circ|/\hat{\sigma}_N \geq c_\alpha^{\theta_1, \theta_2}\left(\sqrt{N}/\hat{\sigma}_N\right) \end{cases} \tag{A.24}$$

with $\theta_\circ \equiv (\theta_1 + \theta_2)/2$, we can be sure that $(\phi_N)_{N \in \mathbb{N}}$ is asymptotically valid at level $\alpha \in (0, 1)$ for $H : \theta(\boldsymbol{F}) \in \Theta \setminus (\theta_1, \theta_2)$ versus $K : \theta(\boldsymbol{F}) \in (\theta_1, \theta_2)$.

Proof. First we consider an arbitrarily fixed $\boldsymbol{F} \in \mathcal{H}$ such that $\theta(\boldsymbol{F}) \geq \theta_2$ and write for brevity $\theta(\boldsymbol{F}) = \theta$, $\sigma(\boldsymbol{F})/\sqrt{N} = \tau_N$, $\hat{\sigma}_N/\sqrt{N} = \hat{\tau}_N$. By definition of $\phi_N(\cdot)$, we have

$$\begin{aligned} E_{\boldsymbol{F}}^{(N)}(\phi_N) &= P_{\boldsymbol{F}}^{(N)}\left[(T_N - \theta_\circ)/\hat{\tau}_N < c_\alpha^{\theta_1, \theta_2}(1/\hat{\tau}_N)\right] - \\ &\quad P_{\boldsymbol{F}}^{(N)}\left[(T_N - \theta_\circ)/\hat{\tau}_N \leq -c_\alpha^{\theta_1, \theta_2}(1/\hat{\tau}_N)\right] \\ &\leq P_{\boldsymbol{F}}^{(N)}\left[(T_N - \theta)/\hat{\tau}_N + (\theta - \theta_\circ)/\hat{\tau}_N - c_\alpha^{\theta_1, \theta_2}(1/\hat{\tau}_N) < 0\right] \\ &\leq P_{\boldsymbol{F}}^{(N)}\left[(T_N - \theta)/\hat{\tau}_N + (\theta_2 - \theta_1)/2\hat{\tau}_N - c_\alpha^{\theta_1, \theta_2}(1/\hat{\tau}_N) < 0\right] \tag{A.25} \\ &\text{by} \quad \theta \geq \theta_2, \quad \theta_\circ = (\theta_1 + \theta_2)/2 \ . \end{aligned}$$

By assumption (A.23) and consistency of $(\hat{\sigma}_N)_{N \in \mathbb{N}}$ for $\sigma(\boldsymbol{F})$ we can write:

$$P_{\boldsymbol{F}}^{(N)}\left[(T_N - \theta)/\hat{\tau}_N < w\right] \to \Phi(w) \quad \text{as} \quad N \to \infty \quad \forall w \in \mathbb{R} \tag{A.26}$$

and

$$N^{1/2}\hat{\tau}_N \xrightarrow{P_{\boldsymbol{F}}^{(N)}} \sigma^* \quad \text{as } N \to \infty \quad \text{for some } \sigma^* \in (0, \infty). \tag{A.27}$$

In view of (A.20) and (A.21) all the conditions of Lemma A.3.3 are satisfied if we put $P_N = P_{\boldsymbol{F}}^{(N)}$, $S_N = \left(N^{1/2}\hat{\tau}_N\right)^{-1}$, $c = 1/\sigma^*$, $q(s) = c_\alpha^{\theta_1, \theta_2}(s) - s\,(\theta_2 - \theta_1)/2$, $y^* = u_\alpha$, and $a_N = N^{1/2}$. Hence, it follows that

$$(\theta_2 - \theta_1)/2\hat{\tau}_N - c_\alpha^{\theta_1, \theta_2}(1/\hat{\tau}_N) \xrightarrow{P_{\boldsymbol{F}}^{(N)}} -u_\alpha \quad \text{as } N \to \infty. \tag{A.28}$$

Combining (A.28) with (A.26) gives

$$P_{\boldsymbol{F}}^{(N)}\left[(T_N - \theta)/\hat{\tau}_N + (\theta_2 - \theta_1)/2\hat{\tau}_N - c_\alpha^{\theta_1, \theta_2}(1/\hat{\tau}_N) < w\right]$$
$$\to \Phi(w + u_\alpha) \quad \text{as } N \to \infty \quad \forall w \in \mathbb{R}. \tag{A.29}$$

Taking $w = 0$ in (A.29) shows that the expression on the right-hand side of (A.25) converges to α as $N \to \infty$ which completes the $\theta \geq \theta_2$ half of the proof.

Let us now choose $\boldsymbol{F} \in \mathcal{H}$ such that $\theta = \theta(\boldsymbol{F}) \leq \theta_1$. Then $E_{\boldsymbol{F}}^{(N)}(\phi_N)$ can be bounded above in the following way:

$$E_{\boldsymbol{F}}^{(N)}(\phi_N) \leq 1 - P_{\boldsymbol{F}}^{(N)}\left[(T_N - \theta_\circ)/\hat{\tau}_N \leq -c_\alpha^{\theta_1, \theta_2}(1/\hat{\tau}_N)\right]$$
$$= 1 - P_{\boldsymbol{F}}^{(N)}\left[(T_N - \theta)/\hat{\tau}_N + (\theta - \theta_\circ)/\hat{\tau}_N + c_\alpha^{\theta_1, \theta_2}(1/\hat{\tau}_N) \leq 0\right]$$
$$\leq 1 - P_{\boldsymbol{F}}^{(N)}\left[(T_N - \theta)/\hat{\tau}_N - (\theta_2 - \theta_1)/2\hat{\tau}_N + c_\alpha^{\theta_1, \theta_2}(1/\hat{\tau}_N) \leq 0\right] \tag{A.30}$$

by $\theta \leq \theta_1$, $\theta_\circ = (\theta_1 + \theta_2)/2$.

Since relations (A.26) and (A.28) hold true for any $\boldsymbol{F}$ with $0 < \theta(\boldsymbol{F}) < 1$ we get in direct analogy to (A.29)

$$P_{\boldsymbol{F}}^{(N)}\left[(T_N - \theta)/\hat{\tau}_N - (\theta_2 - \theta_1)/2\hat{\tau}_N + c_\alpha^{\theta_1, \theta_2}(1/\hat{\tau}_N) \leq w\right]$$
$$\to \Phi(w - u_\alpha) \quad \text{as } N \to \infty \quad \forall w \in \mathbb{R}. \tag{A.31}$$

Specifying $w = 0$ in this latter relation shows that the right-hand side of (A.30) converges to $1 - \Phi(-u_\alpha)$ as $N \to \infty$ so that the $\theta \leq \theta_1$ part of the proof is complete as well. ∎

List of special computer programs

Program Name	Objective	Language	→ p.
bi2ste1	Power of the exact Fisher type test for noninferiority	Fortran	23
bi2ste2	Sample sizes for the exact Fisher type test for noninferiority	Fortran	24
bi2ste3	Increased nominal significance level for the nonrandomized version of the exact Fisher type test for noninferiority	Fortran	26
postmys	Bayesian posterior probability of the alternative hypothesis $\varepsilon_1 < \delta/\sigma_D < \varepsilon_2$ in the setting of the one-sample t-test	SAS	35
exp1st	Critical constants and power against the null alternative of the UMP test for equivalence of the hazard rate of a single exponential distribution to some given reference value	SAS	53
bi1st	Critical constants and power against the alternative $p = (p_1 + p_2)/2$ of the UMP test for equivalence of a single binomial proportion to some given reference value	SAS	56
powsign	Nonconditional power of the UMPU sign test for equivalence and its nonrandomized counterpart against the alternative $p_+ = p_-$	SAS	67
mcnemasc	Corrected nominal significance level for the asymptotic test for equivalence of two paired binomial proportions with respect to the difference of their expectations (McNemar setting)	SAS	75

Program Name	Objective	Language	→ p.
mcnempow	Exact rejection probability of the asymptotic test for equivalence of two paired binomial proportions with respect to the difference of their expectations (McNemar setting) at any nominal level under an arbitrary parameter configuration	*SAS*	77
tt1st	Critical constants and power against the null alternative of the one-sample *t*-test for equivalence with an arbitrary, maybe nonsymmetric choice of the limits of the equivalence range for δ/σ_D	*SAS*	82
sgnrk	Signed rank test for equivalence of an arbitrary continuous distribution of the intraindividual differences to a distribution satisfying $q_+ \equiv P[D_i + D_j > 0] = 1/2$: Test statistic and critical upper bound	*SAS*	84
srktie_d	Generalized signed rank test for equivalence for tied data: Test statistic and critical upper bound	*SAS*	94
srktie_m	Analogue to srktie_d for settings where the distribution of the D_i is concentrated on a finite lattice	*SAS*	95
tt2st	Critical constants and power against the null alternative of the two-sample *t*-test for equivalence with an arbitrary, maybe nonsymmetric choice of the limits of the equivalence range for $(\xi - \eta)/\sigma$	*SAS*	104
mawi	Mann-Whitney test for equivalence of two continuous distributions of arbitrary shape: Test statistic and critical upper bound	*SAS*	108
mwtie_xy	Distribution-free two-sample equivalence test for tied data: Test statistic and critical upper bound	*SAS*	118
mwtie_fr	Analogue to mwtie_xy for settings with grouped data	*SAS*	119

Program Name	Objective	Language	→ p.
fstretch	Critical constants and power against $\sigma^2 = \tau^2$ of the UMPI test for dispersion equivalence of two Gaussian distributions	SAS	128
bi2st	Critical constants for the exact Fisher type UMPU test for equivalence of two binomial distributions with respect to the odds ratio	SAS	135
bi2aeq1	Power of the exact Fisher type test for equivalence	Fortran	135
bi2aeq2	Sample sizes for the exact Fisher type test for equivalence	Fortran	135
bi2aeq3	Increased nominal significance level for the nonrandomized version of the exact Fisher type test for equivalence	Fortran	138
bi2diffac	Corrected nominal significance level for the asymptotic test for equivalence of two unrelated binomial proportions with respect to the difference of their population counterparts	SAS	142
bi2dipow	Exact rejection probability of the asymptotic test for equivalence of two unrelated binomial proportions with respect to the difference of their expectations at any nominal level under an arbitrary parameter configuration	SAS	144
gofsimpt	Establishing goodness of fit of an observed to a fully specified multinomial distribution: Test statistic and critical bound	SAS	180
gofind_t	Establishing approximate independence in a two-way contingency table: Test statistic and critical bound	SAS	187

Program Name	Objective	Language	→ p.
pow_abe	interval inclusion test for average bioequivalence: exact power against an arbitrary specific alternative	*SAS*	212
po_pbibe	Bayesian posterior probability of the alternative hypothesis of individual bioequivalence	*SAS*	225

Frequently used special symbols and abbreviations

BE	bioequivalence
cdf	cumulative distribution function
iff	if and only if
df	number of degrees of freedom
λ_{nc}^2	noncentrality parameter
STP_r	strictly totally positive of order r, with $r \in \mathbb{N}$ or $r = \infty$
$\phi(\cdot)$	critical function of a test
UMP	uniformly most powerful
UMPU	uniformly most powerful unbiased
UMPI	uniformly most powerful invariant
$\mathbb{N}$	set of natural numbers
$\mathbb{N}_0$	" " nonnegative integers
$\mathbb{R}$	" " real numbers
$\mathbb{R}_+$	" " positive real numbers
$\mathbb{Z}$	" " integers
$\# A$	number of elements of an arbitrary finite set A
$I_A(x)$	indicator function of a given subset $A \subseteq \mathbb{R}$ at $x \in \mathbb{R}$
$\mathbf{1}_{(r,s)}$	$r \times s$ matrix with all elements equal to 1.
$d^2(\boldsymbol{u}, \boldsymbol{v})$	squared Euclidean distance between any two vectors $\boldsymbol{u}$, $\boldsymbol{v}$ of the same dimension
$\equiv$	equal by definition
$\stackrel{d}{=}$	equal in distribution
$\times$	Cartesian product of sets
$\stackrel{P}{\to}$	convergence in probability
$\stackrel{\mathcal{L}}{\to}$	convergence in law
$X \sim \mathcal{D}$	random variable X follows distribution $\mathcal{D}$
$\mathcal{U}(a,b)$	uniform distribution over the interval $(a,b) \subseteq \mathbb{R}$

$\mathcal{B}(n,p)$	binomial distribution with parameters $n \in \mathbb{N}_0$ and $p \in [0,1]$
$b(k\,;n,p)$	probability mass function of $\mathcal{B}(n,p)$ evaluated at $k \in \{0,1,\ldots,n\}$
$h_s^{m,n}(x;\rho)$	probability mass function at x of the conditional distribution of $X \sim \mathcal{B}(m,p_1)$ given $X+Y=s$, with $Y \sim \mathcal{B}(n,p_2)$ independent of X and $\rho = p_1(1-p_2)/(1-p_1)p_2$
$\mathcal{E}(\sigma)$	exponential distribution with scale parameter $\sigma \in \mathbb{R}_+$
$\Gamma(x)$	gamma function (complete gamma integral) at $x > 0$
$\mathcal{N}(\xi,\sigma^2)$	normal distribution with expectation $\xi \in \mathbb{R}$ and variance $\sigma^2 \in \mathbb{R}_+$
$\varphi(\cdot)$	density function of $\mathcal{N}(0,1)$
$\Phi(\cdot)$	cdf of $\mathcal{N}(0,1)$
$\Phi^{-1}(\cdot)$	quantile function of $\mathcal{N}(0,1)$
$u_{1-\alpha}$	$\Phi^{-1}(1-\alpha)$, for arbitrary $\alpha \in (0,1)$
$\chi^2_{\nu;\gamma}$	γ-quantile $(0 < \gamma < 1)$ of a central χ^2-distribution with ν degrees of freedom
$C_\alpha(\psi)$	square root of the α-quantile $(0 < \alpha < 1)$ of a noncentral χ^2-distribution with a single degree of freedom and $\lambda^2_{nc} = \psi^2$ $(\psi \in \mathbb{R}_+)$
$C_{\alpha;\tilde{\varepsilon}}$	$= C_\alpha(\tilde{\varepsilon})$, with $(-\tilde{\varepsilon},\tilde{\varepsilon})$ as the equivalence range for the expectation of a Gaussian distribution with unit variance
$\chi^2_{\nu;\gamma}(\psi^2)$	γ-quantile $(0 < \gamma < 1)$ of a noncentral χ^2-distribution with ν degrees of freedom and $\lambda^2_{nc} = \psi^2$
$g_\nu(\cdot)$	density of a χ-distribution with ν degrees of freedom
$F^T_\nu(\cdot)$	cdf of a central t-distribution with ν degrees of freedom
$t_{\nu;\gamma}$	γ-quantile $(0 < \gamma < 1)$ of a central t-distribution with ν degrees of freedom
F_{ν_1,ν_2}	cdf of a central F-distribution with ν_1, ν_2 degrees of freedom
$F_{\nu_1,\nu_2;\gamma}(\psi^2)$	γ-quantile of a noncentral F-distribution with ν_1, ν_2 degrees of freedom and $\lambda^2_{nc} = \psi^2$
$\mathcal{F}_{\nu_1,\nu_2}(\psi^2)$	random variable following a noncentral F-distribution with ν_1, ν_2 degrees of freedom and $\lambda^2_{nc} = \psi^2$
p_+	$P[D_i > 0]$, with D_i as the ith intra-subject difference obtained from a sample of paired observations
p_0	$P[D_i = 0]$, with D_i as above
p_-	$P[D_i < 0]$, " " "

q_+	$P[D_i + D_j > 0]$, with D_i, D_j as the intra-subject difference for two different observational units in a paired-data setting
q_0	$P[D_i + D_j = 0]$, with D_i, D_j as above
q_-	$P[D_i + D_j < 0]$, " " " "
U_+	U-statistic estimator of q_+
U_0	U-statistic estimator of q_0
π_+	$P[X_i > Y_j]$, with X_i and Y_j as independent observations from two different univariate distributions under comparison
π_0	$P[X_i = Y_j]$, with X_i and Y_j as above
W_+	U-statistic estimator of π_+
W_0	U-statistic estimator of π_0
$\|S_1 - S_2\|$	$\sup_{t>0} |S_1(t) - S_2(t)|$, with $S_1(\cdot)$, $S_2(\cdot)$ as two survivor functions of the continuous type
$\lambda_\nu(t)$	hazard function at $t \geq 0$ of the νth sample ($\nu = 1, 2$)
$I_N(\hat{\beta})$	observed information evaluated at the maximum likelihood estimate of the regression coefficient $\beta \in \mathbb{R}$
ϕ_T, ϕ_R	"direct" effect of drug formulation T ($\leftrightarrow$ "Test") and R ($\leftrightarrow$ "Reference"), respectively
π_k	kth period effect in a 2×2 crossover trial ($k = 1, 2$)
σ_S^2	between-subject variance in a standard BE trial
$\sigma_{eT}^2, \sigma_{eR}^2$	within-subject variance associated with drug formulation T and R, respectively
$\sigma_{TT}^2, \sigma_{TR}^2$	total variance of the bioavailability of drug formulation T and R, respectively
X_{ki}	bioavailability measured in the ith subject ($i = 1, \ldots, m$) of sequence group T/R during the kth period ($k = 1, 2$) of a standard bioequivalence trial
X_i^-	$X_{1i} - X_{2i}$
μ^-	$E(X_i^-)$
Y_{kj}	bioavailability measured in the jth subject ($j = 1, \ldots, n$) of sequence group R/T during the kth period ($k = 1, 2$) of a standard bioequivalence trial
Y_j^-	$Y_{1j} - Y_{2j}$
ν^-	$E(Y_j^-)$
$\lambda^{(1)}, \lambda^{(2)}$	carryover effect of the treatment administered in the first period of a 2×2 crossover trial for the 1st ($\leftrightarrow T/R$) and 2nd ($\leftrightarrow R/T$) sequence group

References

Abramowitz, M.x and Stegun, I.(1965) *Handbook of Mathematical Functions.* New York: Dover Publications, Inc.

Andersen, P.K., Borgan, Ø., Gill, R.D. and Keiding, N.(1991) *Statistical Models Based on Counting Processes.* New York: Springer-Verlag.

Andersen, P.K. and Gill, R.D. (1982) Cox's regression model for counting processes: A large sample study. *Ann. Statist.* **10**, 1100–1120.

Anderson, S. and Hauck, W. W. (1983) A new procedure for testing equivalence in comparative bioavailability trials. *Commun. Statist. Theory Methods* **12**, 2663–2692.

Anderson, S. and Hauck, W. W. (1990) Consideration of individual bioequivalence. *J. Pharmacokin. Biopharm.* **18**, 259–73.

Anderson, T.W. (1984) *An Introduction to Multivariate Statistical Analysis. Second Edition.* New York: John Wiley & Sons, Inc.

Armitage, P. (1955) Tests for linear trends in proportions and frequencies. *Biometrics* **11**, 375–386.

Bailey, C.C., Gnekow, A., Wellek, S., Jones, M., Round, C., Brown, J., Philips, A., Neidhardt, M.K. (1995) Prospective randomized trial of chemotherapy given before radiotherapy in childhood medulloblastoma. International Society of Paediatric Oncology (SIOP) and the (German) Society of Paediatric Oncology (GPO): SIOP II. *Med. Pediatr. Oncol.* **25**, 166–178.

Berger, J.O. (1985) *Statistical Decision Theory and Bayesian Analysis. Second Edition.* New York: Springer-Verlag.

Bickel, P.J. and Doksum, K.A. (1977) *Mathematical Statistics: Basic Ideas and Selected Topics.* San Francisco: Holden-Day, Inc.

Bishop, Y.M.M., Fienberg, S.E. and Holland, P.W. (1975) *Discrete Multivariate Analysis: Theory and Practice.* Cambridge, Mass.: MIT Press.

Blackwelder, W.C. (1982) "Proving the null hypothesis" in clinical trials. *Control. Clin. Tr.* **3**, 345–53.

Bondy, W.H. (1969) A test of an experimental hypothesis of negligible difference between means. *Amer. Statist.* **23**, 28–30.

Boschloo, R.D. (1970) Raised conditional level of significance for the $2 \times 2-$table when testing the equality of two probabilities. *Statist. Neerlandica* **24**, 1-35.

Box, G.P.E. and Tiao, G.C. (1973) *Bayesian Inference in Statistical Analysis.* Reading, Mass.: Addison-Wesley.

Brown, B.Wm. (1980) The crossover experiment for clinical trials. *Biometrics* **36**, 69–79.

Brown, L.D., Hwang, G.T.J. and Munk, A. (1997) An unbiased test for the bioequivalence problem. *Ann. Statist.* **25**, 2345–67.

Casella, G. and Berger, R.L. (1987) Reconciling Bayesian and frequentist evidence in one-sided testing problems. *J. Amer. Statist. Assoc.* **82**, 106–11.

Chan, I.S.F. (1998) Exact tests of equivalence and efficacy with a non-zero lower bound for comparative studies. *Statist. Med.* **17**, 1403–13.

Chan, I.S.F. and Zhang, Z. (1999) Test-based exact confidence intervals for the difference of two binomial proportions. *Biometrics* **55**, 1202–09.

Chen, M.-L. (1997) Individual Bioequivalence - A Regulatory Update. *J. Biopharm. Statist.* **7**, 5–11 (1997).

Chester, S.T. (1986) Review of equivalence and hypothesis testing. *ASA Proceedings of the Biopharmaceutical Section*, 177–82.

Chinchilli, V.M., Elswick, R.K. Jr. (1997) The multivariate assessment of bioequivalence. *J. Biopharm. Statist.* **7**, 113–123 (1997).

Chow, S.-C. and Liu, J.-P. (1992) *Design and Analysis of Bioavailability and Bioequivalence Studies.* New York: Marcel Dekker.

Cox, D.R. (1958) Some problems connected with statistical inference. *Ann. Math. Statist.* **29**, 357–72.

Cox, D.R. and Hinkley, D.V. (1974) *Theoretical Statistics.* London: Chapman and Hall.

Dannenberg, O., Dette, H. and Munk, A. (1994) An extension of Welch's approximate *t*-solution to comparative bioequivalence trials. *Biometrika* **81**, 91–101.

Davis, P.J. and Rabinowitz, P. (1975) *Methods of Numerical Integration.* New York: Academic Press.

Devlin, B. and Roeder, K. (1999) Genomic control for association studies. *Biometrics* **55**, 997–1004.

Dunnett, C.W. and Gent, M. (1977) Significance testing to establish equivalence between treatments, with special reference to data in the form of 2 × 2 tables. *Biometrics* **33**, 593–602.

Feller, W. (1968) *An Introduction to Probability Theory and Its Applications. Volume I. Third Edition.* New York: John Wiley & Sons, Inc.

Feller, W. (1971) *An Introduction to Probability Theory and Its Applications. Volume II. Second Edition.* New York: John Wiley & Sons, Inc.

Firle, E.A. (1998) *Asymptotically Distribution-Free Tests for Equivalence for Paired Observations Allowing for Ties.* Diploma Thesis, Department of Mathematics, University of Mainz. [In German.]

Fisher, R.A. (1934) *Statistical Methods for Research Workers. 5th Edition.* Edinburgh: Oliver & Boyd.

Flühler, H., Grieve, A.P., Mandallaz, D., Mau, J. and Moser, H.A. (1983) Bayesian approach to bioequivalence assessment: An example. *J. Pharm. Sci.* **72**, 1178–1181.

Food and Drug Administration (FDA) (1997). *Bioequivalence Studies–II. Gender Studies with non-replicate Designs.* Center for Drug Evaluation and Research at http://www.fda.gov/bioequivdata.

Food and Drug Administration (FDA). (2001) *Guidance for Industry: Statistical Approaches to Establishing Bioequivalence.* Rockville, MD: Center for Drug Evaluation and Research (CDER).

Frick, H. (1987) On level and power of Anderson and Hauck's procedure for testing equivalence in comparative bioavailability trials. *Commun. Statist. Theory*

Methods **16,** 2771–2778.

Giani, G. and Finner, H. (1991) Some general results on least favorable parameter configurations with special reference to equivalence testing and the range statistic. *J. Statist. Plann. Inference* **28,** 33–47.

Giani, G., Straßburger, K., Seefeldt, F. (1997) SEPARATE, Version 2.0B. Düsseldorf: Diabetesforschungsinstitut an der Heinrich-Heine–Universität, Abt. Biometrie & Epidemiologie.

Grizzle, J.E. (1965) The two-period change-over design and its use in clinical trials. *Biometrics* **21,** 467–80.

Guilbaud, O. (1993) Exact inference about the within-subject variability in 2×2 crossover trials. *J. Amer. Statist. Assoc.* **88,** 939–946.

Halmos, P.R. (1974) *Measure Theory.* New York/Heidelberg/Berlin: Springer-Verlag.

Harkness, W.L. (1965) Properties of the extended hypergeometric distribution. *Ann. Math. Statist.* **36,** 938–45.

Hájek, J. and Šidák, Z. (1967) *Theory of Rank Tests.* New York: Academic Press.

Hauck, W.W., Hauschke, D., Diletti, E., Bois, F.Y., Steinijans, V.W. and Anderson, S. (1997) Choice of student's t- or Wilcoxon-based confidence intervals for assessment of average bioequivalence studies. *J. Biopharm. Statist.* **7,**179–189.

Hauschke, D., Steinijans, V.W. and Diletti, E. (1990) A distribution-free procedure for the statistical analysis of bioequivalence studies. *Int. J. Clin. Pharmacol. Ther. Toxicol.* **28,** 72–78.

Hauschke, D., Steinijans, V.W. and Hothorn, L. (1996) A note on Welch's approximate t-solution to bioequivalence assessment. *Biometrika* **83,** 236–7.

Hocking, R.R. (1996) *Methods and Applications of Linear Models. Regression and the Analysis of Variance.* New York: John Wiley & Sons, Inc.

Hodges, J.L. and Lehmann, E.L. (1954) Testing the approximate validity of statistical hypotheses. *J. Roy. Statist. Soc. Ser. B* **16,** 262–8.

Holder, D.J. and Hsuan, F. (1993) Moment-based criteria for determining bioequivalence. *Biometrika* **80,** 835–46.

Holzgreve, H., Distler, A., Michaelis, J., Philipp, T. and Wellek, S. (1989) Verapamil versus hydrochlorothiazide for the treatment of hypertension. Results of a long-term double-blind comparative trial. *Brit. Med. J.* **299,** 881–6.

Hsu, J.C., Hwang, J.T.G., Liu, H.-K., and Ruberg, S.J. (1994) Confidence intervals associated with tests for bioequivalence. *Biometrika* **81,** 103–14.

Jeffreys, H. (1961) *Theory of Probability. Third Edition.* Oxford: Clarendon Press.

Johnson, N.L., Kotz, S. and Balakrishnan, N. (1994) *Continuous Univariate Distributions. Volume 1. Second Edition.* New York: John Wiley & Sons, Inc.

Johnson, N.L., Kotz, S. and Balakrishnan, N. (1995) *Continuous Univariate Distributions. Volume 2. Second Edition.* New York: John Wiley & Sons, Inc.

Johnson, N.L., Kotz, S. and Balakrishnan, N. (1997) *Discrete Multivariate Distributions.* New York: John Wiley & Sons, Inc.

Johnson, N.L, Kotz, S. and Kemp, A.W. (1992) *Univariate Discrete Distributions. Second Edition.* New York: John Wiley & Sons, Inc.

Jones, B. and Kenward, M.G. (1989) *Design and Analysis of Cross-Over Trials.* London: Chapman and Hall.

Kalbfleisch, J.D. and Prentice, R.L. (1980) *The Statistical Analysis of Failure*

Time Data. New York: John Wiley & Sons, Inc.

Kallenberg, W.C.M., et al. (1984) *Testing Statistical Hypotheses: Worked Solutions.* Amsterdam: Centrum voor Wiskunde en Informatica.

Karlin, S. (1956) Decision theory for Pólya type distributions. Case of two actions, I. In J. Neyman (ed.), *Proceedings of the Third Berkeley Symposium on Mathematical Statistics and Probability, Vol.I*, 115–28. Berkeley, Calif.: University of California Press.

Karlin, S. (1957a) Pólya type distributions, II. *Ann. Math. Statist.* **28**, 281–308.

Karlin, S. (1957b) Pólya type distributions, III: Admissibility for multi-action problems. *Ann. Math. Statist.* **28**, 839–60.

Karlin, S. (1968) *Total Positivity. Volume I.* Stanford, Calif.: Stanford University Press.

Kingman, J.F.C. and Taylor, S.J. (1973) *Introduction to Measure and Probability.* Cambridge: Cambridge University Press.

Kloos, T. (1996) *Sufficient Conditions for Maintaining the Significance Level in Bayesian Tests for Equivalence.* Diploma thesis, Department of Mathematics, University of Mainz. [In German].

Lee, A.J. (1990) *U-Statistics. Theory and Practice.* New York: Marcel Dekker Inc.

Lehmann, E.L. (1963) Nonparametric confidence intervals for a shift parameter. *Ann. Math. Statist.* **34**, 1507–12.

Lehmann, E.L. (1975) *Nonparametrics: Statistical Methods Based on Ranks.* San Francisco: Holden-Day, Inc.

Lehmann, E.L. (1986) *Testing Statistical Hypotheses. 2nd Edition.* New York: John Wiley & Sons, Inc.

Lindley, D.V. (1970) *Introduction to Probability and Statistics from a Bayesian Viewpoint. Part 2: Inference.* Cambridge: Cambridge University Press.

Little, R.J.A. (1989) Testing the equality of two independent binomial proportions. *Amer. Statist.* **43**, 283–88.

Liu, J.-P. and Chow, S.-C. (1992) On assessment of variability in bioavailability/bioequivalence studies. *Commun. Statist. Theory Methods* **21**, 2591–607.

Makuch, R.W. and Simon, R. (1978) Sample size requirements for evaluating a conservative therapy. *Cancer Treat. Rep.* **62**, 1037–40.

Mandallaz, D. and Mau, J. (1981) Comparison of different methods for decision-making in bioequivalence assessment. *Biometrics* **37**, 213–22.

Martín Andrés, A. (1998) Fisher's exact and Barnard's tests. In S. Kotz, C. Reid and D.L. Banks (eds.), *Encyclopedia of Statistical Sciences, Update-Volume 2*, 250–58. New York: John Wiley & Sons, Inc.

Mau, J. (1987) On Cox's confidence distribution. In R. Viertl (ed.), *Probability and Bayesian Statistics*, 346–56. New York: Plenum.

Mau, J. (1988) A statistical assessment of clinical equivalence. *Statist. Med.* **7**, 1267–77.

McDonald, L.L., Davis, B.M. and Milliken, G.A. (1977) A nonrandomized unconditional test for comparing two proportions in a 2×2 contingency table. *Technometrics* **19**,, 145–50.

McDonald, L.L., Davis, B.M., Bauer, H.R. III. and Laby, B. (1981) Algorithm AS161: critical regions of an unconditional non-randomized test of homogeneity in 2× contingency tables. *Appl. Statist.* **30**, 182–89.

McNemar, I. (1947) Note on the sampling error of the difference between correlated proportions or percentages. *Psychometrika* **12**, 153–7.

Mehring, G. (1993) On optimal tests for general interval hypotheses. *Commun. Statist. Theory Methods* **22**, 1257–97.

Mehta, C.R., Patel, N.R. and Tsiatis, A.A. (1984) Exact significance testing to establish treatment equivalence with ordered categorical data. *Biometrics* **40**, 819–25.

Metzler, C.M. (1974) Bioavailability - a problem in equivalence. *Biometrics* **30**, 309–17.

Michaelis, J., Wellek, S. and Willems, J.L. (1990) Reference standards for software evaluation. *Methods Inf. Med.* **29**, 289–97.

Miller, K.W., Williams, D.S., Carter, S.B., Jones, M.B. and Mishell, D.R. (1990) The effect of olestra on systemic levels of oral contraceptives. *Clin. Pharmacol. Ther.* **48**, 34–40.

Morgan, W. A. (1939) A test for the significance of the difference between the two variances in a sample from a normal bivariate population. *Biometrika* **31**, 13–9 (1939).

Moses, L.E. (1953) Non-parametric Methods. In H.M. Walker, J. Lev (eds.), *Statistical Inference.* New York: Holt, Rinehart and Winston, 426–50.

Müller-Cohrs, J. (1988) Size and power of the Anderson-Hauck test and the double t-test in equivalence problems. *Proceedings of the SAS European Users Group Internations Conference,* 30–8. Copenhagen.

Munk, A. (1993) An imporovement on commonly used tests in bioequivalence assessment. *Biometrics* **49**, 1225–30.

Neyman, J. and Pearson, E.S. (1936) Contributions to the theory of testing statistical hypotheses. I. Unbiased critical regions of type A and type A_1. *Statist. Res. Mem.* **1**, 1–37.

Pearson, E.S. (1947) The choice of statistical tests illustrated on their interpretation of data classified in a 2×2 table. *Biometrika* **34**, 139–67.

Pfeiffer, N., Grehn, F., Wellek, S. and Schwenn, O. (1994) Intraocular thymoxamine or acetylcholine for the reversal of mydriasis. *Ger. J. Ophthalmol.* **3**, 422–6.

Philipp, T., Anlauf, M., Distler, A., Holzgreve, H., Michaelis, J. and Wellek, S. (1997) Randomised, double blind multicentre comparison of hydrochlorothiazide, atenolol, nitrendipine, and enalapril in antihypertensive treatment: results of the HANE study. *Brit. Med. J.* **315**, 154–9.

Pitman, E.J.G. (1939) A note on normal correlation. *Biometrika* **31**, 9–12.

Pratt, J.W. (1960) On interchanging limits and integrals. *Ann. Math. Statist.* **31**, 74–7.

Racine-Poon, A., Grieve, A.P., Flühler, H. and Smith, A.F.M. (1987) A two-stage procedure for bioequivalence studies. *Biometrics* **43**, 847–56.

Randles, R.H. and Wolfe, D.A. (1979) *Introduction to The Theory of Nonparametric Statistics.* New York: John Wiley & Sons, Inc.

Rao, C.R. (1973) *Linear Statistical Inference and Its Applications. Second Edition.* New York: John Wiley & Sons, Inc.

Rodary, C., Com-Nougue, C. and Tournade, M.-F. (1989) How to establish equivalence between treatments: A one-sided clinical trial in paediatric oncology. *Statist. Med.* **8**, 593–8.

Rodda, B.E. (1990) Bioavailability: Designs and analysis. In D.A. Berry (ed.), *Statistical Methodology in the Pharmaceutical Sciences,* 57–81. New York: Marcel Dekker.

Rodda, B.E. and Davis, R.L. (1980) Determining the probability of an important difference in bioavailability. *Clin. Pharmacol. and Ther.* **28**, 247–52.

Roebruck, P. and Kühn, A. (1995) Comparison of tests and sample size formulae for proving therapeutic equivalence based on the difference of binomial probabilities. *Statist. Med.* **14**, 1583–94.

Röhmel, J. (1998) Therapeutic equivalence investigations: statistical considerations. *Statist. Med.* **17**, 1703–14.

Röhmel, J. and Mannsmann, U. (1999a) Unconditional non-asymptotic one-sided tests for independent binomial proportions when the interest lies in showing non-inferiority and/or superiority. *Biom. J.* **41**, 149–70.

Röhmel, J. and Mannsmann, U. (1999b) Letter to the Editor on "Exact tests of equivalence and efficacy with a non-zero lower bound for comparative studies" by S.F. Chan. *Statist. Med.* **18**, 1734–35.

Roy, S.N. (1953) On a heuristic method of test construction and its use in multivariate analysis. *Ann. Math. Statist.* **24**, 220–38.

SAS (1999) *SAS Language Reference: Dictionary, Version 8.* Cary/North Carolina: SAS Institute, Inc.

Sasieni, P.D. (1997) From genotype to genes: Doubling the sample size. *Biometrics* **53**, 1253–61.

Scaglione, F. (1990) Comparison of the clinical and bacteriological efficacy of clarithromycin and erythromycin in the treatment of streptococcal pharyngitis. *Curr. Med. Res. Opin.* **12**, 25–33.

Schall, R. (1995) Assessment of individual and population bioequivalence using the probability that bioavailabilities are similar. *Biometrics* **51**, 615–26.

Schall, R. and Luus, H.G. (1993) On population and individual bioequivalence. *Statist. Med.* **12**, 1109–24.

Schoenfeld, D. (1981) The asymptotic properties of nonparametric tests comparing survival distributions. *Biometrika* **68**, 316–9.

Schuirmann, D.J. (1987) A comparison of the two one-sided tests procedure and the power appoach for assessing equivalence of average bioavailability. *J. Pharmacokin. Biopharm.* **15**, 657–80.

Schumann, G., Rujescu, D., Szegedi, A., Singer, P., Wiemann, S., Klawe, C., Anghelescu, I., Giegling, I., Wellek, S., Heinz, A., Spanagel, R., Mann, K., Henn, F.A. and Dahmen, N. (2002) No association of alcohol dependence with a NMDA-receptor 2B gene variant. *Mol. Psychiatry* **7**, 000–000. [To appear.]

Searle, S.R. (1987) *Linear Models for Unbalanced Data.* New York: John Wiley & Sons, Inc.

Selwyn, M.R., Dempster, A.P. and Hall, N.R. (1981) A Bayesian approach to bioequivalence for the 2x2 changeover design. *Biometrics* **37**, 11–21.

Selwyn, M.R. and Hall, N.R. (1984) On Bayesian methods for bioequivalence. *Biometrics* **40**, 1103–8.

Sheiner, L.B. (1992) Bioequivalence revisited. *Statist. Med.* **11**, 1777–88.

Steinijans, V.W. and Diletti, E. (1983) Statistical analysis of bioavailability studies: Parametric and nonparametric confidence intervals. *Eur. J. Clin. Pharmacol.* **24**, 127–36.

Steinijans, V.W. and Diletti, E. (1985) Generalisation of distribution-free confidence intervals for bioavailability ratios. *Eur. J. Clin. Pharmacol.* **28**, 85–8.

Steinijans, V.W., Neuhauser, M., Hummel, T., Leichtl, S., Rathgeb, F. and Keller, A. (1998) Asthma management: the challenge of equivalence. *Int. J. Clin. Pharmacol. Ther. Toxicol.* **36**, 117–25.

Stuart, A. and Ord, K. (1994) *Kendall's Advanced Theory of Statistics. Volume I - Distribution Theory. Sixth Edition.* London: Edward Arnold.

Suissa, S. and Shuster, J.J. (1985) Exact unconditional sample sizes for the 2×2 binomial trial. *J. Roy. Statist. Soc. A* **148**, 317–27.

Ungersböck, K. and Kempski, O.S. (1992) A study of the effect of increased intracranial pressure on the cortical microcirculation of New Zealand white rabbits. *Department of Neurosurgery, University of Mainz.* (Unpubl. Techn. Report).

Victor, N. (1987) On clinically relevant differences and shifted nullhypotheses. *Methods Inf. Med.* **26**, 155–62.

Wang, W. (1997) Optimal unbiased tests for equivalence in intrasubject variability. *J. Amer. Statist. Assoc.* **92**, 1163–70.

Welch, B.L. (1938) The significance of the difference between means when the population variances are unequal. *Biometrika* **29**, 350–62.

Wellek, S. (1990) Vorschläge zur Reformulierung der statistischen Definition von Bioäquivalenz. In G. Giani, R. Repges (eds.), *Biometrie und Informatik - neue Wege zur Erkenntnisgewinnung in der Medizin*, 95–9. Berlin: Springer-Verlag.

Wellek, S. (1991) Zur Formulierung und optimalen Lösung des Bioäquivalenznachweis-Problems in der klassischen Theorie des Hypothesentestens. In J. Vollmar (ed.), *Bioäquivalenz sofort freisetzender Arzneiformen*, 91–109. Stuttgart: Gustav Fischer Verlag.

Wellek, S. (1993a) Basing the analysis of comparative bioavailability trials on an individualized statistical definition of equivalence. *Biom. J.* **35**, 47–55.

Wellek, S. (1993b) A log-rank test for equivalence of two survivor functions. *Biometrics* **49**, 877–81.

Wellek, S. (1994) *Statistische Methoden zum Nachweis von Äquivalenz.* Stuttgart: Gustav Fischer Verlag.

Wellek, S. (1996) A new approach to equivalence assessment in standard comparative bioavailability trials by means of the Mann-Whitney statistic. *Biom. J.* **38**, 695–710.

Wellek, S. (2000a) Bayesian construction of an improved parametric test for probability-based individual bioequivalence. *Biom. J.* **42**, 1039–52.

Wellek, S. (2000b) On a reasonable disaggregrate criterion of population bioequivalence admitting of resampling-free testing procedures. *Statist. Med.* **19**, 2755–67.

Wellek, S. (2002) Power approximation and sample size calculation for the log-rank test for equivalence. *In preparation.*

Wellek, S. and Hampel, B (1999) A distribution-free two-sample equivalence test allowing for tied observations. *Biom. J.* **41**, 171–86.

Wellek, S. and Michaelis, J. (1991) Elements of significance testing with equivalence problems. *Methods Inf. Med.* **30,** 194–8.

Westlake, W.J. (1972) Use of confidence intervals in analysis of comparative bioavailability trials. *J. Pharm. Sci.* **61,** 1340–1.

Westlake, W.J. (1976) Symmetrical confidence intervals for bioequivalence trials. *Biometrics* **32,** 741–4.

Westlake, W.J. (1979a) Design and statistical evaluation of bioequivalence studies in man. In J. Blanchard (ed.), *Principles and Perspectives in Drug Bioavailability,* 192–210. Basel: S. Karger.

Westlake, W.J. (1979b) Statistical aspects of comparative bioavailability trials. *Biometrics* **35,** 273–80.

Westlake, W.J. (1981) Response to T.B.L. Kirkwood: bioequivalence testing - a need to rethink. *Biometrics* **37,** 591–3.

Willems, J.L., Abreu-Lima, C., Arnaud, P., Brohet, C.R., Denis, B., Gehring, J., Graham, I., van Herpen, G., Machado, H., Michaelis, J. and Moulopoulos, S.D. (1990) Evaluation of ECG interpretation results obtained by computer and cardiologists. *Methods Inf. Med.* **29,** 308–16.

Windeler, J. and Trampisch, H.J. (1996) Recommendations concerning studies on therapeutic equivalence. *Drug Inf. J.* **30,** 195–200.

Witting, H. (1985) *Mathematische Statistik I.* Stuttgart: B.G. Teubner.

Zinner, D.D., Duany, L.F. and Chilton, N.W. (1970) Controlled study of the clinical effictiveness of a new oxygen gel on plaque, oral debris and gingival inflammation. *Pharmacol. Therapeut. Dentist.* **1,** 7–15.

Author index

Subject index